Field's
ANATOMY, PALPATION & SURFACE MARKINGS

FIFTH EDITION

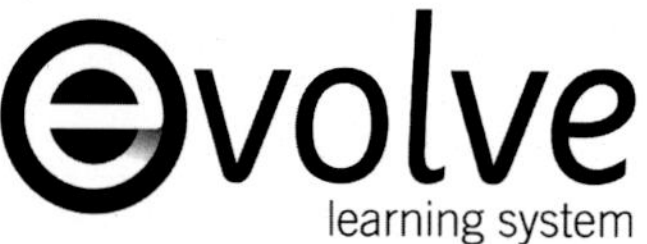

For Elsevier:
Commissioning Editor: Rita Demetriou-Swanwick
Development Editor: Sheila Black
Project Manager: Andrew Riley
Designer: Miles Hitchen
Illustration Manager: Bruce Hogarth

Field's
ANATOMY, PALPATION & SURFACE MARKINGS

FIFTH EDITION

Derek Field **Grad Dip Phys, FCSP, Dip TP, SRP**
Former Vice Principal, North London School of Physiotherapy,
City University, London, UK

Jane Owen Hutchinson **MA(Ed), MCSP, SRP, Cert Ed, Dip TP, Dip Rehab Counselling**
Manager, Allied Health Professions Support Service,
Royal National Institute of Blind People, London, UK

Illustrations by Derek Field and Antbits

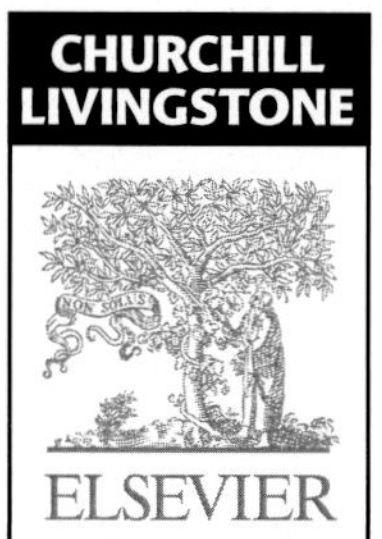

Edinburgh London New York Oxford Philadelphia St Louis Sydney Toronto 2013

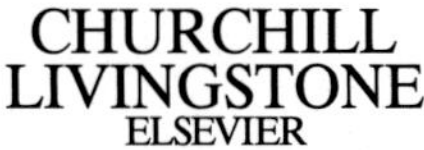

First edition 1994
Second edition 1997
Third edition 2001
Fourth edition 2006
Fifth edition 2013

ISBN 978-0-7020-4355-0

British Library Cataloguing in Publication Data
A catalogue record for this book is available from the British Library

Library of Congress Cataloging in Publication Data
A catalog record for this book is available from the Library of Congress

Notices
Knowledge and best practice in this field are constantly changing. As new research and experience broaden our understanding, changes in research methods, professional practices, or medical treatment may become necessary.

Practitioners and researchers must always rely on their own experience and knowledge in evaluating and using any information, methods, compounds, or experiments described herein. In using such information or methods they should be mindful of their own safety and the safety of others, including parties for whom they have a professional responsibility.

With respect to any drug or pharmaceutical products identified, readers are advised to check the most current information provided (i) on procedures featured or (ii) by the manufacturer of each product to be administered, to verify the recommended dose or formula, the method and duration of administration, and contraindications. It is the responsibility of practitioners, relying on their own experience and knowledge of their patients, to make diagnoses, to determine dosages and the best treatment for each individual patient, and to take all appropriate safety precautions.

To the fullest extent of the law, neither the Publisher nor the authors, contributors, or editors, assume any liability for any injury and/or damage to persons or property as a matter of products liability, negligence or otherwise, or from any use or operation of any methods, products, instructions, or ideas contained in the material herein.

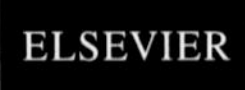

Printed in China

Contents

Preface to the fifth edition

The anatomy of the human body has changed very little over many thousands of years. The nomenclature does, however, change from time to time and the use of high powered microscopes facilitates the discovery of minute structures which contribute to an increased understanding of what Descartes would classify as this fascinating 'machine'. Additionally, educational methods and technological advances have radically changed the way human anatomy is now studied, at undergraduate, graduate and postgraduate levels. As well as attending lectures and practical sessions, students also benefit from a variety of other study methods: study guides, DVDs and numerous interactive online resources. All these methods enrich the learning experience and encourage the development of self-directed learning strategies which are essential for independent practice and successful patient management.

In view of these educational and technological advances, we considered it important to update both the style and content of this fifth edition of *Field's Anatomy, Palpation & Surface Markings*, (formerly *Anatomy, Palpation and Surface Markings*) and to produce a resource that reflects current trends in academic and clinical practice.

The aim of this text and the accompanying online resource is to familiarize the student of anatomy with a basic outline of the human body and to provide practical guidance to assist in the development of palpation skills. We believe that the combination of scientific, anatomical knowledge, together with the art of palpation, is vital if practitioners are to gain a true appreciation of the crucial relationship between structure and function, which, in turn, is essential for accurate diagnosis and treatment. We recognize, however, that the acquisition of this discipline will take considerable time. It is important for students to understand the relationship between internal and external structures by being able to visualize this through touch. This will require many hours of dedicated practice, with regular encouragement from tutors and colleagues.

The resource does not pretend to replace other methods of tuition. Rather, it should be regarded as an adjunct to anatomical study: only details of bone, joint structure, muscle attachments, nerve origins and distributions which can be palpated or determined from the surface are included. We hope, however, that the text, bullet point instructions, photographs and diagramatic illustrations will provide learners with a source of information which is clear and easy to understand. We also hope that it will encourage a genuine interest in the subject of anatomy and an enthusiasm for the development of good palpation skills. All kinds of subcutaneous structures can be identified through sensitive touch, as well as the quality of movement in joints, tension and texture in tissues. With practice, we hope that therapists will gain the expertise to identify anomalies in fine movements, tissue and joint damage which will facilitate patient assessment and treatment.

After the introductory chapter, the text comprises five sections: the upper limb, the lower limb, the head and neck, the thorax and the abdomen. Each is divided into the following subsections: bones, joints, muscles, nerves, arteries and veins. The lymphatic system has been excluded as it is normally impossible to palpate, although the drainage routes can be seen from time to time, particularly when there is an infection in the region drained. The lymph nodes are also difficult to palpate unless they are enlarged as a consequence of pathological reaction.

While the success of the four previous editions of this book has been considerable, it was deemed appropriate, when preparing this fifth edition, to undertake a complete re-evaluation of the text in the light of current professional educational philosophy and clinical practice.

In the fourth edition, Chapter 1 was re-written with a view to reflecting current trends in relation to the underpinning principles of medical practice. Furthermore, it attempted to provide a more detailed analysis of the nature of touch and its significance in relation to the practice of the art of palpation. Throughout the remainder of that edition, a different approach to the study of anatomy and palpation skills was adopted which more accurately reflected the study methods undertaken by students on many professionally validated programmes throughout the UK.

Because this approach is based on the principle that individuals learn best when they play an active part in the learning process, students are required to become more self-directed than before, to take a greater responsibility for their own learning and to engage in exploring the practical significance of their theoretical knowledge. To date, our experience indicates that while learners often find these methods more challenging initially, they eventually regard them as extremely rewarding and more enjoyable than the rather traditional approaches to teaching which might have been encountered during previous educational programmes.

It is worth emphasising that a sound knowledge of anatomy and physiology are essential to the successful practice of palpation techniques. To become skilled in the art of palpation requires the practitioner to be able to identify and locate the various anatomical structures of the body and to engage in regular practice, evaluation and modification of techniques. Students are encouraged to undertake regular evaluation of theoretical knowledge and its practical application. The fourth edition therefore included a self-assessment section which followed each separate anatomical area of the body. This consisted of a series of questions, diagrams and photographs relating to the text of each section. The questions followed each of these sections, followed by page numbers and a space below for the answer indicating the page on which the answer could be found. This provided a quick reference system for students who identified a gap in knowledge.

The success of of the self-assessment section, and the increasing use of Virtual Learning Environments, prompted us to transfer the self-assessment component to an online resource in the fifth edition. Here, questions and answers enable students to evaluate their knowledge by obtaining a score. Undertaken regularly, this should act as an incentive to learning. Identification of errors should encourage learners to return to the relevant part of the text and re-read that particular section. It should be noted, however, that, while students may have answered a question correctly, the terminology used may not match that provided online. This is inevitable because in many cases an anatomical question can be answered in a variety of ways. In such instances, students should be encouraged in the knowledge that the original answer was correct.

Additionally, the line drawings have been enhanced by the addition of colour while the photographs have been re-rendered. The text has been extensively reviewed, modified and condensed. The use of bullet points in sections where students are required to undertake specific palpation techniques is designed for ease of reference and to facilitate learning.

We hope that all these changes will encourage practitioners to use the text and online resource in their anatomical studies. We believe that this resource is an essential component in the ever increasing range of educational options now available to students and practitioners in the following disciplines: chiropractic, medicine, nursing, occupational therapy, osteopathy, physiotherapy, podiatry, remedial massage, sports medecine and other health-related professions concerned with rehabilitation. People involved in other disciplines such as art, dance, design, drama and industry may also find this resource of interest.

Whatever your reason for purchasing *Field's Anatomy* we hope that you will find it interesting, easy to understand, useful, but most of all, enjoyable.

Derek Field
Jane Owen Hutchinson
July 2012

Acknowledgements

I would like to thank Jane Owen Hutchinson MA (Ed), MCSP, SRP, Dip TP, for all her help and hard work in producing the fifth edition of this book. We hope that this edition will become an even more popular addition to the student's bookshelf than the fourth. In view of the changes we have made, it should become an an essential component of the student's self-assessment programme.

I would also like to take this opportunity to thank my colleagues, friends and readers from all over the world who assisted me in the production of the original version of *Field's Anatomy, Palpation & Surface Markings*, formerly *Anatomy, Palpation and Surface Markings*.

My thanks go to Anthony B. Ward LBIPP of Churchill Ward Associates, Long Hanborough, for shooting the many photographs used in the third, fourth and fifth editions. My thanks also go to Tim Brown and Sally Ede for posing for the many photographs.

I must express a special 'thank you' to Rita Demetriou-Swanwick, Sheila Black and Andrew Riley, who, together with their colleagues at Elsevier, made our task more enjoyable by easing our workload wherever possible. I would also like to thank Antbits for the upgrading of many of the drawings and photographs.

Derek Field
July 2012

Dedication

I would like to dedicate this fifth edition of *Field's Anatomy* to the memory of my late wife Yvonne, who spent many hours organizing schedules and work sessions, reading and editing all manner of information and research, helping to collate the dots on the photographs with the labels and, most importantly, for her encouragement.

Derek Field

Palpation: definition, application and practice

1

Contents

SOME DEFINITIONS AND CONCEPTS

Palpation: some definitions

The Oxford Dictionary of English defines the verb to palpate as: 'to examine (a part of the body) by touch, especially for medical purposes'. Its derivative noun is 'palpation' (from the Latin verb 'palpare': to 'feel or touch gently'). According to *The Chambers Dictionary*, the term 'palp' means 'to feel, examine or explore by touch'; 'palpare' is defined as 'to touch softly, stroke, caress or flatter'. *Churchill's Medical Dictionary* defines palpation as 'to stroke, caress; to explore or examine by touching and probing with the hands and fingers'.

Whilst 'stroking', 'caressing' or (tactile) 'flattering' represent practices (through 'gentle touch') that are essentially designed to give physiological and psychological 'healing' to the recipient, palpation, for the purposes of this text, is primarily a purposeful activity requiring considerable skill. It is associated with methodical exploration and detailed manual examination, the aim of which is to acquire objective information that will eventually lead to a reasoned medical diagnosis upon which a subsequent treatment regimen can be based. *Gould's Medical Dictionary* makes the direct link between the activity of palpation and diagnosis by gentle touch which involves the detection of the 'characteristics and condition of local tissues of the underlying organs or tumors'.

In *The Oxford Dictionary of English*, to examine is defined as 'to test; to inquire into; to question; to look closely at or into; to inspect'. According to *The Chambers Dictionary*, to examine is to 'inspect (someone or something) thoroughly in order to determine the nature of a condition'. The activity involves critical, reflective thinking: the systematic weighing up of evidence in an attempt to arrive at a balanced conclusion.

General characteristics of palpation

Palpation is a highly complex and sophisticated manual skill. Citing Frymann, Chaitow (2003) draws attention to the potential which palpation offers members of the healing professions:

> *The human hand is equipped with instruments to perceive changes in texture, surface texture, surface humidity, to penetrate and detect successively deeper tissue textures, turgescence, elasticity and irritability. The human hand, furthermore, is designed to detect minute motion, motion which can only be detected by the most sensitive electronic pick-up devices available. This carries the art of palpation beyond the various modalities of touch into the realm of proprioception, of changes in position and tension within our own muscular system.*
>
> ***(Chaitow 2003)***

As Frymann emphasizes, the hand is particularly well equipped to play the key role in this activity. With reference to palpation of the human body, Chaitow reminds us that different parts of the hand possess the ability to discriminate between variations in tissue features: '... relative tension, texture, degree of moisture, temperature and so on'. He then makes the important point that 'This highlights the fact that an individual's overall palpatory sensitivity depends on a combination of different perceptive (and proprioceptive) qualities and abilities' (Chaitow 2003).

TOUCH

Some general characteristics

Palpation involves the use of one of the primary senses, that of touch, in order to investigate and obtain information or to supplement that already gained by other means, such as by visual and auditory input. As Poon (1995) points out:

> *The act of touching and the feeling of being touched are very powerful experiences ... (and touch) is the earliest and most primitive form of communication.*
>
> ***(Poon 1995)***

Montague (1978) reminds us that:

> *Touch is the first of the senses to develop in the embryo and it plays a very important role in the birth process itself and in the early life of the individual.*
>
> ***(Montague 1978)***

Not only is it the earliest system to become functional in the human being but also touch is thought to be the last of the senses to be lost immediately prior to death.

Touch plays a very significant part in our everyday experience:

> *When the other senses are not wholly effective, we return to the sense of touch to rediscover reality. Clothing is felt to determine its quality, fruit is squeezed to determine its ripeness and paint is touched to test for dryness.*
>
> ***(Mason 1985)***

Experience suggests, however, that there are instances when touch is often subjugated in favour of reliance upon other sensory modalities. Only when an awareness of an alteration in incoming stimuli occurs do we become conscious of the sense of touch. An example of this phenomenon might be when picking up a garment, we recognize its unfamiliarity through its texture or 'feel'; another example might be an awareness of the material of trousers touching the legs immediately after a long period of wearing shorts.

Touch may be divided into two distinct categories: instrumental and expressive. Touch is described as instrumental when it is associated with a deliberate action: locating an anatomical structure for the purposes of examination during a clinical assessment, for example. Touch is identified as expressive when it is associated with spontaneous, affective actions: touching a distressed person's arm in order to convey sympathy and offer comfort (MacWhannell 1992, Poon 1995).

Touch can be experienced as safe or unsafe; physically comfortable or uncomfortable. It can be used to establish rapport: hand-shaking as a formal greeting at the beginning of a clinical interview or as a means of ending a treatment session. Communication by touch is specifically permitted within particular interpersonal relationships (see later). In certain contexts, however, permission to touch may be required, for example, at the commencement, and during the various stages of a clinical examination and treatment session. Touch is associated with psychological reactions: it is difficult to touch or be touched by those who elicit negative responses. The anticipation of touching or being touched can increase stress levels and these reactions may be influenced by personality, cultural and social factors: some female patients may deliberately avoid consulting a male therapist; some patients may be reluctant to remove clothing. It is important to remember that professional personnel are placed in an extremely powerful and privileged position in relation to others: they are given a license to touch and this power and privilege should never be abused.

The physiology of touch

All areas of the skin supplied with appropriate receptors are normally able to perceive a variety of sensations (pain, degrees of pressure, temperature changes, etc.) to a greater or lesser degree. Some areas, however, are more sensitive to stimuli than others because:

> *The degree of tactile sensitivity in any area is in direct proportion to the number of sensory units present and active in that area, as well as to the degree of overlap of their receptive fields, which vary in size. Small receptive fields with many*

sensory units therefore have the highest degree of discriminatory sensitivity.

(Chaitow 2003)

Sensitivity to spatial discrimination is poor in the lumbar region, the legs and the back of the hands. In the back of the hands, for example, two points can only be perceived separately if they are more than 50–100 mm apart. The lips, tongue and fingertips, however, rate high (1–3 mm). Thus individuals with normal sensation in the fingertips should be able to distinguish between two points even when they are less than 6 mm apart. This is referred to as the 'Two Point Discrimination Test' (see Chaitow 2003, Evans 2000, Magee 1997). The significance of this is that only relatively large objects can be recognized by the receptors in the lumbar region, whereas fine point discrimination can be achieved when employing the fingertips.

Chaitow makes the further point that:

Not only is there a difference of perception relating to spatial accuracy, but also one relating to intensity. An indentation of 6 micrometers is capable of being registered on the finger pads, while 24 micrometers is needed before the sensors in the palm of the hand reach their threshold and perceive the stimulus.

(Chaitow 2003)

Additionally, Evans (2000) contends that:

Under normal conditions, touch is an exploratory sense rather than purely receptive, and it is becoming increasingly evident that tactile acuity is enhanced in active exploration when compared with passive reception.

(Evans 2000)

Citing Meyers, Etherington and Ashcroft (1958), Evans suggests that:

An early indication of the phenomenon may be seen in an examination of the parameters of perception required to read Braille. The dots are separated by 2.3 mm, which is close to the threshold value for two-point discrimination at the pad of the index finger. Reduction of the inter-dot space to 1.9 mm only moderately reduces the legibility of the Braille text.

(Evans 2000)

While sighted Braille transcribers, relying solely on visual input, have been known to become proficient at reading Braille by the end of only three weeks, experience confirms that individuals attempting to conquer the system by touch are estimated to take an average of 1½–2 years to reach a speed suitable for serious study, even with regular practice. This is not due to lack of knowledge of the system; rather it is because the palpation and recognition of the signs using tactile input requires a considerable amount of dedicated time and practice in which to develop. As with all skills, the speed and quality of reading depends upon the frequency and amount of use. The ability to palpate with any finger or fingers can usually be developed, the use of the index finger being the most popular. Reading speed is further enhanced by using the fingers of both hands. In some cases, this skill never develops if the individual has not learnt to employ touch from an early age. In rare instances, people who have been unable to use their fingers have developed the same ability to read Braille by using their toes or even their lips! (see above). This means that regardless of the method by which this skill is acquired, the ability to increase the information received through sensory input can be improved, given time and serious dedication to regular practice. This can be of great benefit to the clinical practitioner who wishes to 'read' information that lies deep to the skin. The controlled use of pressure and movement, coupled with feedback and experience, unlocks a vast quantity of information that is often unavailable to the eye.

Obtaining information through touch is a skill, the practical significance of which is often not fully appreciated or valued until it is needed, perhaps to compensate for the impairment or loss of one of the other senses: sight or hearing, for example. Because of this, considerable practice is often required before the skill of palpation becomes developed to the point where it is of practical use to the individual concerned (see above). Initially, new techniques have to be devised and then undertaken slowly and carefully, with regular practice and evaluation, often involving feedback from other observers with consequent modification of behaviour. Efforts to recognize and accurately interpret tactile sensory input demand high levels of concentration which necessarily cause anxiety and additional stress to an individual who is unaccustomed to placing such reliance on this variety of incoming stimuli. These reactions are likely to be experienced by the novice clinical practitioner as well as by the recently disabled person and should be regarded as normal responses to the process of acquiring a new range of sophisticated psychomotor skills and personal strategies (Owen Hutchinson, Atkinson and Orpwood 1998).

In other non-medical contexts, touch-related skills are used to acquire general information about the environment such as establishing the temperature of water. A thermometer could be employed for this purpose, but it is often easier (and quicker) to test water temperature by utilizing the input from the sensory endings in the skin. While the results of this method of temperature testing are likely to be far less accurate than if a thermometer were to be used, they provide a range of potentially significant information upon which subsequent action could be based. The water temperature, for example, might be experienced as burning, scorching, boiling, extremely hot, very hot, fairly hot, hot, quite hot, very warm, blood heat, warm, fairly warm, slightly warm, cool, cold, quite cold, very cold, bitterly cold, freezing and icy cold. A temperature of 42°C read from a thermometer has little practical meaning as to whether something is too hot or too cold to touch.

The social significance of touch

The concept of the novice engaged in learning to interpret incoming stimuli received through touch extends, of course, into the realm of social interaction. As suggested above, touch can represent a powerful means of expressive communication (Nathan 1999). The way in which this communication is interpreted will be contingent upon such variables as personality, upbringing, culture and social situation and, in these contexts, it seems unhelpful to separate touch into mechanical and psychosocial categories. Referring to a medical intervention, Nathan contends that:

Touching a person's body in a non-therapeutic context is not normally considered an act of merely mechanical significance. Nor is it a procedure of a technique – rather it is an act of self-expression, or occasionally self-assertion, or preservation.

(Nathan 1999)

The degree to which people will engage in touching will be dictated by the nature of the interpersonal relationship in which they are involved at the time. Nathan continues:

In the main, frequent touching is reserved for parent–child relationships, lovers and close friends. In these contexts it both signifies emotional intimacy and is emotionally significant.

(Nathan 1999)

Touch can be employed to communicate a variety of emotions. For example, affection may be conveyed by a gentle squeeze of the hand, whereas a loose handshake may imply indifference or even dislike. Touching and being touched can be extremely therapeutic. Montague summarizes the observations of many researchers who conclude that:

Cutaneous stimulation in the various forms in which the newborn and young receive it is of prime importance for their healthy physical and behavioural development .... It appears probable that for human beings, tactile stimulation is of fundamental significance for development of healthy, emotional and affectional relationships.

(Montague 1978)

Montague quotes examples of cases that were studied by Lorna Marshall, a researcher who spent much time between 1950 and 1961 living among the Bushmen of the Kalahari Desert in Botswana, South West Africa. He observed that, within this society, the development of the newborn, infant, adolescent and adult appeared to be influenced by the way in which the child was handled in early life. Montague also refers to accounts by Margaret Mead, who studied the Arapesh and Mundugumor societies in New Guinea during the 1930s and documented the characteristics of their respective social practices. In the former tribe, the child was in contact with the mother for most of the day. The adults of this tribe were observed to be kind, happy and peace-loving people. In the latter tribe, the child had little human contact, being kept in a rough plaited basket which was usually suspended from the mother's forehead. The adults of this tribe were observed to become unattractive, aggressive and cannibalistic.

The tendency to avoid close physical contact can be demonstrated in adults from certain cultures and within some social backgrounds of particular nationalities. Montague comments that 'There exists not only cultural and national differences in tactile behaviour but also class differences.' He cites the English upper class as a an example of a social group that is characterized by non-tactile social behaviour when compared with social groups of other nationalities: French and Italian people display more demonstrative behaviour when greeting one another and are observed to engage in more physical interpersonal contact.

When considering the practice of palpation skills, the significance of Montague's observations cannot be underestimated. Not only is it crucial for us to recognize the relevance of culture, nationality and social class on the degree to which people communicate by touch, but also the impact of living in a multicultural society in which we are likely to encounter unfamiliar and potentially disconcerting practices. Additionally the effect of globalization on our patterns of non-verbal communication has been considerable.

In contrast to the somewhat reserved behaviour of English people in the 19th and early 20th centuries, we now regularly witness overt instances of emotion (love and friendship, happiness and sadness) through physical contact. Behaviour such as mutual embracing, hand-holding and kissing is frequently to be observed in public places. Sportspeople will leap in the air and hug each other following a winning achievement such as the scoring of a goal in football; equally, it is not uncommon for athletes to display tears of misery and frustration and to engage in mutually sympathetic embraces after a failure to attain high standards of performance.

Touch and clinical practice

Palpation, then, would seem to be a practice which involves a combination of many other skilled activities: the appropriate use of touch, the application of methodical investigatory techniques, accurate interpretation of sensory feedback (based upon sound general knowledge), the ability to draw on previous experience, to reflect, critically, upon findings and arrive at a reasoned conclusion.

Palpation is the art of feeling tissues with your hands in such a manner that changes in tension and position within these tissues can be readily noticed, diagnosed and treated.

(Mitchell, Moran and Pruzzo (1979) cited in Chaitow 2003)

A skill is attained and retained by its continual use, evaluation and modification of practice (Phillips 2004). The study and practice of manual contact techniques over a long period of time enables the practitioner to become highly skilled in the art of palpation. The development of this skill provides valuable supplementary information to that which can be obtained through observation and verbal questioning and is crucial to arriving at a meaningful clinical diagnosis. After many years experience of practising palpation skills, the moving, stretching and compression of tissues will be undertaken with precise control. This will enable the therapist to receive and interpret vital information from the patient and to apply and modify techniques as appropriate. Small changes in tension, temperature, dampness, movement and swelling will be identified by the sense of touch; these will then be noted and the appropriate course of action taken. Grieve states:

Of the entire objective examination of the vertebral column, the palpation examination of accessible tissues is probably the most informative and therefore the most valuable.

(Grieve 1986)

As has been noted above, however, learning to palpate is also associated with acquiring the skills to 'read', accurately, the patient's problem. Citing Ford (1989) Chaitow reminds us that:

In days gone by, when a physician had to diagnose by touch a good practitioner did not feel a tumour at his fingertips but he projected his vibratory and pressure sensations into the patient. So we regularly project our sense of touch beyond our physical being and ... merely make the ordinarily unconscious process available to our conscious mind. In so doing, we cross the delicate boundary between self and other, to explore, to learn, and ultimately to help.

(Chaitow 2003)

Personal experience confirms that patients can easily distinguish between a novice and an expert practitioner. During the initial examination, both the practitioner and the person being palpated progress through a learning process in which each is engaged in assessing the other by the giving and receiving of information. Relatively little significant information can be obtained if one of the participants in this relationship is reluctant to communicate. This learning process takes time and it is often the case that an accurate picture of the underlying issues does not appear until much later in the treatment session. The reason for this is partly due to the need for each participant to become comfortable with the other, so permitting mutual reduction in anxiety and the relaxation of tension. It is also due to the need for both parties to become familiar with the learning process itself, so that each can benefit from the knowledge gained as a result of their participation in this two-way event. The skill of palpation, therefore, should not be regarded merely as an arbitrary form of physical intervention; rather it must be respected as a highly skilled investigative process which elicits specialized information to both participants. In our experience, the skill of palpation is estimated to be only 10% innate: the other 90% is acquired through dedicated practice.

EFFECTS OF PALPATION ON THE PATIENT

Patient and person

It is far beyond the scope of this book to enter into the complexities of the mind–body debate, but its significance in relation to clinical diagnosis and management cannot be ignored. Traditionally, medical practice has been characterized by the biomedical model of health. This model is underpinned by the philosophical principles of dualism: the mind and body are regarded as separate and distinct entities that do not interact and, essentially, the practitioner is engaged in treating one or the other. The manual therapist would, in this context therefore, be regarded as being concerned only with the treatment of the patient's body. Indeed, it is not uncommon to hear therapists refer to a patient as 'a neck' or 'a back'. The body is considered to resemble a sophisticated machine; if part of that machine is malfunctioning, physical intervention is required in order to rectify the fault (Chaitow in Nathan 1999, Christensen, Jones and Edwards 2004, Owen Hutchinson 2004).

The 1990s, however, have witnessed significant changes in the approach towards illness and disability with the consequent development of the biopsychosocial model of disability which 'is a way of conceptualizing the multifactorial and complex system that shapes a person's experiences of pain and disability' (Christensen, Jones and Edwards 2004). Citing various sources, Christensen, Jones and Edwards explain the biopsychosocial theory:

> *... the degree of disability a person develops will be based upon the reactions of that person to the pain experienced far more than on the physical experience of the pain itself. The biopsychosocial model places a complaint of pain into a more holistic context, and views the pain as important not in isolation, but in relation to any disability the person with pain is experiencing as a result of that pain.*
>
> ***(Christensen, Jones and Edwards 2004)***

(See also Ramsden 1999, Stevenson, Grieves and Stein-Parbury 2004.)

The last decade has also witnessed a growth in the popularity of complementary medicine, whose underlying holistic principles stand in direct contrast to those of orthodox medical practice. This trend would suggest that patients prefer to be treated as whole persons rather than as bodies requiring cures. When they seek consultation with a therapist, patients are asking for help with more than just a painful neck or back: they want far more than to be the passive recipient of skillfully performed physical techniques. Indeed, patients regard a satisfactory healing experience as one that acknowledges the inextricable links between mind and body and which therefore treats the whole person who is more than just the sum of a collection of constituent parts. Recognizing this, the therapist must adopt an empathic and sensitive approach to all input from the patient, both in terms of verbal and non-verbal communication. Social and cultural factors must also be taken into account.

The quality of all clinical interventions will improve dramatically if the person-centred approach to patient management is adopted. The therapist, however, should not underestimate the degree to which patients have learned the conventions associated with society in general and medicine in particular. During the session, patients will often choose to use language to conceal as well as to reveal emotional states: 'That movement does not hurt any more'; 'I feel much freer now'. It must always be remembered that the patient has this choice. It must also be borne in mind that some patients may not have recognized the link between physical and psychological states and may need to be encouraged to reflect upon their choice of language in order to gain insight into certain aspects of their emotional lives.

As has been suggested above, the act of touching and the feeling of being touched are very powerful experiences and the degree to which people engage in touching is largely contingent upon personality, cultural and social factors. Both patient and therapist may experience an increase in stress levels due to unfamiliarity within particular therapeutic contexts. The practitioner must demonstrate a respect for the patient as a person. Permission to touch should be obtained at the commencement, and during the various stages of a clinical intervention. Abuse of power and the privilege of being licensed to touch must be avoided.

The consultation process

For a variety of physical and psychosocial reasons, many patients remain reluctant to consult professional personnel on matters associated with their personal issues, especially those problems relating to their own bodies. Barriers may be erected by one or both participants in the therapist–patient relationship, although both must contribute to the dismantling of these barriers if effective communication and co-operation are to be achieved. Experience suggests that each patient usually presents with a combination of issues which are revealed by the identification of problems, the giving of information and the posing of a number of questions during the consultation process. Typically, no particular order of priority emerges except perhaps that associated with the overriding presence of pain. Some of the information provided by the patient may appear to be somewhat peripheral in relation to the practitioner's objective of establishing a clinical diagnosis, but it nevertheless represents a vital component of the overall clinical picture and must be thoroughly evaluated before it can be discounted.

The practitioner must be sympathetically receptive to all forms of information offered by the patient. Standards governing all areas of professional practice demand that the clinician must objectively evaluate all clinical evidence and attempt to produce a comprehensive analysis of the presenting situation. On some occasions, a prescribed plan will be used to facilitate the compilation and evaluation of data; at other times, the practitioner will be expected to tailor the procedure according to the patient's individual circumstances. The use of such strategies will enable the practitioner to arrive at a reasoned clinical diagnosis. Care must be taken, however, that any prescribed plan does not preclude the practitioner from obtaining relevant information from the patient; adherence to such standard pro forma can sometimes adversely affect the practitioner's judgement and thus lead to an incorrect clinical assessment of the patient's current problem.

It is crucial that the practitioner should manage the initial investigation with great care and sensitivity as this process is likely to have a significant influence on both parties during the subsequent clinical examination. The practitioner should exercise the same degree of tact and diplomacy when conducting the subsequent physical examination, which should be undertaken with equal care, precision and gentleness. Physical or verbal clumsiness at this stage of the proceedings could lead to a complete breakdown of the interpersonal relationship between the therapist and patient, who may become reluctant to communicate vital information. The therapist employs palpation techniques during the first contact with the patient and it is vital that efficient methods of obtaining information are employed at this time. Experience suggests that most patients have an expectation that a clinical examination involving the use of palpation techniques will take place; indeed, they would consider it to be unprofessional practice if such a procedure were not undertaken. Inevitably, each person will exhibit different reactions to being touched and it is important that the practitioner should establish and evaluate the patient's unique reaction to such interventions at the earliest opportunity. An initial indication of the patient's reaction to physical contact can be obtained by the act of hand-shaking at the commencement of the session. Additionally, information gained by the act of assisting the patient to and from a chair can provide the practitioner with valuable feedback relating to the patient's degree of willingness or reluctance to accept help. Of course, such strategies represent only part of the range of techniques being employed during this initial session. The use of visual, auditory and olfactory input can also provide useful sources of relevant clinical information.

During the period of questioning, the practitioner is recommended to make sensitive and careful physical contact with the area of the patient's pain. When these techniques are performed successfully, this encourages both parties to focus attention on the patient's motivation in seeking the consultation. All movements should be tested carefully, palpation skills being employed simultaneously with continual observation of the ongoing situation, the therapist monitoring any reluctance on the part of the patient to perform movements due to tension, muscle spasm, joint anomalies and pain. Inadvertently eliciting symptoms of acute pain will inevitably destroy the patient's confidence, resulting in an unwillingness to offer potentially significant information.

In most cases, the patient will gradually gain confidence and learn to trust the practitioner. Much of the apprehension of meeting will have passed during the initial contact. When the time comes for the therapist to undertake an objective physical examination of the patient's movements, rapport should have been well established which overcomes that initial reluctance to seeking of medical advice.

Palpation continues throughout the examination and subsequent treatment. If it is carried out carefully and sympathetically, it reveals valuable information concerning the patient's physical and psychological condition. Indeed, palpation has the potential to 'unlock' psychological issues which had hitherto been deliberately ignored or unrecognized by the patient as having any relevance to the presenting physical problem. Many practitioners will have experience of patients who seek medical consultation for a relatively minor physical ailment which, during the examination or treatment, will be found to be masking much deeper and more complex issues. All practitioners should be sensitive to this possibility and should note any incongruous sentiments that the patient may express during the session. Experience suggests that it is the physical contact with the patient which appears to facilitate the unveiling of these underlying issues, but the importance of recognizing this phenomenon is contingent upon the quality of the practitioner's professional training.

That the patient must have confidence in the practitioner cannot be over-emphasized. This will promote the offering of information through both verbal and non-verbal communication methods. Throughout the consultation, the practitioner should be receptive to the patient; as the session progresses, continual evaluation of the patient's verbal and non-verbal reactions to events should take place. Whether complex or simple, all treatment sessions should promote mutual trust and understanding. Experience indicates that the degree to which a patient contributes to the treatment session is directly proportional to the practitioner's input; this reciprocal relationship is, however, contingent on the practitioner's willingness to impart information and the patient's genuine interest in receiving it.

TECHNIQUES OF PALPATION

It is not enough merely to place the hands on the patient's body and hope to receive the information required. Positive steps must be taken to search for the data. As has been noted above, palpation is associated with the seeking of information and all techniques must be approached in a rational and logical manner. The practitioner can gain very little by contacting a surface with the hands and remaining stationary. Movement of the hands is required so that structures can pass under the fingers in a controlled manner so that any alterations in skin temperature, surface tension, and bone structure can be evaluated and recorded. The practitioner's speed of movement can be adjusted to facilitate the full interpretation of information. The importance of regularly modifying the speed of movement can be demonstrated by the following example. If the fingers are run over Braille script too quickly, dots can be felt but no information is obtained; if the individual adapts the speed accordingly, however, what initially appeared to be an incomprehensible mass of dots now becomes an intelligible text.

Sometimes palpation techniques need to be performed slowly and at considerable depth; at other times they should be carried out quickly and at a superficial level. For example, palpation of the transverse processes of the spines of the lumbar region or the hook of the hamate needs careful application of deep pressure, combined with slow movement and sensitivity to the patient's reactions. Palpation of the spines of the thoracic vertebrae – particularly when counting downwards – is much easier if the fingertips are gently moved up and down three or four centimetres at a time, marking each spine with the finger of the other hand and holding it until the position of the next spine is confirmed. This type of palpation works in a similar way to a scanner using a beam to build up a clearer picture. The technique can be used to obtain a clearer picture of the rib cage, particularly from the posterior aspect.

In our experience, using one or even two complete palms and fingertips conveys more information regarding movement below the skin surface and about the patient's general reaction to physical contact than if the fingertips alone were used. The application of the fingertips alone, for example, would be used for palpating a pulse. Generally, if the structures below the surface are stationary, the hands will have to be used in a controlled movement, whereas if the structures are mobile, the hands should remain stationary. The finer the movement below the surface, the more delicate the palpation technique must be: this is clearly demonstrated when searching for a faint pulse.

If joints are being manipulated to examine the quality of movement and to assess limiting factors, the hands should be moved as little as possible so as to avoid any feedback from the palpator's own tissues which would obscure information from those of the patient. In fact, with this kind of palpation, a minimum of all other movements – with the exception of the joint being examined – is required. This involves adopting a stance which will avoid movement of the feet, applying a hold that will allow the full range of movement without change and also reducing all skin sliding by firm contact. Finally, the palpator must be absolutely sure that the patient's position is stable and that the movement being tested is localized to the joint being examined and is in the plane around the axis required. It is not uncommon, when testing the movements of the upper or lower limb, for a 'clicking' or crepitus to occur and neither the patient nor the examiner are able to locate its source. Conversely, if the examiner's thumb nails touch when pressure is being applied to the posterior aspect of the lateral mass of the atlas (C1), the patient may, erroneously, report a grinding sound located in the atlanto-occipital joint.

When examining the end-range of a joint, all variations must be known in advance so that movement, physiological and accessory, is tested accurately, noting the range available and the limiting factors. This is a highly skilled form of palpation, requiring a great deal of practice on normal joints in order to perfect the technique, considerable experience with abnormal joints to be able to recognize the variations and an expert knowledge of the various conditions to assess how much or how little testing should be undertaken. It is not suggested that this form of palpation should be employed by an expert only; on the contrary, the technique should be practised at the earliest opportunity and based on palpation of normal anatomy. Gradually, if care is taken and limits set, considerable skill can be gained.

Experience suggests that some palpators either under-employ the use of touch and try to compensate by observation, or they tend to palpate over-enthusiastically but fail to interpret the significance of what they feel. Some may also feel what they believe they are meant to feel. It is easy to be persuaded by an eager patient, by prior knowledge or by a more experienced observer that one can feel changes that are not actually present. An open and honest interpretation of what is beneath the fingertips is essential: remember Hans Andersen's story of the Emperor's new clothes!

IMPROVING THE ART OF PALPATION

Returning to the example of the Braille reader, improvement in palpation techniques can only be achieved with practice. As with all areas of knowledge, the motivation to learn is crucial. In relation to clinical practice, the learning of good palpation skills is contingent upon the need to know what lies beneath the surface of the body and the desire to find some means of offering help to patients. Practitioners frequently express the wish to be able to 'see what is happening beneath the surface'. These sentiments confirm the importance of developing appropriate palpation techniques which can then be employed as a means of providing assistance. Inextricably linked with this process is the development of manual dexterity and sensitivity.

It is worth noting that, when practising any technique that necessarily involves the use of the hands, the quality of the information that is received through the sense of touch can often be enhanced by reducing the input from the other senses. Closing the eyes and using the hands to recognize different textures, weights, surfaces, liquids, coins, etc., often reveals hitherto unrecognized characteristics of what are regarded as familiar objects. The palpator must endeavour to obtain as much information from the sense of touch as possible. In order to develop this skill, different objects can be placed in a bag and identified only by using the hands. As the skill improves, less familiar objects can be chosen so that they are less recognizable: their shape might be more unusual and/or they may be smaller. All of these objects should be handled sensitively by the palpator who should attempt to identify their distinctive features (such as blemishes). Progression of this exercise would be to require the palpation and identification of the same objects through the material of the bag. The material of the bag could be chosen so that the exercise becomes progressively more difficult: beginning with a relatively thin surface such as fine plastic and gradually changing to a thicker material. Practise should be undertaken regularly during the course of everyday activities, the practitioner always noting the technique which is most suitable for the identification of each object. One suggestion would be habitually to identify the loose change in a pocket or purse before removing the correct amount to make a purchase. Recognition of coins is a relatively easy task and it should be unnecessary to use vision in order to verify the amount tendered. Take care: this could prove to be an expensive way to learn the art of palpation if adequate practice is not undertaken! Another exercise might be to select clothing on a daily basis using tactile and not visual input. It is a salutary point that all visually impaired people necessarily employ these tactual skills every day.

The development of the sense of touch needs to be nurtured. It is recommended that each contact with an object should be treated as if no visual or auditory input is available whilst attempting to obtain the maximum amount of information. Those who have the privilege of handling patients professionally possess a constant source of practice in their study of structure and function and examination of normal and abnormal phenomena. Those professionals are even more fortunate if they specialize in the use of massage, movement, mobilization and manipulation techniques as part of clinical practice. Individuals who have undertaken formal study and practice of the art of massage are indeed already well versed in the appropriate knowledge and skills relating to palpation. Their contribution to the increased public recognition of palpation as a crucial element in the diagnosis and treatment of clinical conditions cannot be underestimated. Indeed it is gratifying to note the increased status of all the manual therapies during the past decade: people are deliberately selecting practitioners who possess skills that rely on touch for their efficacy. It should never be forgotten, however, that all such therapists are required to demonstrate a serious commitment to Continuing Professional Development (CPD): they are required to revise and update their anatomical and physiological knowledge on a regular basis in order to maintain the high standards of professional practice demanded by their respective professional organizations.

CARE OF THE HANDS

All skills in which complex manual techniques are employed in the performance of precise movements necessarily rely on the regular care and maintenance of the hands: their mobility, sensitivity and dexterity. Prior to engaging in any form of manual contact, however, the practitioner should ensure that the temperature of the skin is warm; patients do not appreciate being touched by therapists whose hands are cold!

Cleanliness is essential and its positive contribution to the quality of tactile input cannot be underestimated. Traces of grease, cream, dirt, dust, etc., effectively create an additional intervening layer between the sensory receptor organs and nerve endings in the hand and the object or subject to be palpated. It is significant that most Braille readers will make every effort to keep their hands clean while reading Braille; many tend to avoid eating anything sticky in order to prevent their fingers from losing sensitivity. A routine of washing the hands in warm water using a mild soap and drying them thoroughly after washing should be adopted; the use of additional creams or ointments is not recommended unless this is absolutely necessary. A good, oil-based hand cream can be used at night in order to maintain a smooth, soft condition of the skin; some authorities also recommend the regular use of Vaseline and sugar. Whichever maintenance routine is adopted, the hands must always be washed thoroughly prior to attempting palpation techniques. In addition, the nails should be kept clean and short so that the risks of injury or infection are avoided. No wrist or hand jewellery should be worn. The quality of the palpation depends, to a great extent, upon the texture and suppleness of the hands. They should look and feel good, thus promoting the patient's confidence in the palpator. Poorly maintained hands which are dirty, stiff and with hard skin will be off-putting to patients: a reluctance to be touched will act as a barrier to the passage of information from the body of the patient to the receptors of the palpator.

The joints of the hands must be maintained in a supple condition with the musculature being firm and strong. Regular exercises should be practised in order to maintain joint mobility and increase muscle strength. Contact with all abrasive surfaces and detergents should be avoided as far as possible and gloves should be worn at all times when manual work is performed, particularly during activities such as washing-up, cleaning, gardening, car maintenance and building work. Many liquids, certain soaps and detergents, tend to remove the natural greases from the skin and the use of these should, therefore, be minimal. Any activity that is likely to lead to the production of blisters, finger calluses or general hard skin should also be minimized: examples might include such pastimes as rowing, playing a stringed musical instrument, rope-climbing and woodwork. Additionally, great care must be taken when using sharp instruments or engaging in any activity that is likely to cause trauma and/or skin infection. Lack of vigilance whilst performing any of these activities may prejudice the ability to perform high-quality palpation techniques.

PALPATION OF DIFFERENT TISSUES

Experience suggests that normal palpation when performed by the lay person – and even when undertaken by some professionals – is sometimes ineffective. It may enable the operator to differentiate between such tissues as bone, muscle or tendon, etc., but often does little more. By contrast, the skilled student practitioner will be able to distinguish different parts of bones, contrasting shapes and texture of muscles, identify their connections to tendons and trace them to their attachments. Such students will also be able to count vertebrae, palpate lumbar transverse processes and other deep bony structures, locate certain ligaments, palpate elusive pulses and determine abnormalities such as different types of swelling, misalignment and rupture. The expert clinician must progress far beyond this concept in order to complete the picture that lies hidden within the body. Bony landmarks should be studied, linking them together and obtaining a clear mental image of the skeletal layout. This programme should include studying rib angles, transverse processes and spines of all vertebrae including their differing features. For example, the bifid spinous processes of the cervical region contrast with the pointed spines in the thoracic and the rectangular-shaped spines of T12 and in the lumbar region. Alignment of one bone to another is relatively easily examined in the upper and lower limbs, whereas this is much more difficult to examine in the vertebral column. Defects in the contour of a bone can also be located and possible avulsions recognized.

Variations in muscle texture should be identifiable and note taken of differences occurring in normal muscle, enabling the examiner to recognize any abnormal variations. Some muscles, such as gluteus maximus and the middle fibres of deltoid, have a coarse structure due to the type of muscle fibres involved, whereas muscles such as the oblique abdominals and quadratus lumborum have a smoother texture. Fibrous tissue between the muscle fibres may give a stringy feel, while local areas of spasm are hard but regular in shape. The former tend to remain in the same position irrespective of what technique is performed on them; the latter will often disappear on applying either heat or massage. Both types of muscle spasm can be found in the rhomboid muscles between the scapula and spinous processes of the vertebral column.

Careful palpation will reveal where each muscle joins its tendon and where and how the tendon is attached. Palpation can also determine how tightly the muscle is bound down by fascia and whether the tendon is maintained in its position by a retinaculum. The extent of the retinacula can be examined and a study made of those structures which pass under or over them.

Swellings in muscle are often caused by bruising (contusion) and bleeding (haematoma) between the muscle fibres. These are normally contained within a localized area and become hard and painful, often warm to the touch and sometimes produce redness over the area. There is nearly always a history of trauma to the region. Care should be taken, however, when palpating any area of swelling as this symptom could be caused by other more serious conditions. It is important to be sensitive to local changes in temperature, noting whether these are higher or lower than expected. The condition of the underlying structures must be recorded and a knowledge of the possible causes of such variations will contribute to the establishment of a clinical diagnosis and subsequent treatment of the condition.

When palpating joints, other considerations must be taken into account. The precise location of the joint line is essential, the quality of this technique being based on the accurate identification of bony landmarks and measurements, taking into account the general size and shape of other bones and the patient's posture at the time. A detailed knowledge of the structure and extent of the adjacent joint surfaces, as well as where ligaments may obscure the joint space, is essential. The presentation of tissue-filled joint spaces under differing circumstances – for example, whether fluid is contained within the joint capsule or within a bursa – together with a detailed knowledge of the surrounding tendons is also a necessary pre-requisite when examining joints. As Chaitow points out:

> *There are many important features to note during the examination of joints: the range and smoothness of movement, whether the axis varies according to the position of the joint and to what degree movement may be limited. Employing great care and skill, movement of joints can be examined indirectly through the bones of either side of that joint. The movement between the joint surfaces may be experienced as smooth or grinding; the restriction felt at 'the end of a joint's range of motion may be described as having a certain feel and this is called (the) 'end-feel'.*
>
> **(Chaitow 2003)**

In his discussion of barriers to joint movement Chaitow continues:

> *If there is, for any reason, a restriction in the range of motion then a pathological barrier would be apparent on active or passive movement in that direction. If the reason for the restriction involved interosseous changes (arthritis, for example) the end-feel would be sudden or hard. However, if the restriction involved soft tissue dysfunction the end-feel would have a softer nature.*
>
> **(Chaitow 2003)**

Most joints possess additional movements which are of small range and not under voluntary control: these are essential for the efficient functioning of the joint. These are known as 'accessory' movements.

> *Accessory or joint play movements are those movements of a joint that cannot be performed actively by the individual. Such accessory movements include the roll, spin and slide which accompany a joint's physiological movements.*
>
> **(Hengeveld and Banks 2005)**

A simple example of this type of movement would be found in the axle of a bicycle wheel. On each side, the axle is surrounded by a ring of ball-bearings maintained in position by a cone which screws on to the axle. When the cones are loose, they allow the wheel to be moved slightly from side to side; when the cones are tight, there is no side-to-side or accessory movement. When there is side-to-side movement, the wheel is free to turn; as the cones are tightened, the ball-bearings become 'close packed' and more difficult to turn so finally locking the wheel. The side-to-side (or accessory) movement is thus essential for the free turning of the wheel, since its elimination results in no movement.

Accessory movements are most demonstrable in human joints within a certain range of the joint movement: when the ligaments allow joint surfaces to be parted or when the surfaces are not congruent. This is termed the 'loose packed' position. When the ligaments of a joint become taut and its surfaces are congruent, no further movement is possible, either physiological or accessory. The joint is now said to be in a 'close packed' position (Standring 2004). If the accessory movements of a joint are lost, the joint becomes extremely difficult to move, similar to the cones of the bicycle wheel being tightened (see above). If, however, accessory movement is restored, as in loosening the cones in the bicycle wheel, normal movement is also restored. The restoration of accessory movements is an important principle underlying the practice of mobilization and manipulation techniques to restore normal movement in joints. With care and expertise, by using a combination of accessory and normal movements, joint function can be assessed and the treatment varied accordingly. The use of 'quadrant' techniques (combined movements at the end of range) is a good example of this testing. (For further information on the application of these types of examination and techniques, see Grieve 1986, Hengeveld and Banks 2005.)

Chaitow's definition of 'joint play' is also useful:

> *Joint play refers to the particular movements between bones associated with either separation of the surfaces (as in*

traction) or parallel movement of joint surfaces (also known as translation or translatoric gliding).

(Chaitow 2003)

This information is important in establishing the joints' condition.

Swelling around a joint deforms its shape and contour, the extent of the deformity being dependent upon the degree of swelling involved. The bony features can usually be identified between the areas of swelling. In some instances, the swelling is so profuse that it is difficult to locate bony landmarks; on other occasions, the amount of fluid is so small that precise techniques have to be employed to palpate the swelling which is interfering with normal joint function. Most joint swelling is contained within the capsule, causing a build-up of pressure which results in increasing pain. The swelling may have to be removed surgically, although this is usually deferred until absolutely necessary because of the risk of infection into the joint. Blood can also escape into a joint space (haemarthrosis), resulting in a similar appearance, but this is usually accompanied by some discoloration and an increased local temperature. Any swelling can lead to severe damage to the mechanics of the joint; this damage may vary according to the type of fluid involved.

Careful palpation of the swelling can produce more information than at first thought. The swelling may appear soft and movable with the application of pressure; this often gives a fluid feel as it passes from one part of the joint cavity to another. Alternatively it may appear thick and pliable although difficult to move unless sustained pressure is applied. Swelling may appear to be a solid mass, pitting under pressure from the fingers but taking a considerable time before signs of movement are evident.

SUMMARY

Palpation is a detailed examination using the hands as tools to enable the palpator to elicit information about structures beneath the skin and fascia. It is, in our opinion, still under-used and undervalued, mainly because of lack of practise and appreciation of its intrinsic value. In addition, its teaching and practice are time-consuming, requiring expert instruction from experienced practitioners, genuine interest, patience and commitment from students. While its techniques can be practised and developed, however, expertise, takes time and dedication to acquire.

Palpation is more than just a desire to 'see' through the skin and interpret the underlying anatomy. It can be developed in such a way that information can be imparted to the patient through the practitioner's hands. It is not difficult to appreciate the ways in which the expert palpator can employ the art of instrumental and expressive touching in combination to obtain clinical diagnosis and establish sympathetic communication. Indeed, the philosophy that underpins the practice of many therapists emphasizes the intrinsic therapeutic qualities of touch per se (see for example Charman 2000, Dennis, Jones and Holey 1995, Everett 1997, Nathan 1999). Healers who practise the 'laying on of hands' and Therapeutic Touch also share this belief (see Krieger 1986, 1993, 1997, 2002, Macrae 1987, Sayre-Adams and Wright 2001). The increasing popularity of complementary therapies amongst the general public further confirms the general tendency to place considerable value in a holistic approach to patient care. Rather than relying solely on orthodox medical practice, patients and therapists alike are now recognizing the importance of healing in the management of chronic physical and psychological problems (Charman 2000, Nathan 1999).

Palpation must be learned, practised and developed before it can be applied professionally. The study of anatomy, physiology and the human sciences, together with the additional information obtained through the appropriate use of touch, are excellent ways of learning the art of palpation. Anatomy will become clearer and more understandable as the hands become more sensitive to what lies below the skin, leading to an enhancement of knowledge and improvement in assessment: an asset in therapeutic application. Finally, and perhaps most importantly, the skilled palpator should be aware of the patient's reaction to movement. By observing the patient's face, listening to the patient's comments and being sensitive to all reactions in muscle and joint movement, a total picture of the patient's condition becomes available. With care and sensitivity, a great deal of information can easily be obtained.

The following pages contain a detailed study of the surface markings of many of the body's structures, including a guide to the palpation of particular areas. It must be remembered, however, that the development of effective palpation skills for the purposes of clinical intervention requires more than the acquisition of sound theoretical knowledge upon which to base practice. As Chaitow emphasizes, expertise in palpation techniques is achieved '... by application (and repetition) of hundreds of carefully designed exercises that are capable of refining palpation skills to an astonishing degree of sensitivity' (Chaitow 2003).

Citing Frymann (1963) he adds:

... palpation cannot be learned by reading or listening; it can only be learned by palpation. This learning process is not just about hard dedicated labour; it should be fun and it should be exciting. The thrills to be experienced when taking this journey of exploration of the tissues of the human body is hopefully contagious ...

(Chaitow 2003)

We hope that readers will take inspiration from this and other related texts and strive to attain expertise in palpation skills in the interests of improving the quality of their clinical practice.

The upper limb 2

Contents

At the end of this chapter you should be able to:

1. Find and recognize the shape and position of the clavicle, scapula, humerus, radius, ulna, carpal, and metacarpal bones and the phalanges
2. Recognize and palpate many of the bony features.
3. Name all the joints of the upper limb and understand their structure.
4. Trace the lines of the joints and where possible indicate their bony landmarks and surface markings.
5. Describe or carry out any accessory movements, possible noting the ranges in which they are most easily performed.
6. Note the ranges of each of the joints and indicate the factors limiting their movement.
7. Give the class and type of each joint, noting the axes of movement where possible.
8. Name and demonstrate the action of all the muscles palpable in the upper limb.
9. Outline the shape of the muscle on the surface and palpate its contraction.
10. Palpate tendons and attachments where possible.
11. Name and trace all the main nerves supplying the upper limb.
12. Demonstrate the course and distribution of each of the main nerves of the upper limb.
13. Name the main arteries of the upper limb, outlining their course and indicating their distribution.
14. Name the main veins of the upper limb, noting their drainage areas and course.

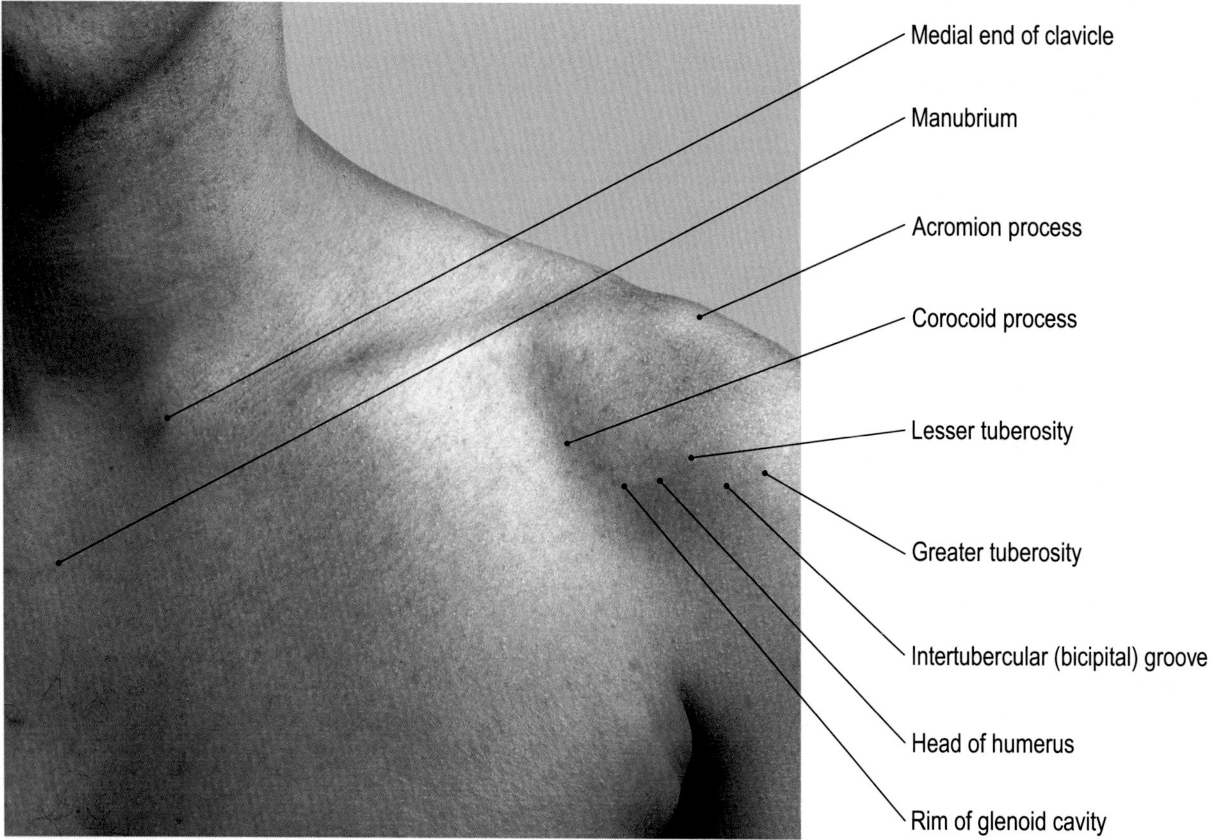

Fig. 2.1 (a) The left shoulder (anterior view)

BONES

The pectoral region

The bones in this region comprise the clavicle and scapula. These bones form the pectoral girdle, with the upper end of the humerus situated vertically under its lateral margin. The clavicle is situated on the upper part of the anterolateral aspect. The scapula is situated on the upper part of the posterolateral aspect of the chest wall. The humerus is the upper bone of the arm articulating with the glenoid [*glene* (Gk) = a socket] cavity of the scapula at the shoulder (glenohumeral) joint.

The clavicle (Fig. 2.1)

The clavicle [*clavis* (L) or *kleis* (Gk) = key; also, *clavis* (L) = an S-shaped bar for striking a gong] is a bone about 10 cm long and situated between the manubrium sterni medially and the acromion process of the scapula laterally (Fig. 2.1). It is a long bone and is a shallow S-shape when viewed from above. It ossifies in membrane, which means that its articular surfaces are covered with fibrocartilage and it has no medullary cavity.

Palpation

For palpation in this region, the model should be in the sitting position.

- The sternal (jugular) notch. Palpate the sternal (jugular) notch which is located centrally, at the lower boundary of the front of the neck. This is formed by the superior border of the manubrium sterni inferiorly and the medial end of each clavicle on either side. Articular cartilage together with an interarticular disc and interclavicular ligament are interposed between the medial ends of the clavicles and the skin.
- The medial third of the clavicle. Move your hands laterally and you will palpate the medial third of the bone which is convex forward with a superior and anterior surface. These features are easily palpable despite giving attachment to the sternocleidomastoid muscle superiorly and pectoralis major muscle anteriorly.
- The anterior end of the first rib. Now move your hands downwards to palpate the anterior end of the first rib. It is easily identifiable where it articulates with the lateral border of the manubrium sterni.
- The middle third of the clavicle. If you move your hands further laterally, you will notice that the middle third of the clavicle begins to curve backwards, being a little more rounded in cross-section.
- The supraclavicular fossa. Posterior to the superior surface of the clavicle you will palpate a depression: the supraclavicular fossa. This fossa contains the cord-like structures of the trunks of the brachial plexus running downwards and laterally towards the upper limb.
- The upper surface of the first rib. If you now apply deep, but careful, pressure in this notch in an inferomedial direction, you will be able to palpate the upper surface of the first rib, over which the trunks of the brachial plexus pass.

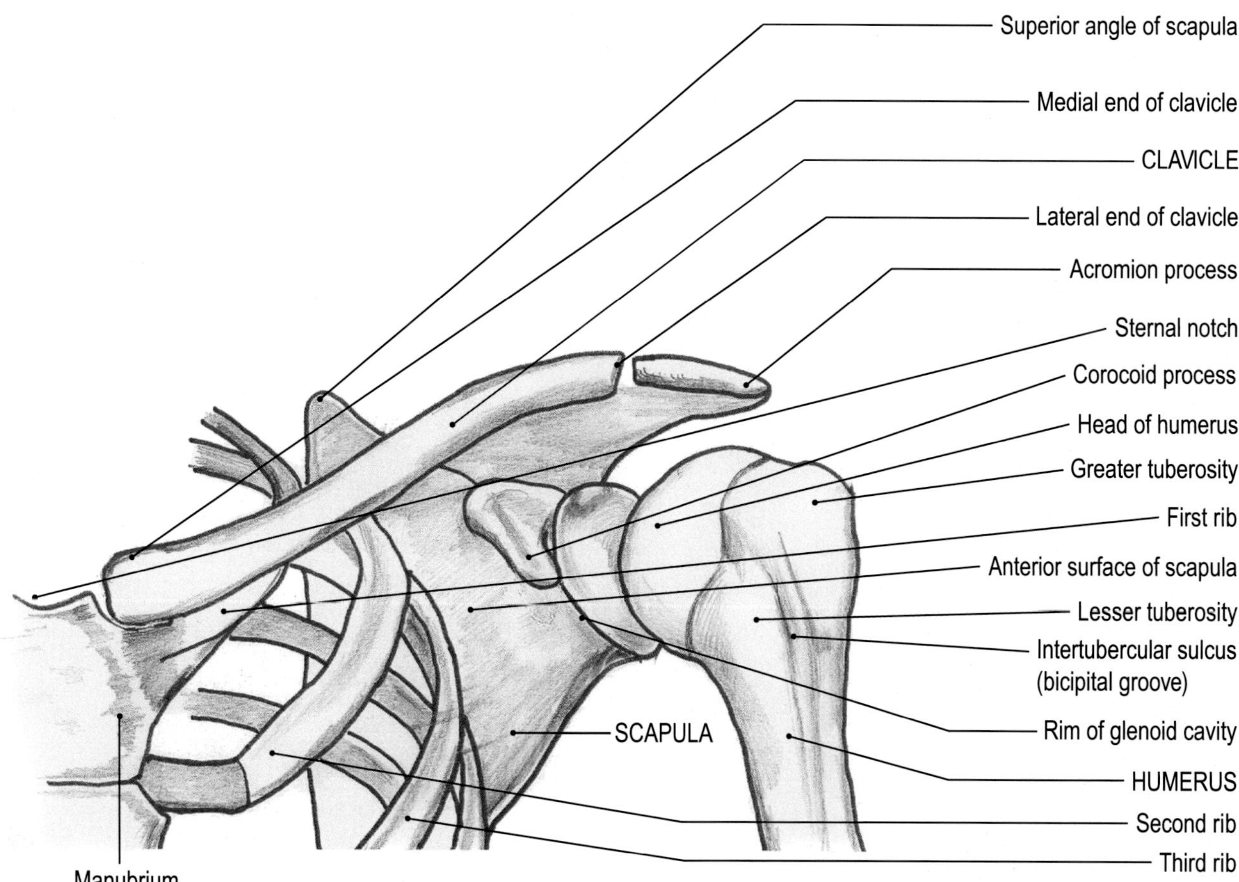

Fig. 2.1 (b) Bones of the left shoulder (anterior view)

- The lateral third of the clavicle. You will notice that the lateral third of the clavicle becomes flattened from above down and that its sharper anterior border is concave forward. Its subcutaneous superior surface can be easily palpated through the skin, becoming thicker at the lateral end toward the acromioclavicular joint.
- The infraclavicular fossa. Below the anterior border of the clavicle you will palpate a depression: the infraclavicular fossa. This fossa is situated between the deltoid muscle laterally and pectoralis major inferomedially.
- The coracoid process of the scapula. The coracoid [*korax* (Gk) = a crow and *oeides* (Gk) = shape] process lies within the infraclavicular fossa and you can palpate its tip lying approximately 3 cm below the junction of the middle and lateral thirds of the anterior border of the clavicle and just medial to the anterior fibres of deltoid muscle.
- Note. Both anterior and posterior borders of the clavicle give attachment to muscles: deltoid anteriorly and trapezius posteriorly.
- The lateral end of the clavicle. This can be identified by a small tubercle on its superior surface which is palpable lying just medial to the acromioclavicular joint (see joints of the upper limb).

The upper end of the humerus

This comprises the head, the greater tuberosity and the lesser tuberosity.

Palpation

- The head of the humerus. On palpation, you will notice that the head is slightly more than half a sphere. It is smooth and is directed medially, slightly backwards and upwards. Its greater tuberosity lies laterally and the lesser tuberosity projects forwards with the intertubercular groove running vertically between the two tuberosities.
- The lesser tuberosity of the humerus. If you now move lateral to the coracoid process, you will palpate a slightly pointed projection. This is the lesser tuberosity of the humerus [*humerus* (L) = the shoulder].
- Note. This forms the medial border of the intertubercular groove, through which passes the tendon of long head of biceps.
- The intertubercular groove of the humerus. This groove can easily be palpated as it runs vertically downwards (Fig. 2.1).
- The greater tuberosity of the humerus. Lateral to the tendon of biceps, the anterior surface of the greater tuberosity may be difficult to palpate as it is covered by deltoid muscle. Place your fingers on the anterior aspect and bring your thumb in, just below and lateral to the angle of the acromion. You should now be able to grasp the greater tuberosity with your thumb and fingers between the fibres of deltoid muscle.
- Note. The greater tuberosity accounts, in part, for the rounded shape of the shoulder region.

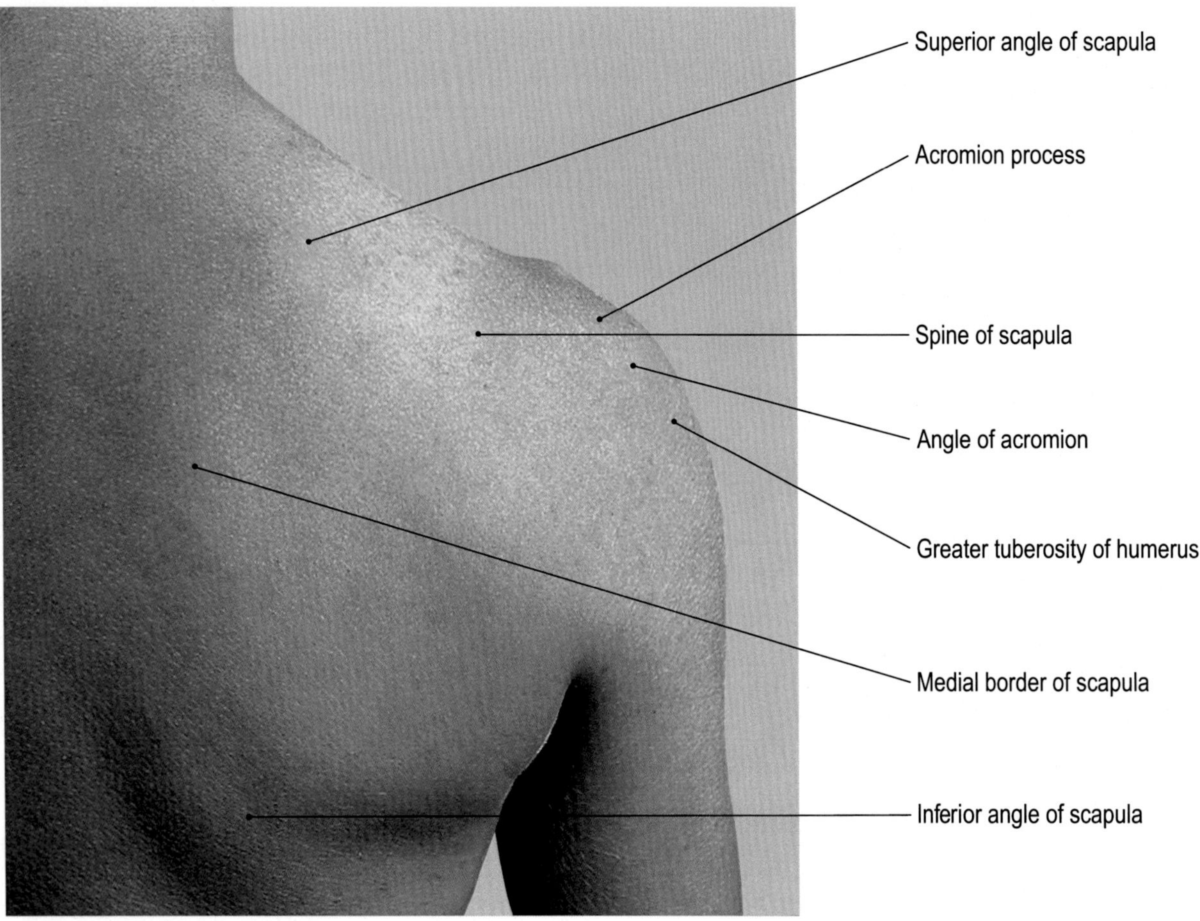

Fig. 2.2 (a) The right shoulder (posterior view)

The scapula (Fig. 2.2)

The scapula [*scapulae* (L) = shoulder blades] (Fig. 2.2) is a flat triangular bone situated on the posterolateral aspect of the upper chest wall. It has three angles, three borders and costal and dorsal surfaces, the latter being marked by a ledge-shaped spine running almost horizontally.

The spine is wider laterally where it joins the acromion process, but narrows as it passes medially. Its upper and lower borders diverge as it meets the medial border forming a small smooth triangular area. Above the spine there is a deep hollow called the supraspinous fossa and below a larger but shallower depression called the infraspinous fossa.

The lateral angle is expanded and forms the glenoid cavity for articulation with the head of the humerus at the shoulder joint. It presents a sharp bony projection passing forward just below the lateral end of the clavicle. This is the coracoid process, which is roughened for the attachment of muscle.

Palpation

- The spine of the scapula. The whole length of the spine can be palpated between the acromion process laterally and the medial border of the scapula. You will be able to recognize its upper and lower lips even though they give attachment to the trapezius and deltoid muscles, respectively. The posterior surface is easily visible and palpable. Notice that it is narrow medially but that it gradually broadens out as it passes laterally to become the superior surface of the acromion.
- Note 1. At this point the spine is covered by a bursa (the supra-acromial bursa), enabling the skin to move easily over the bone.
- Note 2. The bone then appears to form a large quadrilateral surface, which is directed upwards and slightly backwards having posterior, lateral and short anterior borders. On its medial side, the lateral end of the clavicle and the small gap produced by the acromioclavicular joint can be palpated. The smooth triangular area at the medial end of the spine is also covered by a bursa and can be palpated through the tendinous lower fibres of trapezius muscle.
- The medial border of the scapula. The medial border of the scapula is approximately 5 cm lateral to the spines of the second to eighth thoracic vertebrae. Its full length can only be palpated with difficulty, except in lean subjects, as it gives attachment to levator scapulae above and rhomboid major and minor below, as well as being mostly covered by trapezius muscle.
- The superior angle of the scapula. This is buried in muscle and is tender on deep palpation.
- The inferior angle of the scapula. This can be identified lying on the posterolateral parts of the seventh and eighth ribs. Ask the model to raise the arm above the head. You will now be able to see and feel the inferior angle of the scapula moving laterally around the chest wall as far as the mid-axillary line.

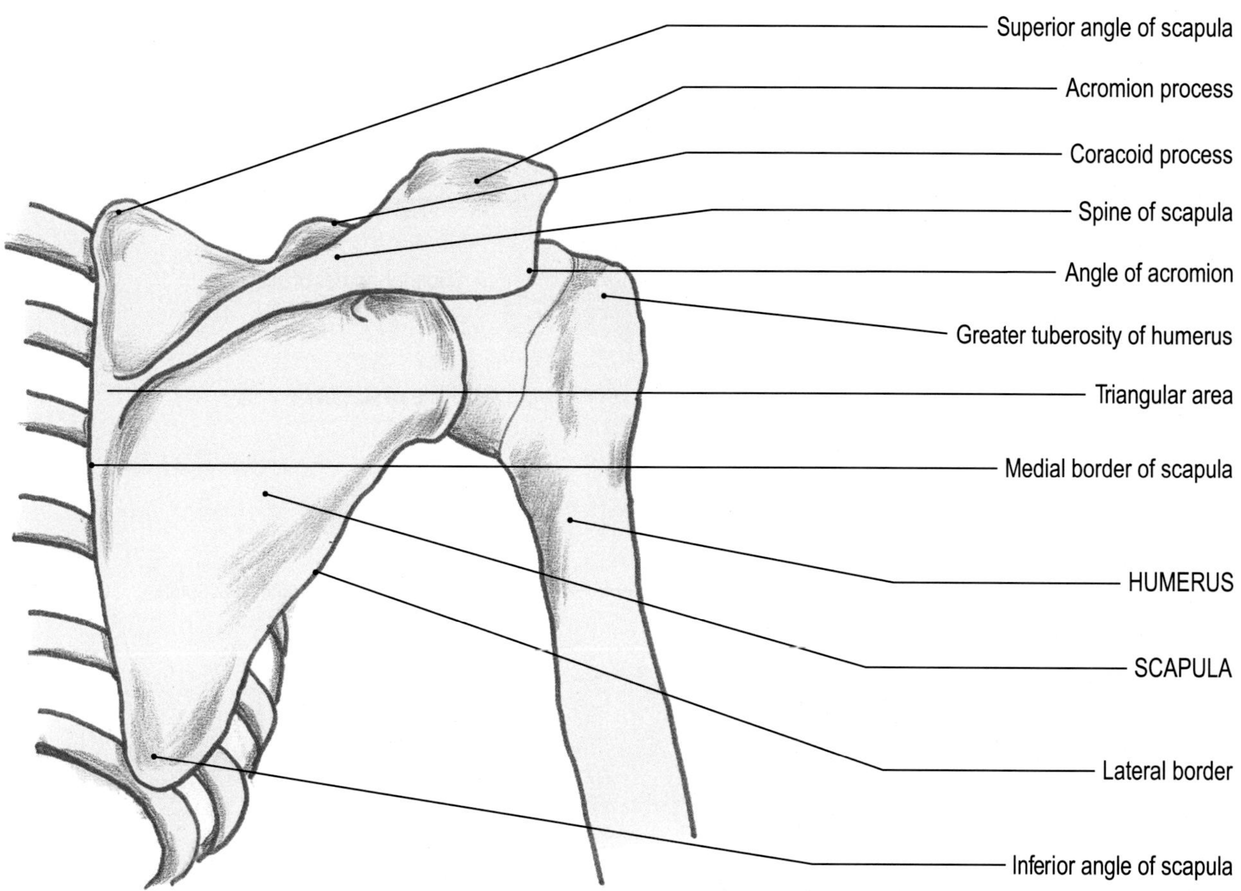

Fig. 2.2 (b) Bones of the right shoulder (posterior view)

- The **lateral border** of the scapula. This is very difficult to palpate as it is embedded in thick muscle (teres major and minor).
- **Note.** The lateral border of the scapula is by far the thickest of the borders and acts as a lever for its strong muscles to pull it laterally in scapula rotation.
- The coracoid process of the scapula. This process can be palpated where it lies anteriorly, in the infraclavicular fossa, 3 cm below the junction of the lateral and middle thirds of the clavicle. This is in spite of the fact that it gives attachment to three muscles: the short head of the biceps, coracobrachialis and pectoralis minor. Care should be taken not to apply very deep pressure as this may elicit tenderness in some subjects.
- The anterior rim of the glenoid cavity. The concave anterior rim of the glenoid cavity can be palpated just lateral to the coracoid process, running downwards and laterally for approximately 3 cm, with the head of the humerus lying on its lateral side.

Palpation on movement

Once you have been able to recognize the boundaries of the scapula by palpation of its various features, it is important to be able to follow its movements around the chest wall during activities of the shoulder girdle and upper limb.

For palpation in this area, the model should be in the standing or sitting position.

- Protrusion. Place your right hand on the point of the model's right shoulder. Now place your left hand on the inferior angle and the lower part of the medial border of the scapula. Ask the model to pull the shoulder girdles forward as in hunching the shoulders (protrusion). You will be able to see and palpate the scapula moving forwards around the chest wall whilst remaining in its vertical position.
- Retraction. Ask the model to brace back the shoulder girdles. You will be able to see and palpate the scapula moving backwards, again not changing its vertical position.
- Elevation and depression. Keep your hands in the same position. Ask the model to raise (elevation) and lower (depression) the shoulder girdles as in shrugging. You will be able to see and palpate the scapula rising and lowering but still holding its vertical position.
- Lateral rotation. Ask the model to raise the right arm above the head. When the upper limb reaches 20°, you will be able to see and palpate the scapula rotating around an axis just below the spine nearer to its medial end. The superior angle will rise, moving medially, and the inferior angle will be observed, moving laterally and slightly upwards around the chest wall (lateral rotation). In fact, the inferior angle will reach as far as the mid-axillary line on full elevation of the humerus.
- Medial rotation. Ask the model to lower the right arm from above the head. As the arm is lowered, you will be able to see and palpate the scapula returning to its original position (medial rotation). If, however, the arm is taken behind the back, medial rotation continues and the inferior angle will come close to the spines of the vertebrae.

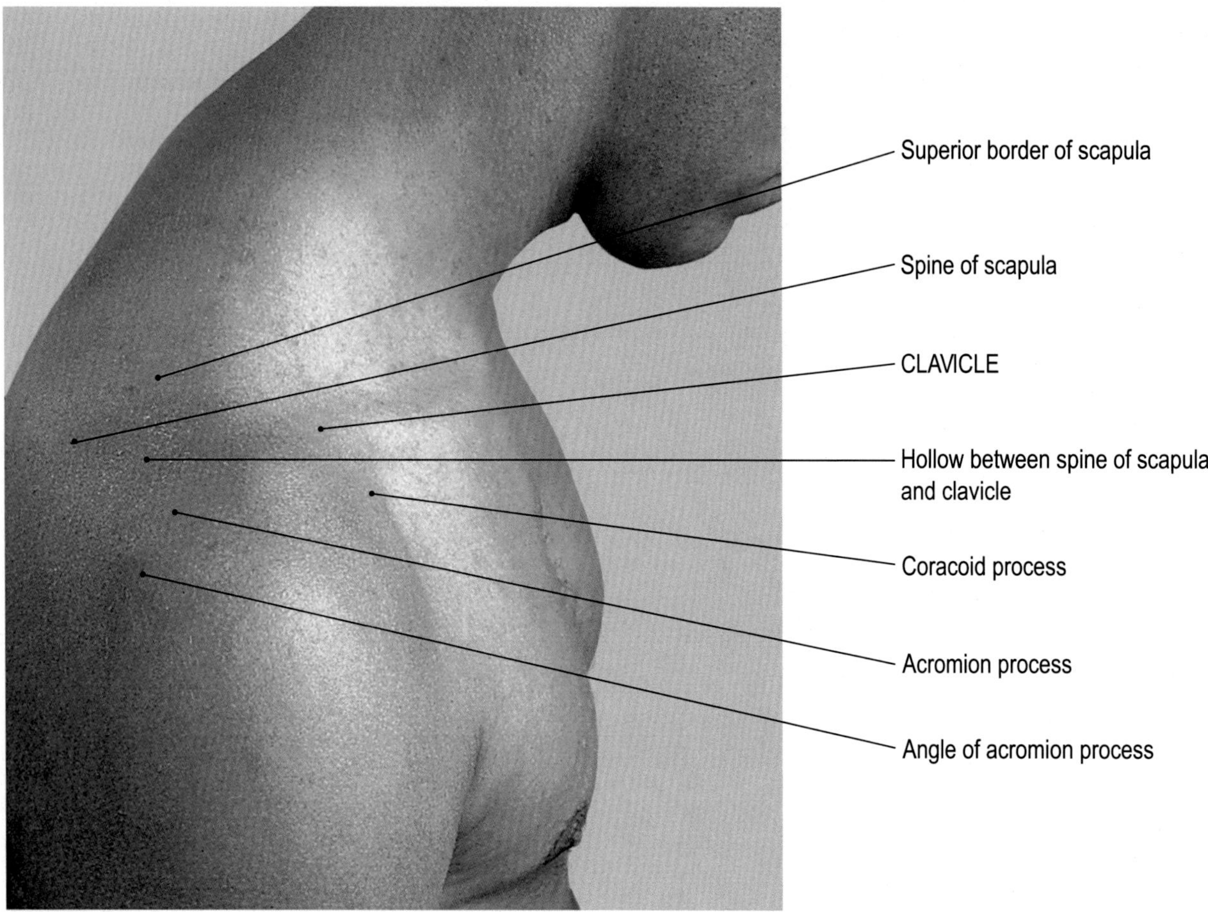

Fig. 2.2 (c) The right shoulder (upper lateral view)

Anatomy

Viewed from above and slightly laterally with the upper limb in about 45° of abduction, the shoulder girdle forms a 'V' shape with the **clavicle** being the anterior and the **spine of the scapula** the posterior stem. They form an angle with each other of approximately 70° and are joined at the acromioclavicular joint. The greater tuberosity of the humerus is now tucked underneath the arch of the **acromion**. Below the junction of the middle with the lateral third of the clavicle lies the **coracoid process** and below the lateral third of the clavicle lies the head of the humerus. The acromion appears quadrilateral from above and continues medially and backwards as the spine of the scapula. The **upper third of the scapula** lies above and anterior to the spine with the superior angle being most medial and the **superior border** passing laterally, presenting the **suprascapular notch** and continuing to the **base of the coracoid process**.

The anterior border of the lateral third of the clavicle continues laterally with the short anterior border of the acromion process. It continues as the lateral and posterior borders, becoming the inferior border of the spine.

Palpation

- The acromion process of the scapula. [*Akros* (Gk) = summit and *omos* = shoulders]. Run your fingers from the anterior border of the clavicle across the acromioclavicular joint where the anterior border of the acromion process of the scapula continues in line for approximately 1.5 cm.
- The lateral border of the acromion process. It then passes backwards as the lateral border of the acromion for a further 5 cm.
- The inferior lip of the spine of the scapula. The border then turns medially (**acromial angle**) to become the inferior lip of the spine of the scapula. You will be able to palpate the whole of this area.
- **Note.** This area gives attachment to deltoid muscle.

Palpation on movement

- Protraction. Place the fingers and thumb of your right hand on the medial end of the right clavicle. Now place the fingers and thumb of your left hand on the lateral end of the right clavicle. Ask the model to draw the shoulder girdle forward

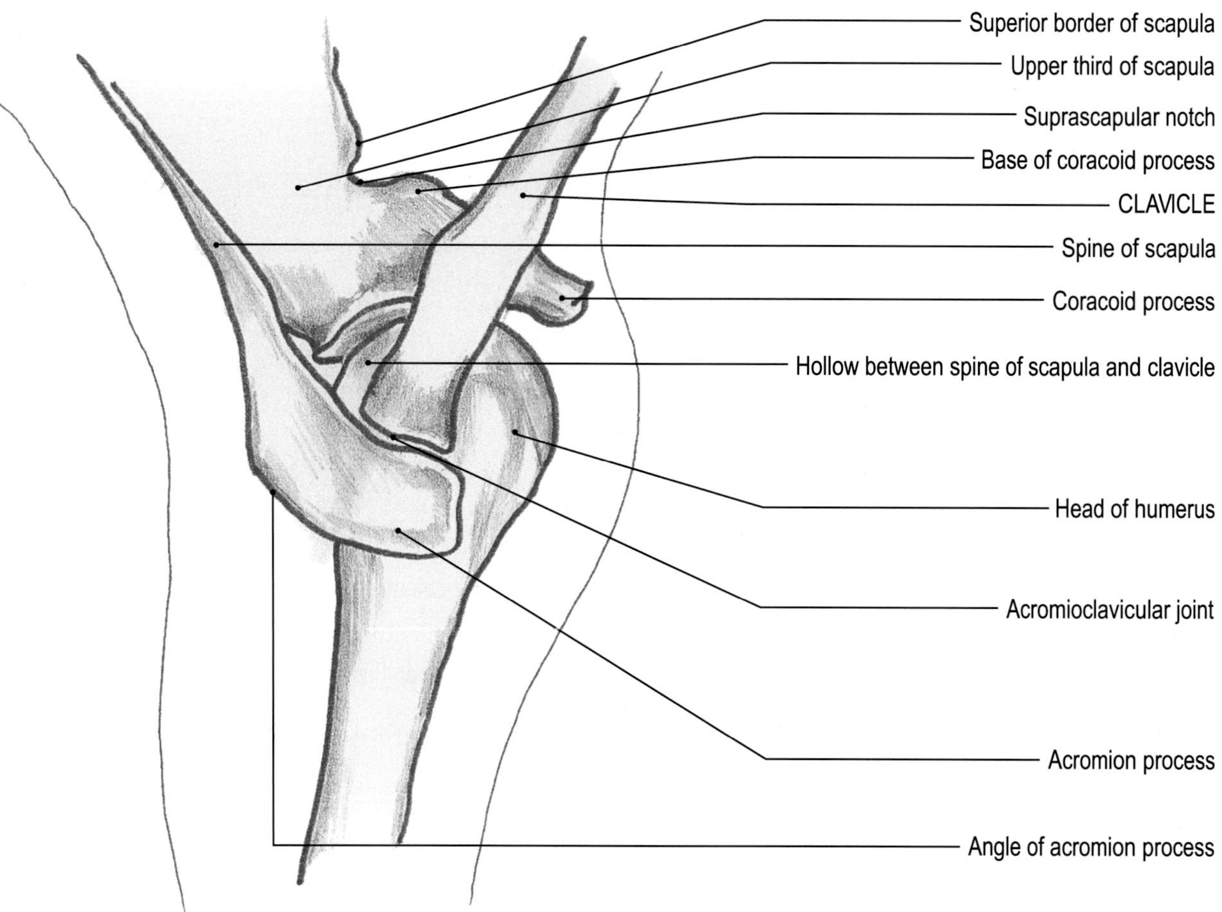

Fig. 2.2 (d) Bones of the right shoulder (upper lateral view)

(protrusion). Palpate the lateral end of the clavicle as it moves forward, accompanied by the gliding of the scapula around the chest wall. Now palpate the medial end of the clavicle and note that it glides backwards in the clavicular notch of the sternum.

- Note. The axis around which this movement occurs is approximately 3 cm from the medial end of the clavicle, where the costoclavicular ligament attaches to the undersurface of the bone.
- Retraction. Ask the model to draw the shoulders backwards (retraction). Palpate the lateral end of the clavicle which will move backwards. Now palpate the medial end of the bone which will move forwards and become proud of the sternum.
- Elevation. Ask the model to raise the shoulder girdle (elevation). Now palpate the lateral end of the clavicle which will rise. Palpate the medial end of the bone which will move down, rolling into the clavicular notch of the sternum using the same fulcrum as above.
- Depression. Ask the model to lower the shoulder girdle. Now palpate the lateral end of the clavicle which will drop. If you palpate its medial end, you will feel this end of the bone rising to its original position. If you now ask the model to depress the shoulder girdle further, you will feel the medial end of the clavicle protruding upwards.
- Elevation of the upper limb. Ask the model to raise the arm above the head. Now palpate the clavicle as, initially, it will move as in the movement of elevation. In the final stage of the movement, however, you will be able to feel the entire bone rotating with its anterior surface moving upwards. You will also be able to palpate the lateral rotation of the scapula which accompanies this movement. If the model now lowers the arm, the shoulder girdle will return to its original position.
- Note. Movements of the clavicle, scapula and humerus and the joints between them are highly complex and should be studied in *Anatomy and Human Movement* (Palastanga et al 2002).

Functional anatomy

The clavicle acts as a rigid lever bracing the shoulder girdle backwards, allowing the upper limb to move freely away from the chest wall. With the powerful upper fibres of trapezius muscle raising or supporting its lateral end and the adjoining acromion process, it helps to transmit weight from the upper limb to the vertebral column via the manubrium sterni and the upper ribs. The clavicle moves around an axis close to its medial end at the attachment of the costoclavicular ligament. It is tightly bound to the coracoid process laterally by the coracoclavicular ligament.

Fractures of the bone may occur due to a fall on the shoulder, as in horse riding, motorcycling and rugby. Normally the fracture will take place where the medial two-thirds joins the lateral third, medial to the coracoclavicular ligament. The shoulder girdle may protrude forwards and a large hard swelling can be palpated and seen at the site of the fracture. Complications can occur following fractures of this bone if it is more central and the sharp bone ends are forced backwards, thus damaging the brachial plexus and/or the subclavian artery.

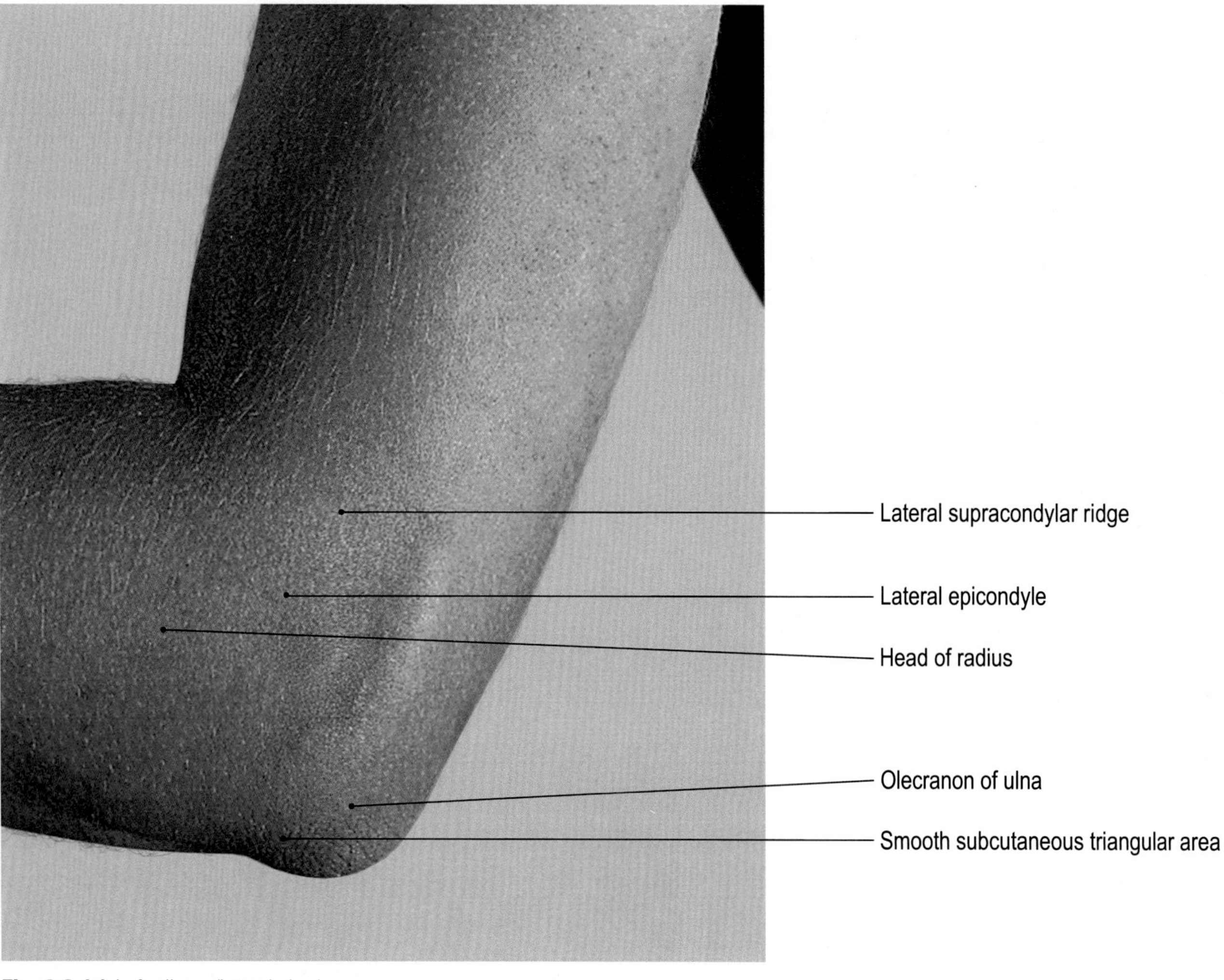

Fig. 2.3 (a) Left elbow (lateral view)

The elbow region (Fig. 2.3)

This region comprises the lower end of the humerus and the upper ends of the radius and ulna.

The lower end of the humerus is composed of a medial and lateral condyle, having two articular surfaces: the trochlea and the capitulum, respectively. Above these surfaces anteriorly are two fossae: the coronoid medially and radial laterally. Posteriorly, there is a larger depression: the olecranon fossa. On the lateral side of the lateral condyle is a prominence: the lateral epicondyle. This lies at the lower end of the lateral supracondylar ridge. The upper end of the radius is composed of a head which is button-shaped and articular on its upper surface, and the medial third of its rim. There is a neck, which is cylindrical, joining the head to the upper end of the shaft. There is also a large tuberosity (bicipital tuberosity), which projects from its medial side at the base of the neck. It is roughened on its posterior aspect for the attachment of the tendon of biceps brachii.

Palpation

For palpation in this area, the model should be in the sitting position.

- The humerus. Find the lower attachment of deltoid muscle which is halfway down the lateral side of the arm. Just below this, you will be able to palpate the humerus.
- Note. The humerus is crossed laterally by the radial nerve running downwards and forwards. Trauma in this area can cause pain, tingling and, sometimes, numbness of the postero-lateral aspect of the hand.
- The lateral supracondylar ridge of the humerus. Inferiorly, you will palpate a sharp border on the bone. This is the lateral supracondylar ridge which terminates at the large lateral epicondyle.
- The lateral epicondyle of the humerus. You will be able to palpate the posterior surface of this epicondyle which is subcutaneous.
- The olecranon fossa of the humerus. Ask the model to flex the elbow. Now you can trace the ridge medially across the back of the humerus to the commencement of the olecranon [*ole-kranon* (Gk) = the point of the elbow] fossa.
- The head of the radius [*radius* (L) = spoke of a wheel]. Ask the model to extend the elbow. Now you will be able to palpate the lateral side of the button-shaped head of the radius situated immediately below the humeral epicondyle. The

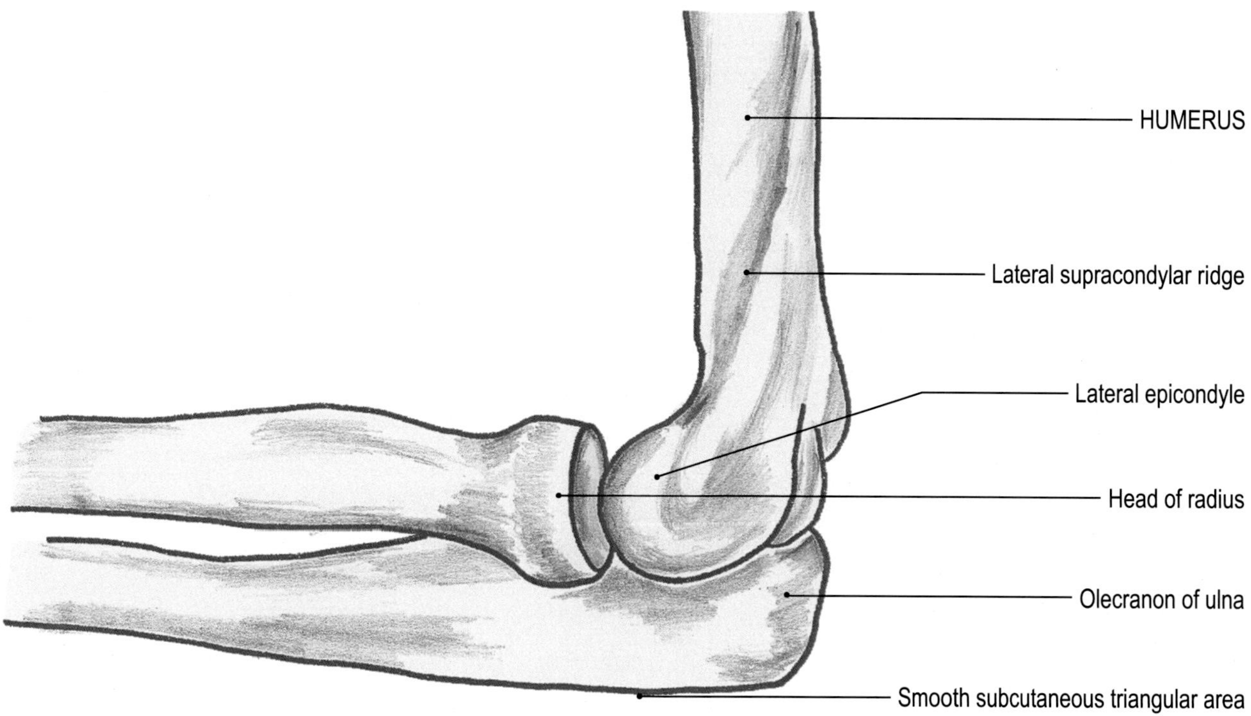

Fig. 2.3 (b) Bones of the left elbow (lateral view)

narrow groove running horizontally between the two is the radiohumeral part of the elbow joint.

- The neck of the humerus. Palpate around the lateral half of the radial head, posteriorly, as far as the posterior aspect of the superior radioulnar joint. Just below the head, laterally, palpate the narrowed radial neck which is hidden by muscles anteriorly and posteriorly.
- The olecranon process of the ulna (Fig. 2.3a, b). Ask the model to extend and then to flex the elbow. Now palpate the large bony formation of the olecranon, particularly when the elbow is flexed. Its superior surface is more difficult to feel because it is covered by the tendon of triceps as the tendon inserts into its posterior aspect.
- The olecranon bursa. Now place your fingers on the posterior triangular surface of the olecranon. You will find that the skin and superficial fascia can easily be moved owing to the presence of the subcutaneous olecranon bursa.
- Note. If pressure is applied for some time to this area, as in leaning on the elbows, the bursa can become inflamed and swollen (bursitis).
- The medial and lateral surfaces of the olecranon process. Palpate the narrow triangular surface which has its apex downwards and is continuous with the posterior border of the ulna. Palpate this border which is subcutaneous as far as its head. Whilst you will be able to palpate the medial and lateral surfaces of the olecranon relatively easily, they are covered by muscle lower down and are more difficult to identify. The olecranon is much more difficult to palpate when the elbow is extended, as it moves into the olecranon fossa of the posterior surface of the distal end of the humerus.

Palpation on movement

- Extension. Ask the model to flex the right elbow joint to 90°. Place the fingers of your left hand on the superior surface of the olecranon, which will be at the back of the elbow. Now place the fingers of your right hand on the medial epicondyle and your thumb on the lateral epicondyle of the humerus. Ask the model to extend the elbow joint. You will be able to palpate the olecranon which will virtually disappear into the olecranon fossa on the posterior aspect of the humerus.
- Pronation and supination. Ask the model to flex the right elbow joint. Now locate the outer edge of the disc-like head of the radius. Ask the model to pronate and supinate the forearm. Note the rotation of the head of the radius beneath your fingers.
- Finally, stand in front of the model. Ask the model to flex the elbow joint fully. Take the arm in your left hand and the forearm in your right. Now ask the model to extend the elbow joint. You will observe that the forearm, which was slightly medial to the line of the humerus, now moves more to the lateral side forming an angle with the upper part of the arm. This is termed 'the carrying angle'.

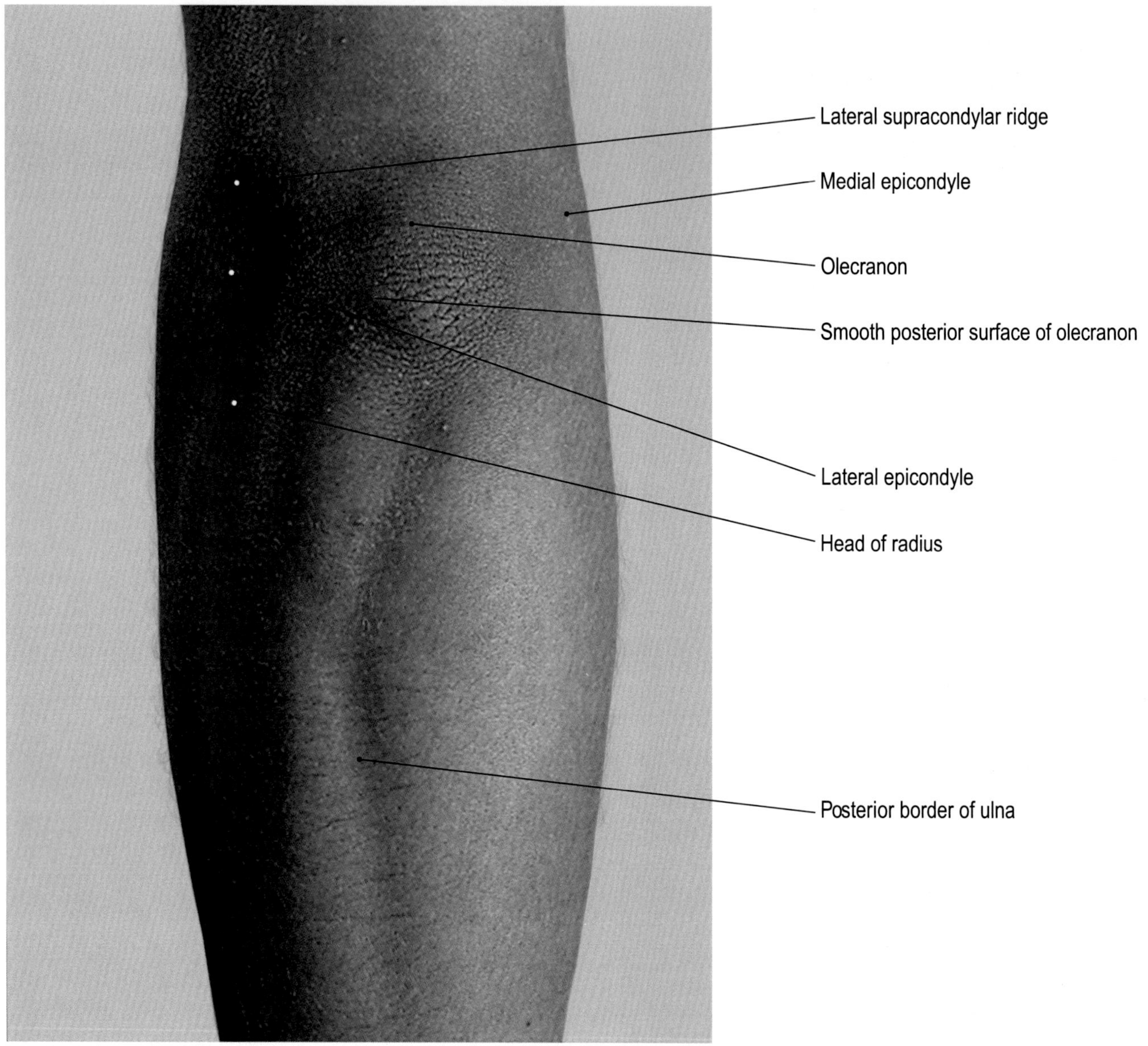

Fig. 2.3 (c) Left elbow (posterior view)

On the medial surface of the medial condyle of the humerus there is a large projection: the **medial epicondyle**. This is slightly hollowed posteriorly. Above this is the **medial supracondylar ridge** which passes up to the medial side of the shaft.

The pulley-shaped trochlea is articular and covers the anterior, inferior and posterior aspect of the bone. Its medial flange is lower than the lateral and accounts for the angle at the elbow joint.

The upper end of the ulna, lying below the trochlea of the humerus, is composed mainly of a hook-shaped process: the **olecranon**. There is a shelf-like process projecting forwards from the upper end of the shaft: the coronoid process. The two form a socket shape facing forwards: the trochlear notch. This articulates with the trochlea of the humerus in the elbow joint.

Palpation

- The medial supracondylar ridge of the humerus. On the medial side of the elbow, you will be able to palpate the sharp medial supracondylar ridge. Trace this ridge upwards for approximately the lower quarter of the humerus.
- The medial epicondyle of the humerus. At the lower end of the medial supracondylar ridge, palpate a large, bony prominence 2 cm above the elbow joint and approximately 1 cm below the level of the lateral epicondyle. This is the medial epicondyle of the humerus, behind which there is a deep groove for the ulnar nerve.
- **Note.** Palpation of this area may be quite tender and could cause tingling or even numbness on the medial side of the hand due to pressure on the ulnar nerve. This is often erroneously referred to as the 'funny bone', owing to the strange sensation when the nerve is compressed.
- The olecranon fossa. Ask the model to flex the elbow joint fully. It is just possible to feel the depression of the olecranon fossa through the tendon of triceps.
- The medial and lateral epicondyles of the humerus. From the posterior aspect, locate the medial and lateral epicondyles.

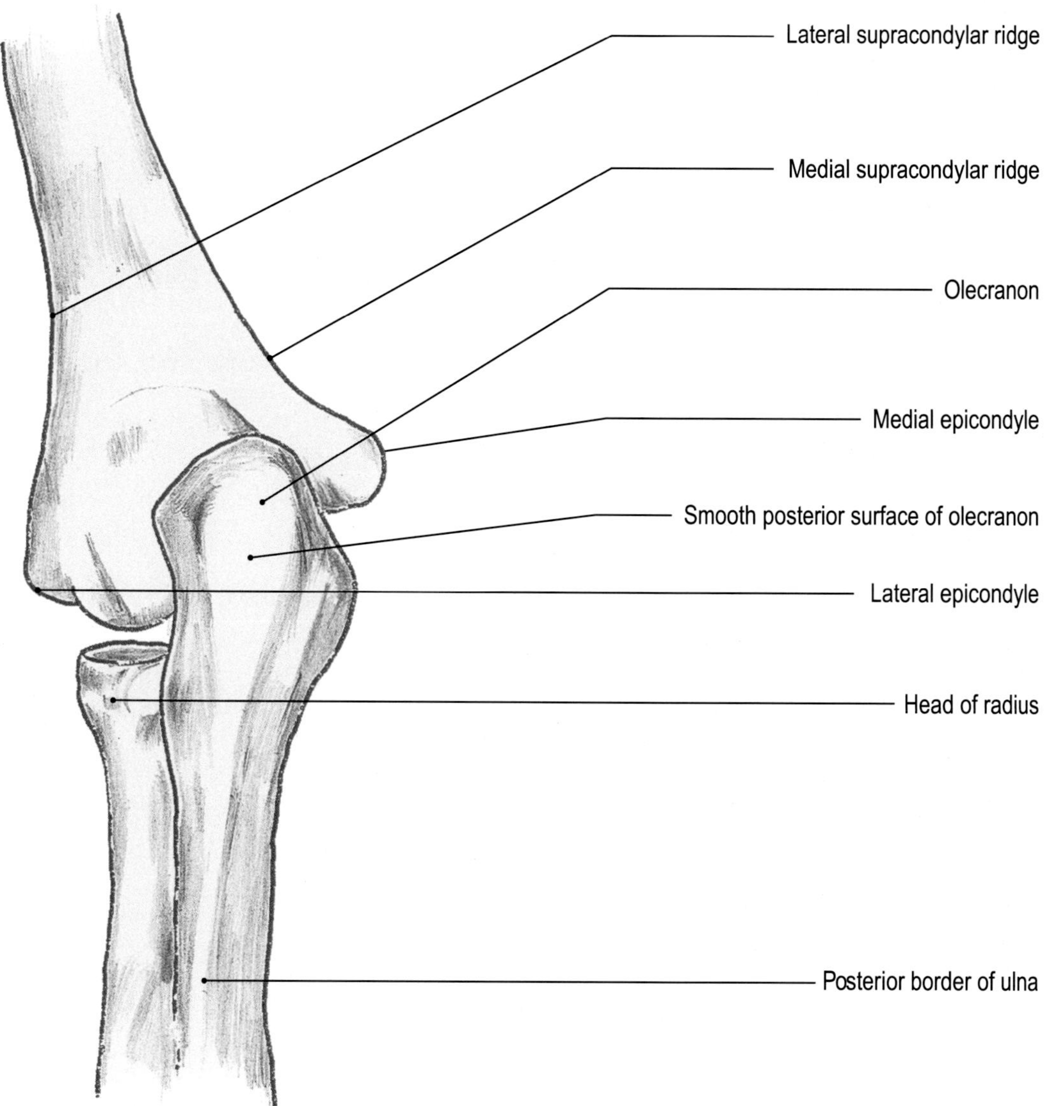

Fig. 2.3 (d) Bones of the left elbow (posterior view)

- The olecranon process of the ulna. At a point midway between the two epicondyles, press your thumb onto the back of the triceps tendon. You will observe that the tendon will sink slightly into the olecranon fossa. Just below your thumb you will palpate the bony olecranon.
- The coronoid process of the ulna (coronoid [*corone* (Gk) = crown; also the name given to the pointed front of a ship or plough]). Ask the model to extend the right elbow joint and and fully supinate the forearm. With the forearm in this fully extended position, examine the anterior aspect of this region. Place the flat surface of your right hand 2.5 cm below and 2.5 cm lateral to the medial epicondyle of the humerus. You will feel a hard bony projection deep to the mass of the flexor muscles. This is the coronoid process of the ulna.

Functional anatomy

- Note 1. The title 'carrying angle' at the elbow joint must have been given when the carrying of pails of water was common. In fact most objects carried in the hand with the elbow extended are normally accompanied by the forearm being held in the mid prone position. This eliminates the angle at the elbow.
- Note 2. When the elbow is fully flexed the hand does not oppose the shoulder joint; it is located in the mid clavicular area.
- Note 3. If the model now flexes the shoulder joint, the hand is taken first to the chin and then to the mouth, thus facilitating feeding. Keep the arm in this position. If the forearm is then fully pronated and the fingers extended, the hand now becomes a protection to the face.

Injuries and degeneration of the elbow and superior radioulnar joint often lead to loss of flexion or extension or both. This results in serious dysfunction of the upper limb, impeding its shortening and positioning of the hand. In one elbow this is perhaps acceptable, but if this dysfunction is present in both elbow complexes it may be devastating to a person's quality of life.

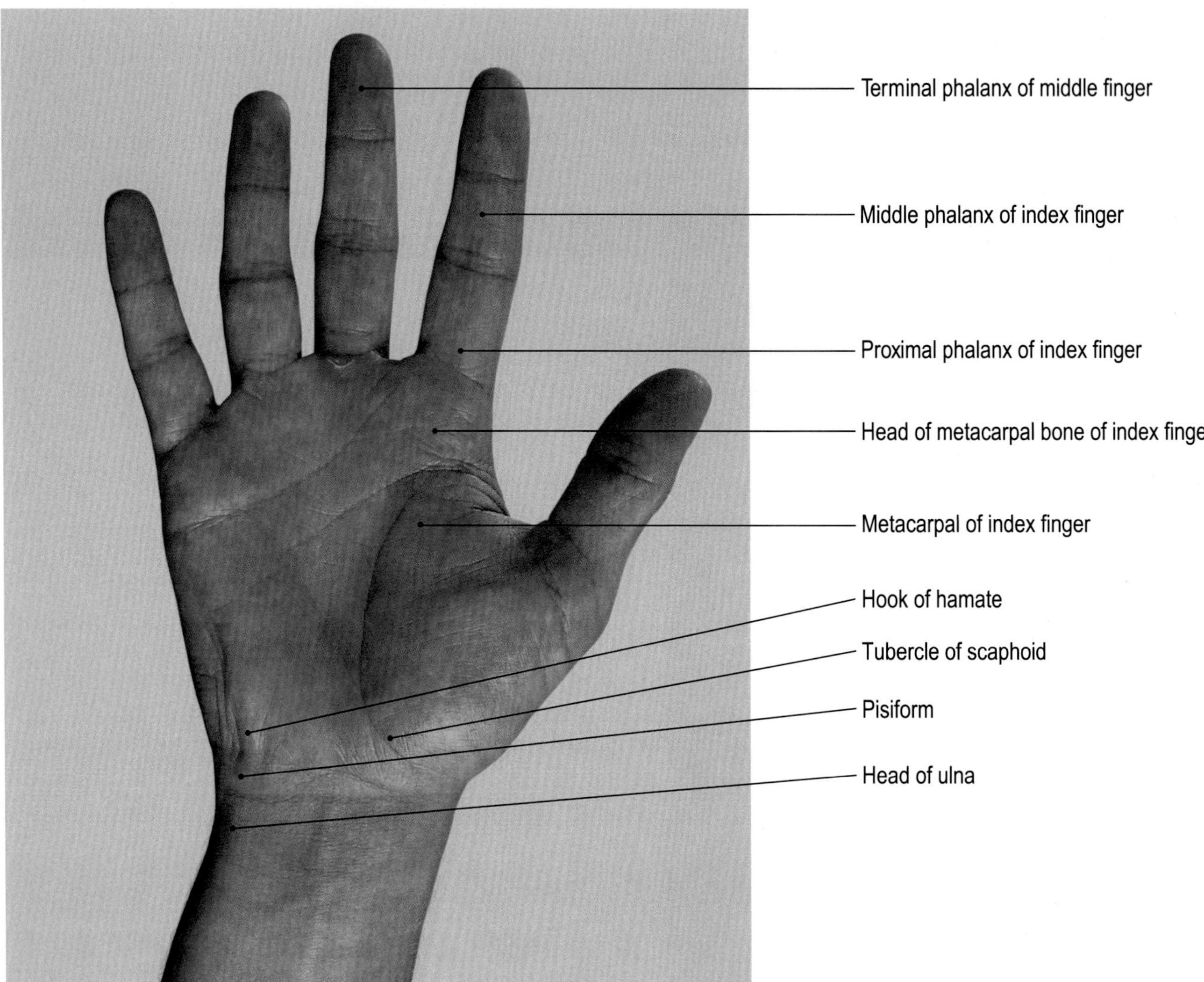

Fig. 2.4 (a) Right hand (anterior view)

The wrist and hand

The **lower ends of the radius and ulna** form a shallow mortice into which three of the four bones of the proximal row of carpals – scaphoid, lunate and triquetral – fit. The fourth bone in the proximal row, the **pisiform**, lies anterior to the triquetral. Distally, the proximal row of carpal bones form another concavity for the reception of the second row of carpal bones: the trapezium, trapezoid, capitate [*capitate* (L) = head-shaped] and hamate. The capitate is the largest of the four and fits snugly into the deepest part of the concavity, being in contact with all the carpal bones except the pisiform, triquetral and trapezium (Fig. 2.4b).

The **metacarpals** are miniature long bones lying distal to the carpals. The metacarpal of the thumb articulates with the trapezium; the second mainly articulates with the trapezoid; that for the middle finger mainly articulates with the capitate and the fourth and fifth articulate with the hamate.

Each metacarpal head articulates with a proximal **phalanx**. Each finger has a middle and a distal phalanx, the thumb has only a distal phalanx.

Anterior, medial and lateral aspects

Palpation

The bones of the wrist and hand are more difficult to locate on the anterior surface as they tend to be hidden by the muscles which arise and insert in the hand.

For palpation in this region, the model should be in the sitting position with the forearm resting on a pillow or an alternative support.

- The triquetral bone [*triquetrus* (L) = having three corners]. Return to the wrist joint. Locate the **head of the ulna** on its medial side (Fig. 2.4). Immediately distal to this, palpate the medial and posterior surfaces of the triquetral bone.
- The pisiform bone [*pisum* (L) = a pea]. On the anterior surface of the triquetral bone, palpate the pea-shaped pisiform bone. This bone is easily recognizable owing to its prominence and by the attachment of the tendon of flexor carpi ulnaris to its proximal side.
- **Note.** Application of deep pressure on the pisiform bone may elicit tenderness.
- The **hook of the hamate bone** [*hamatus* (L) = hooked]. If you now apply relatively deep pressure with the tip of your thumb 1 cm distal and slightly lateral to the pisiform bone, you will be able to feel a small but distinct bony prominence. This is the hook of the hamate bone. Now move your thumb from side to side and palpate two small nerves: the superficial terminal branches of the ulnar nerve. These can be compressed against the prominent hook of the hamate.
- The **tip of the radial styloid process**. On the lateral side of the wrist, locate the tip of the radial styloid process. It lies within a space termed the 'anatomical snuff box'.

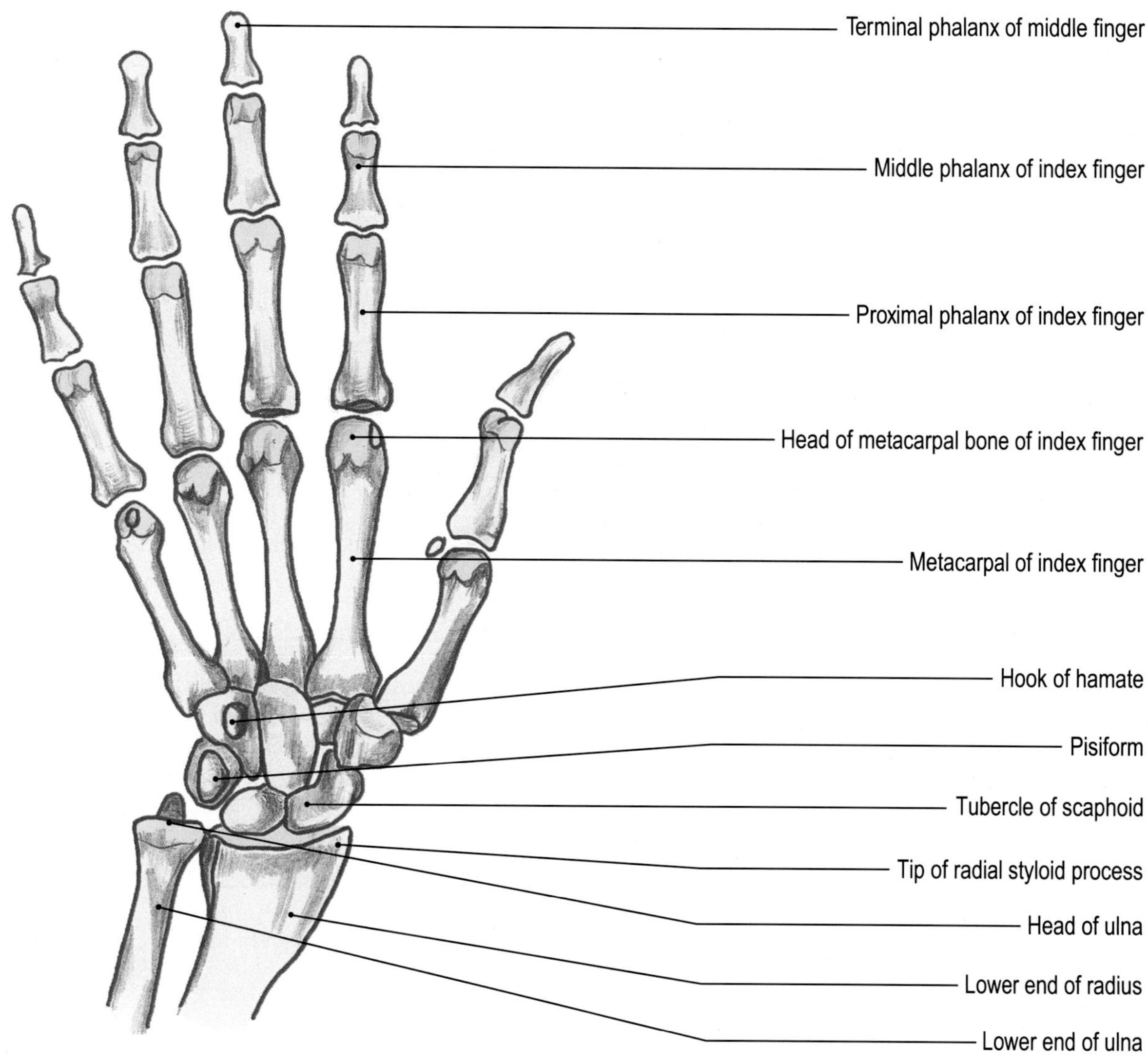

Fig. 2.4 (b) Bones of the right hand (anterior view)

- The anterior border of the radius. From the styloid process, trace upwards for a short distance and palpate the sharp anterior border of the radial shaft. The radial artery lies just medial to the crest of the anterior border.
- The scaphoid bone [*skaphe* (Gk) = a skiff] and the trapezium [*trapezion* (Gk) = an irregular four-sided figure]. Distal to the styloid process of the radius, palpate the lateral surfaces of the scaphoid and trapezium bones.
- The first metacarpal bone and its proximal and distal phalanges. The first metacarpal bone is identified by a small tubercle. Its shaft leads distally to its head. You should find the base, shaft and the head of the proximal phalanx easy to palpate. The base and shaft as far as the nail of the distal phalanx [*phalanx* (Gk) = a band of soldiers] are equally identifiable.
- **Note.** The posterior surface of the bones of the thumb face laterally due to the thumb lying at right angles to the palm. Medially, the anterior surfaces are difficult to palpate due to the presence of muscle and tendon.
- The **tubercle of the scaphoid bone**. To facilitate palpation of the tubercle of the scaphoid bone, ask the model to extend the wrist. The tubercle should then be palpable at the proximal end of the thenar eminence, on the front of the carpal region, 1 cm medial to the tip of the radial styloid process.
- The vertical edge of the trapezium bone. If you apply deep pressure, the vertical ridge of the trapezium is just palpable 1 cm distal to the scaphoid tubercle.
- **Note 1.** This can often be a painful area for deep palpation so it is advisable to limit the number of times this technique is performed.
- **Note 2.** The scaphoid tubercle is prominent enough to be damaged by falls on the outstretched hand leading to a fracture. This is likely to cause pain and dysfunction of the hand for many months due to its poor blood supply leading to a long healing time.
- The second–fifth metacarpal and phalangeal bones. The anterior surfaces of these remaining bones are difficult to palpate as they lie deep to the muscle and fascia. To facilitate palpation, ask the model to extend the fingers fully. The anterior surfaces of the heads of the metacarpals can be felt in line with each finger, 2 cm proximal to the web between the fingers. Ask the model to extend/hyperextend the metacarpophalangeal joints. Now palpate the heads of each phalanx, just proximal to the creases of the interphalangeal joints. If you now grip the lateral sides of the heads between your finger and thumb, you should be able to palpate a small tubercle situated on each side.

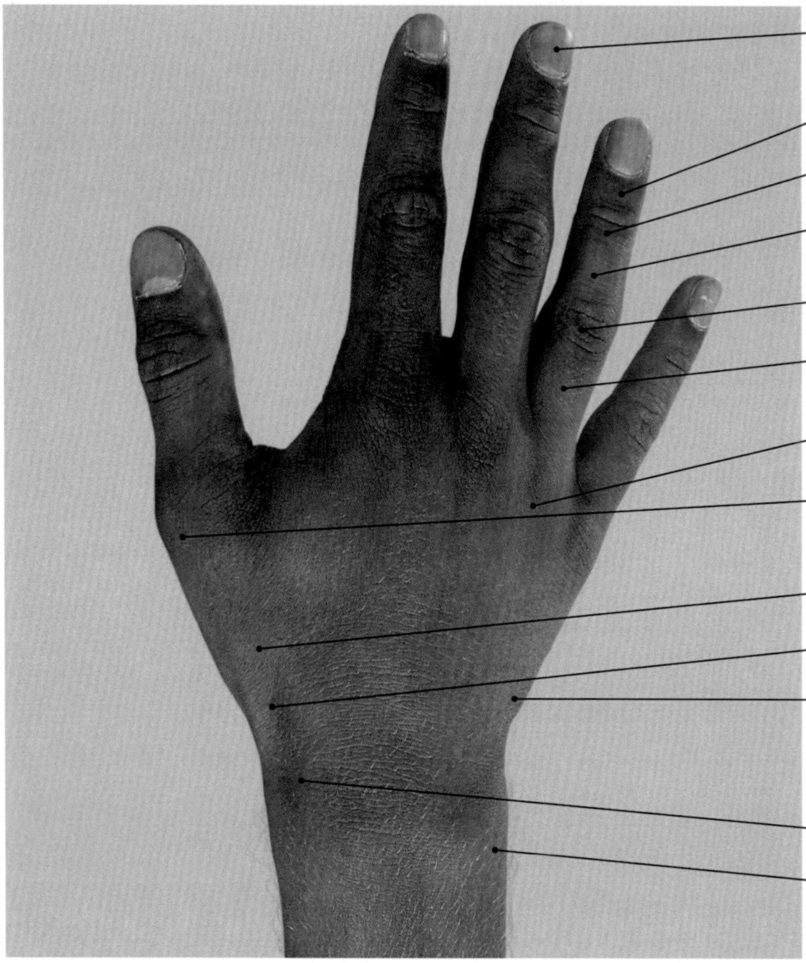

Nail bed of terminal phalanx
Terminal phalanx (shaft)
Head of middle phalanx
Middle phalanx of ring finger
Head of proximal phalanx
Proximal phalanx of ring finger
Head of metacarpal (knuckle)
Head of metacarpal of thumb
Base of first metacarpal
Trapezium (posterior surface)
Base of fifth metacarpal
Styloid process of radius
Head of ulna

Fig. 2.5 (a) Right hand (posterior view)

Posterior aspect (Fig. 2.5)

Palpation

- The styloid process of the ulna. Place your finger on the button-shaped head of the ulna. This is clearly palpable posteromedially, but is hidden by the tendon of flexor carpi ulnaris anteriorly. Palpate the ulna styloid process as a small projection on its posteromedial aspect, although this may be difficult as the bone is partially hidden by the tendon of extensor carpi ulnaris muscle. To facilitate palpation, ask the model to deviate the wrist radially. You will find that the **head of the ulna** and its **styloid process** become much easier to identify.
- The styloid process of the radius. Palpate the **radial styloid process** situated on the lateral side of the wrist, having tendons running in front and behind.
- The lateral side of the lower half of the radius. From the styloid process, trace upwards and palpate the lower half of the lateral side of the radius. From here, palpation becomes more difficult because the bone is covered by the bulk of brachioradialis muscle.
- **Note.** This region may be quite tender to palpate as it is often crossed by the superficial terminal branch(es) of the radial nerve.
- The dorsal tubercle of the radius. On the posterior aspect of the distal end of the radius, just above the level of the styloid process, the **dorsal tubercle of the radius** can be palpated. The tendon of extensor pollicis longus muscle grooves its medial side and uses it as a pulley.
- The posterior surfaces of the scaphoid, lunate [*luna* (L) = the moon] and triquetral bones. Find the dorsal tubercle of the radius. Below the level of this tubercle and the **head of the ulna**, locate a hollow; this is limited 2 cm below by the bases of the metacarpal bones. Ask the model to flex the wrist joint. Now palpate the posterior surfaces of the **scaphoid**, lunate and triquetral bones. They form a line distal to the tips of the radial and ulnar styloid processes.
- The trapezoid, capitate and hamate bones. Move your fingers just distal to the previous line of bones. Grip the bones between your fingers posteriorly and your thumb anteriorly. Just beyond them, palpate the trapezoid bone, which is situated at the base of the second metacarpal. Now palpate the capitate bone, situated at the base of the third metacarpal. Lastly, palpate the hamate, situated at the base of the fourth and fifth metacarpal bones.
- The second–fifth metacarpal and phalangeal bones. The lower limit of this area is marked by the bases of the metacarpal

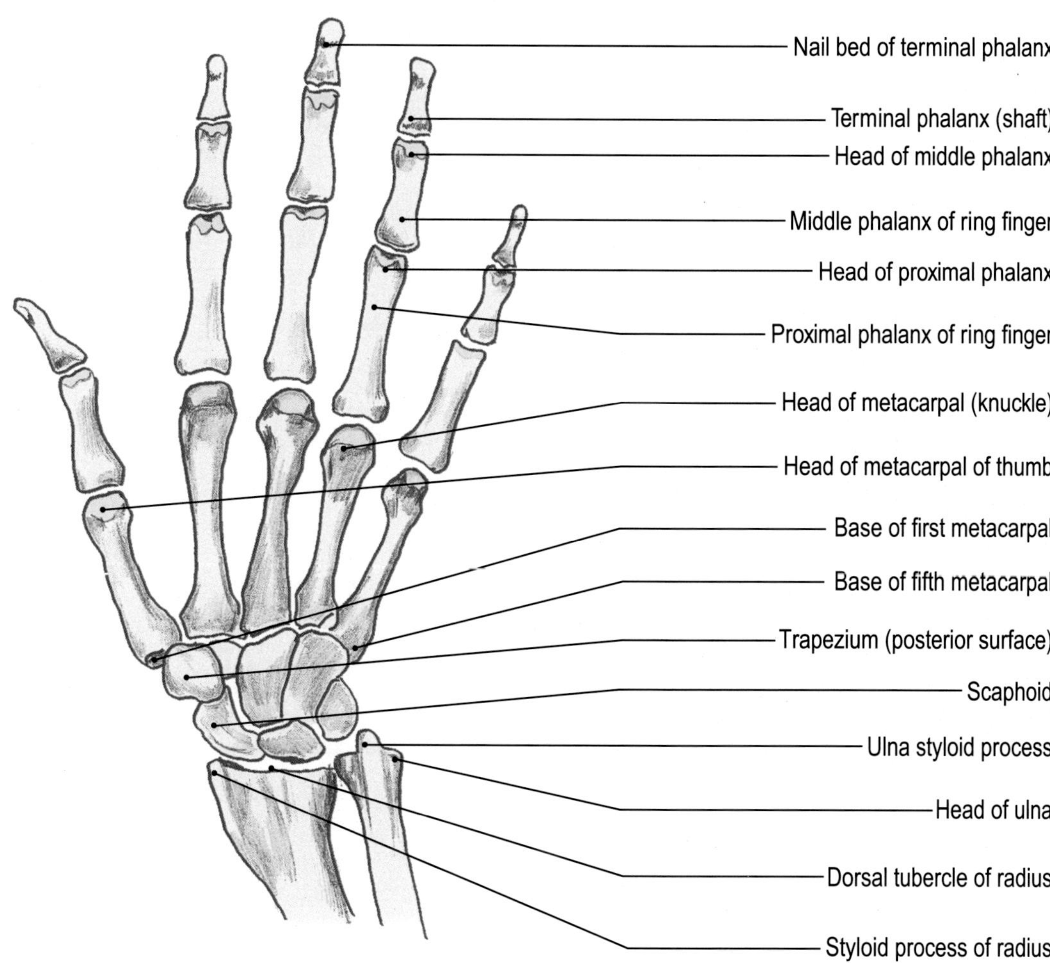

Fig. 2.5 (b) Bones of the right hand (posterior view)

bones with their shafts running distally to end in rounded heads, all of which are easily palpable. To facilitate palpation, ask the model to flex the fingers. The base, shaft and head of each phalanx are now equally easy to palpate posteriorly. Anteriorly, they are hidden by tendons and the pulp of the fingers.

Palpation on movement

- Flexion and extension of the wrist. Ask the model to extend the wrist. Locate the tubercle of the scaphoid and the pisiform bone. Now ask the model to flex the wrist. Palpate the scaphoid and pisiform bones as they appear to move backwards and become indistinct. Keep the model's wrist in flexion. Palpate the posterior aspect of the carpal bones just below the ulna and radius. Ask the model to extend the wrist. Palpate the posterior aspect to the carpal bones as they appear to move forwards and become indistinct.
- Flexion and extension of the fingers. Ask the model to extend the index finger. Now grip the base of the proximal phalanx with your thumb anteriorly and your fingers posteriorly. Ask the model to flex the finger. Palpate the phalanx as it moves round to the front of the head of the metacarpal leaving the head prominent (the knuckle). This is common to all the fingers, but more obvious in the index finger.
- Flexion of the interphalangeal joints. If you apply the technique as described above on the interphalangeal joints, you will palpate the head of the most proximal of the two bones as a small 'knuckle' shape.
- Flexion and extension of the thumb. If you now apply the same procedure as described above to the base of the proximal phalanx of the thumb, you will note that only half the movement is available and the head of the metacarpal is only partially exposed.

Functional anatomy

Fractures of the carpal bones are rare except in the case of the tubercle of the scaphoid, which is sometimes damaged by a fall on the outstretched hand.

Fractures of the metacarpal bones are fairly common at all ages and are often due again to a fall on the outstretched hand or a longitudinal force along the metacarpal, as in punching.

Injuries to the phalanges are usually due to direct violence such as trapping the fingers in a door.

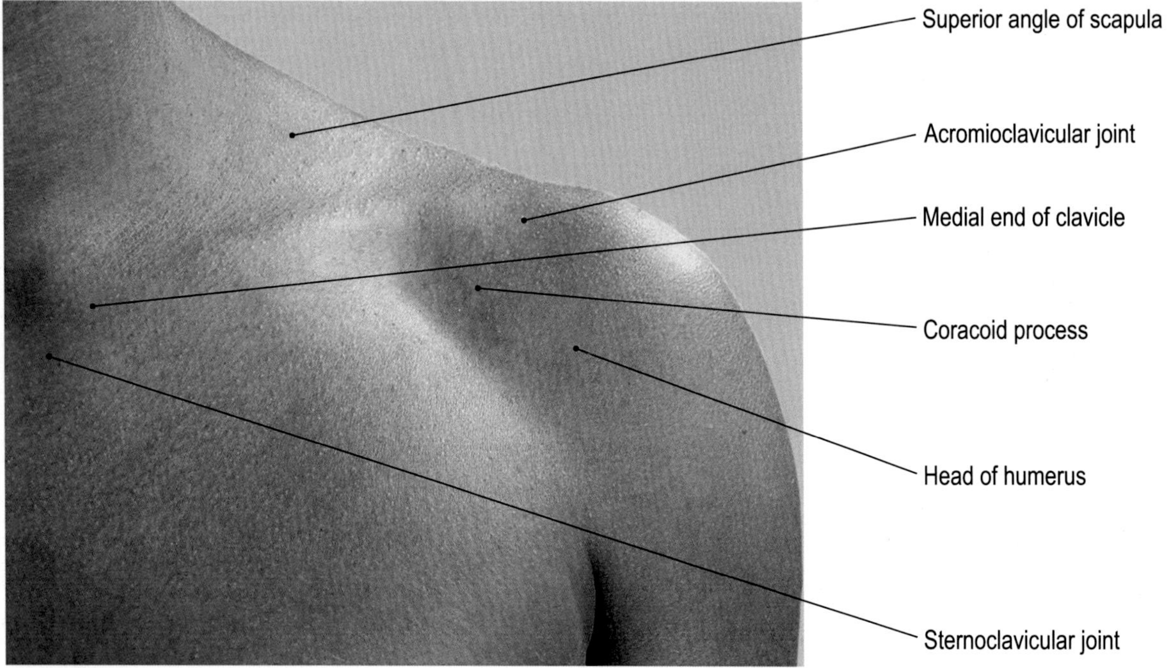

Fig. 2.6 (a) The shoulder region (anterior view)

JOINTS

Joints of the pectoral girdle

The sternoclavicular joint (Fig. 2.6)

At its medial end the clavicle articulates with the clavicular notch of the manubrium sterni. The joint is synovial, being surrounded by a capsule lined with synovial membrane, except where it is attached to the edges of a fibrous disc which divides the joint space into two separate cavities. It is a modified saddle (sellar) joint and its capsule is supported by ligaments, the intercostal above and medially, the costoclavicular laterally below the clavicle and the anterior and posterior across the front and back of the joint. It is subcutaneous, allowing easy palpation of the joint line and a reasonable examination of joint movement.

Palpation: surface marking

For palpation in this region, the model is in the sitting position.

- The sternoclavicular joint. You can palpate this joint at the upper lateral corner of the manubrium sterni. Draw a curved line concave laterally. It is approximately 1 cm in length, extending over the lower half of the medial surface of the clavicle, passing inferolaterally for approximately 0.5 cm. Run your fingers down the front of the neck until you reach the sternal notch. Below you will feel the manubrium sterni and laterally the medial end of the clavicle with the sternoclavicular joint between the two.

Palpation on movement

- Retraction. Immediately lateral to the joint, between the clavicle and the first rib, is the costoclavicular ligament. This is not palpable, but acts as the fulcrum for movements of the clavicle at the joint. Thus when the lateral end of the clavicle is drawn backwards (retraction), the medial end can be observed gliding forward, projecting anterior to the plane of the manubrium.
- Protraction. Similarly, when the lateral end of the clavicle is brought forwards (protraction), you will be able to palpate the medial end moving backwards behind the plane of the manubrium.
- Elevation 1. Ask the model to raise the lateral end of the pectoral girdle. Palpate the medial end of the clavicle as it glides downwards on the clavicular notch of the manubrium sterni until it is level with the superior border of the manubrium sterni.
- Elevation 2. Ask the model to raise the upper limb above the head. The scapula laterally rotates around the chest wall and the lateral end of the clavicle is elevated. During the final few

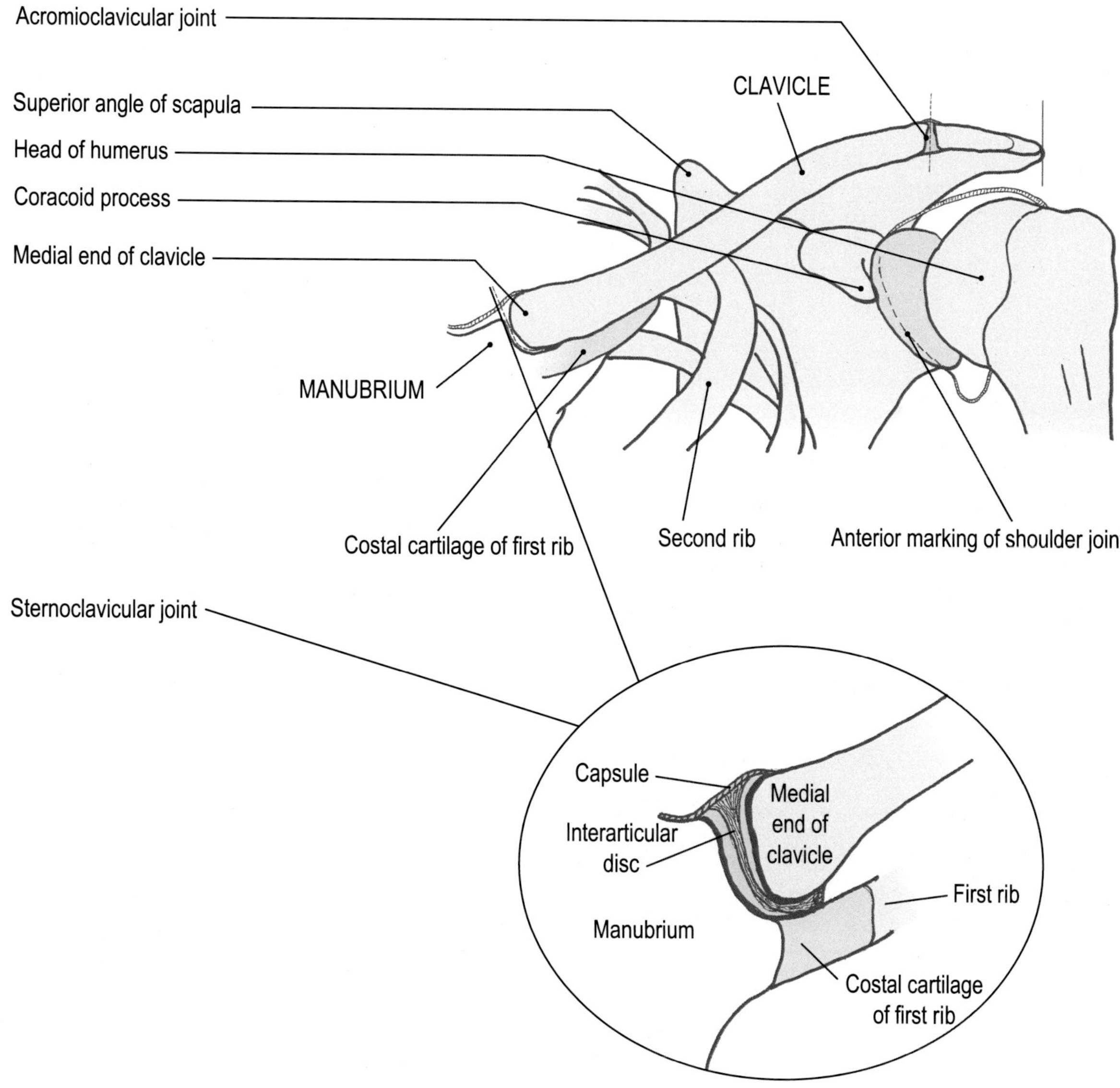

Fig. 2.6 (b) Joints of the shoulder region (anterior view)

degrees of movement, the clavicle rotates around its long axis so that the anterior surface faces more superiorly. This rotation is due to the tension developed in the coracoclavicular ligament.

- Depression. Ask the model to pull the pectoral girdle downwards (depression). Palpate the medial end of the clavicle as it rises on the clavicular notch.
- Note. All these movements can be observed occurring around the attachment of the costoclavicular ligament.

Accessory movements

Palpation

- Gliding movements of the medial end of the clavicle. The forwards, backwards, upwards or downwards, or rotating the clavicle's articular surfaces upwards, are all normal movements. Pressure applied to the medial end of the clavicle will produce little movement, as the stress is taken by the costoclavicular ligament which usually remains taut and reasonably inflexible.
- Movements of the medial end of the clavicle. If you apply similar pressures to the medial end of the clavicle, with the pectoral girdle in an appropriate position to aid the movement, additional movement can be achieved. Ask the model to protrude the shoulder girdle. Now apply pressure anteroposteriorly. This will augment the movement of the medial end of the clavicle. Pressure to raise the anterior surface of the medial end of the clavicle, as in the final stages of elevation, is best applied when the upper limb is as near to full elevation as possible.

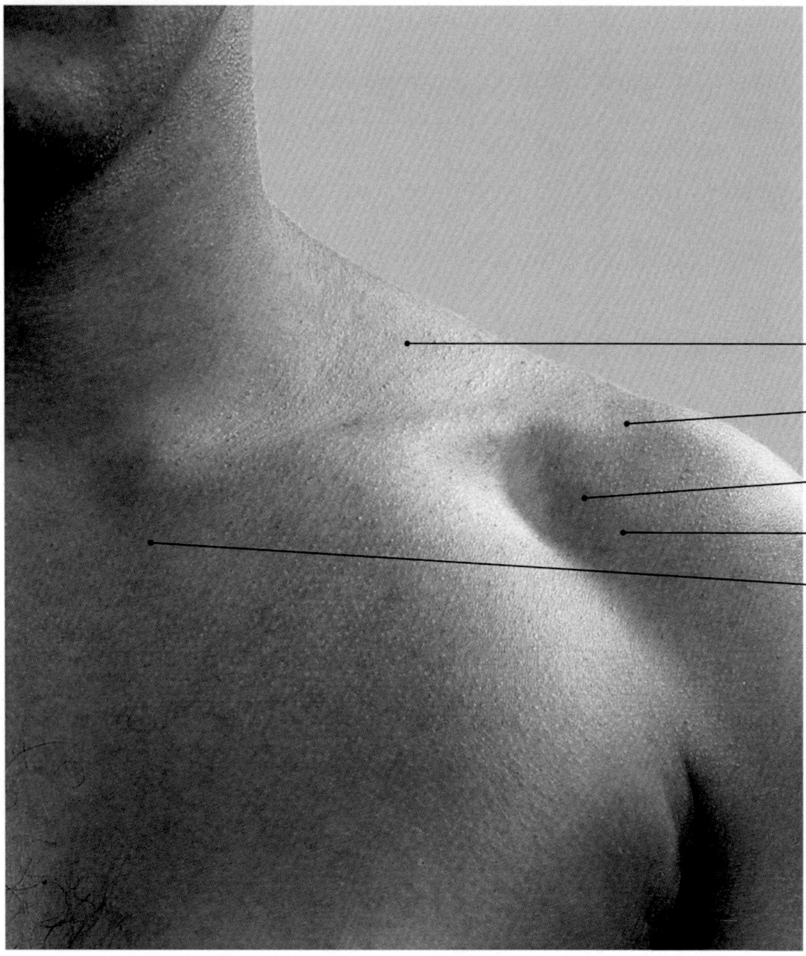

Superior angle of scapula
Acromioclavicular joint
Coracoid process
Shoulder joint
Sternoclavicular joint

Fig. 2.7 (a) The acromioclavicular joint (anterior view)

The acromioclavicular joint (Fig. 2.7)

The acromioclavicular joint is immediately lateral to the anterior concavity of the lateral one-third of the clavicle, approximately 1.5 cm medial to the lateral border of the acromion process.

Palpation: surface marking

- The acromioclavicular joint. From above, draw a line in an anteroposterior direction just lateral to a small tubercle on the upper surface of the lateral end of the clavicle.

The acromioclavicular joint is a plane synovial joint. It lies in a paramedian plane of the body. It is surrounded by a joint capsule supported above by the superior acromioclavicular ligament. It relies for its stability, however, on the costoclavicular and the coracoclavicular ligaments which act as accessory ligaments to this joint. The two oval facets, one on the lateral end of the clavicle and the other on the medial aspect of the acromion process, are not congruent and rely on a small disc or part of a disc which fills the upper part of the joint space.

Palpation

- The angle of the acromion. Stand facing the model's left shoulder. Run your right hand up over deltoid muscle on the lateral aspect of the shoulder. At the top you will feel the lateral border of the acromion process marked posteriorly by its angle.
- The acromial indentations. Now trace along the anterior border of the acromion for 1.5 cm. You will feel a small indentation where the clavicle joins the acromion. A very faint groove passes posteriorly to another small indentation on the posterior surface. The joint is quite difficult to palpate unless movement is occurring.

Palpation on movement

- Twisting or gapping. With careful palpation, you may be able to detect slight twisting or gapping of the acromion against the clavicle with movements of the pectoral girdle.
- Rotation. Ask the model to elevate the upper limb fully. Now palpate the acromion process as it rotates backwards against the lateral end of the clavicle. This occurs until the final few

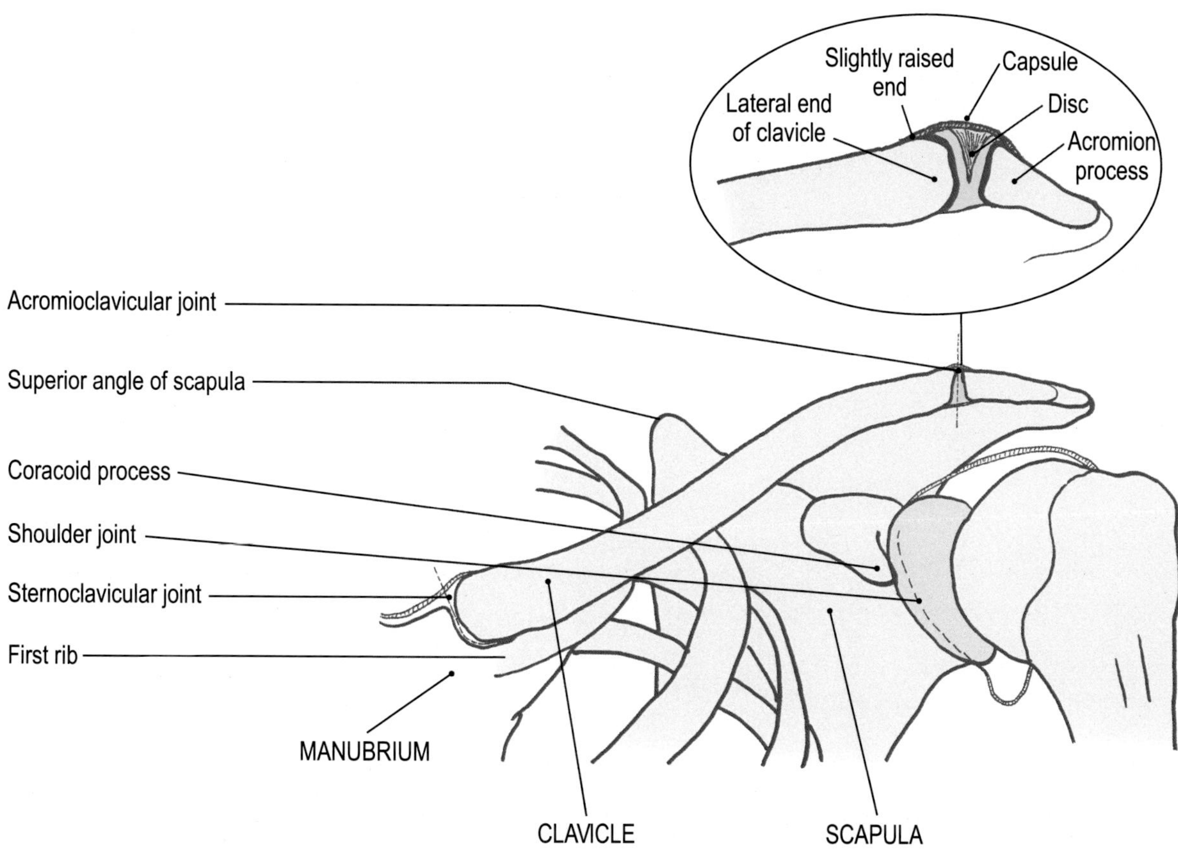

Fig. 2.7 (b, c) The acromioclavicular joint (anterior view)

degrees of elevation when you will feel the clavicle also rotating backwards. This produces an upward movement of the anterior surface of the clavicle in its entire length.

- Note 1. This is partly due to the tension of the conoid part of the coracoclavicular ligament pulling down the posterior aspect of the clavicle, and partly due to the costoclavicular ligament at the medial end of the clavicle attaching to its posterior aspect.
- Note 2. This movement is also facilitated by the thickness of the disc in the sternoclavicular joint allowing a longitudinal rotation to occur.
- Note 3. The superior surface of the acromioclavicular joint is usually quite tender on palpation due to pressure on the superior acromioclavicular ligament. This tenderness is increased after prolonged activity involving the pectoral girdle or after carrying heavy loads on the shoulder.

Accessory movements

This joint is capable of slight gliding movements, these being forwards, backwards, upwards and downwards. It can also rotate, with one surface pivoting on the other, as well as allowing a certain amount of gapping anteriorly and posteriorly.

Palpation

- Note 1. All the above movements are normal but, as with the sternoclavicular joint, the end-range can be increased by addition of pressure in the appropriate direction.
- Note 2. The movements are best performed at the end of normal range.
- Posterior gliding of the acromion. An increase in this movement is facilitated if you ask the model to retract the shoulder girdle. Using your thumbs, now apply pressure, either to the lateral end of the clavicle or the anterior aspect of the acromion. You may find it easier to apply the former technique.
- Note 3. Although the acromioclavicular and sternoclavicular joints may appear to be insignificant, stiffness of either will reduce the range of movement of the pectoral girdle. This may result in serious functional loss in the range of movement of the upper limb and may be misdiagnosed as shoulder joint stiffness.

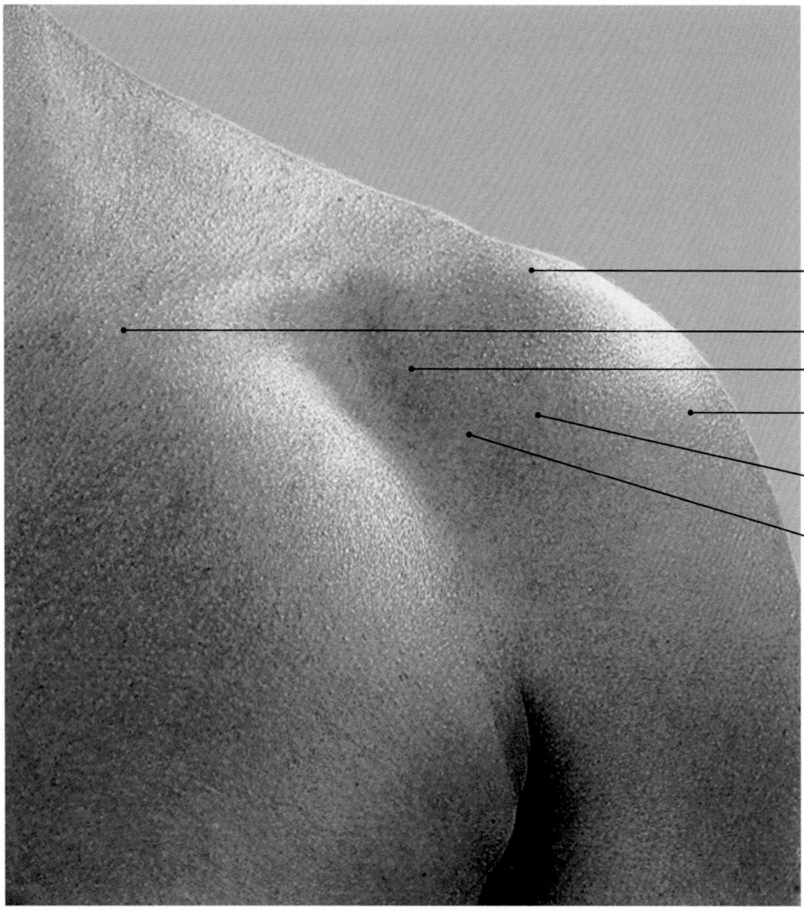

Fig. 2.8 (a) The left shoulder joint (anterior view)

The shoulder joint (Fig. 2.8)

This is a synovial joint of the ball-and-socket type. The **head of the humerus** is slightly less than half a sphere, but is more ovoid in shape. The **glenoid cavity** is shallow and is estimated to contain only one-third the articular surface of the head of the humerus. Both surfaces are covered with articular cartilage. The joint is capable of a large range of movements which are essential for full functional activity of the upper limb. The apparent range of the joint is further increased by the movements of the shoulder (pectoral) girdle, allowing the glenoid cavity to be directed more upwards than laterally.

The joint is surrounded by a loose capsule which is lined by synovial membrane and is supported by ligaments. Anteriorly, it is supported by the glenohumeral, above and posteriorly by the coracohumeral and across the bicipital groove by the transverse ligament. A fibrous ring, triangular in cross section (the glenoidal labrum) is attached to the outer rim of the glenoid cavity, deep to the joint capsule.

Palpation: surface marking

- The anterior joint line. This is identified by a shallow curve concave laterally. Palpate its upper boundary, which is just lateral to, and above the **coracoid process**. It passes downwards and slightly laterally for approximately 2–3 cm.
- The head of the humerus. Palpate the humeral head, which lies lateral to the joint line.

Palpation

The joint is deep, being surrounded by strong, thick muscles, and is therefore not easy to palpate.

For palpation in this region, the model is in the sitting position.

- The anterior part of the head of the humerus. The anterior aspect of the joint is the nearest to the surface. First, palpate the rounded anterior part of the head of the humerus. You should find this relatively easy.

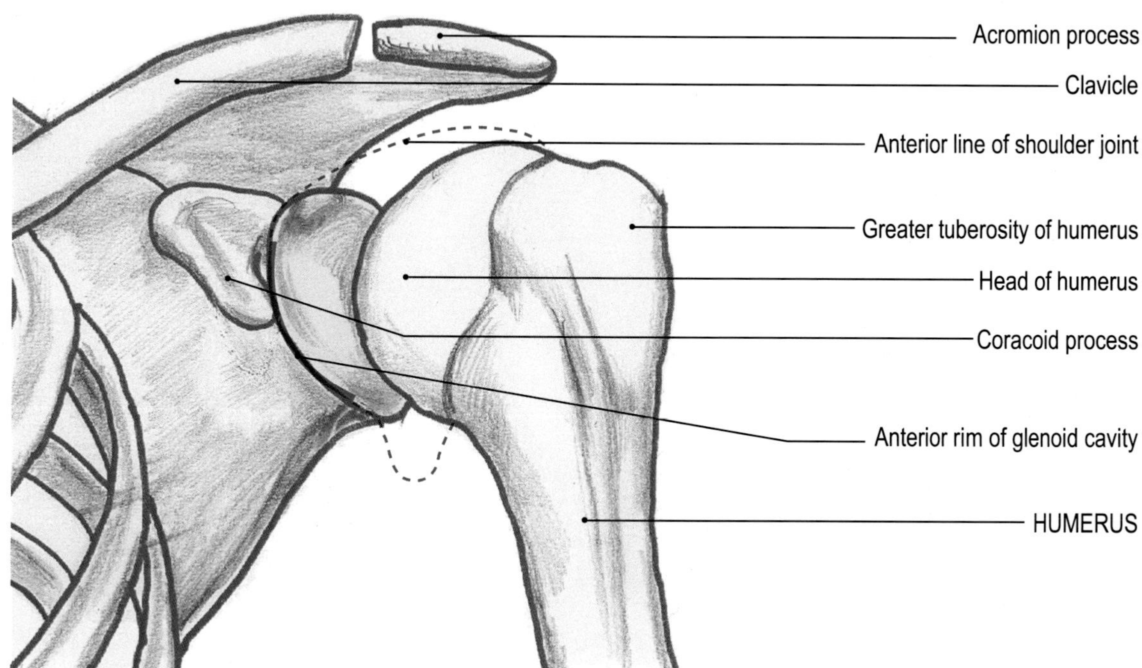

Fig. 2.8 (b) The left shoulder joint (anterior view)

- The anterior rim of the glenoid fossa of the scapula. Now carefully palpate the **anterior rim of the glenoid fossa** lying just medial to the humeral head.
- The head of the humerus. If you trace this bone upwards, you will feel that it is masked by the anterior part of the acromion. If you now move your fingers downwards, you will note that it becomes lost in the axilla. Laterally, you will feel that the head is bounded by the lesser tubercle of the humerus. This projects forwards and forms the medial lip of the bicipital (inter-tubercular) groove.
- The long head of biceps brachii muscle. Now palpate the long head of the biceps brachii muscle running up the groove and on to the anterolateral aspect of the humeral head.

Palpation on movement

- Lateral rotation. Ask the model to rotate the upper limb laterally. In this position, you will be able to palpate more of the humeral head.
- Medial rotation. Now ask the model to medially rotate the upper limb. You will feel the humeral head sliding backwards against the glenoid fossa and eventually disappearing.
- The lesser tubercle of the humerus. You can palpate the lesser tubercle which you will feel moving laterally and medially with the movement of rotation of the humerus.
- Abduction. Ask the model to raise the arm laterally. Now palpate the anterior part of the humeral head gliding downwards.
- Adduction. Now ask the model to lower the arm. Palpate the anterior part of the humeral head gliding upwards.
- **Note 1.** Palpation of the head during the movement of abduction is made more difficult by the contraction of the anterior fibres of deltoid muscle which pass across the anterior aspect of the joint.
- **Note 2.** Posteriorly (see Fig. 2.8e, f), the shoulder joint is estimated to be at the same level and in the same sagittal plane as it is anteriorly, being just below the spine of the scapula 2–3 cm medial to the angle of the acromion.
- **Note 3.** Laterally (see Fig. 2.8c, d), the centre of the joint is approximately 2 cm below the anterior half of the lateral border of the acromion.

Although the spine of the scapula, its inferior angle and medial border arc easily palpable and useful for calculating the position of the shoulder joint from the back, the joint itself is set so deeply in muscle that it is impossible to recognize in normal subjects.

Superior marking of shoulder joint
Angle of acromion process
Lateral border of acromion
Coracoid process
Lesser tuberosity of humerus

Fig. 2.8 (c) The right shoulder joint (upper lateral view)

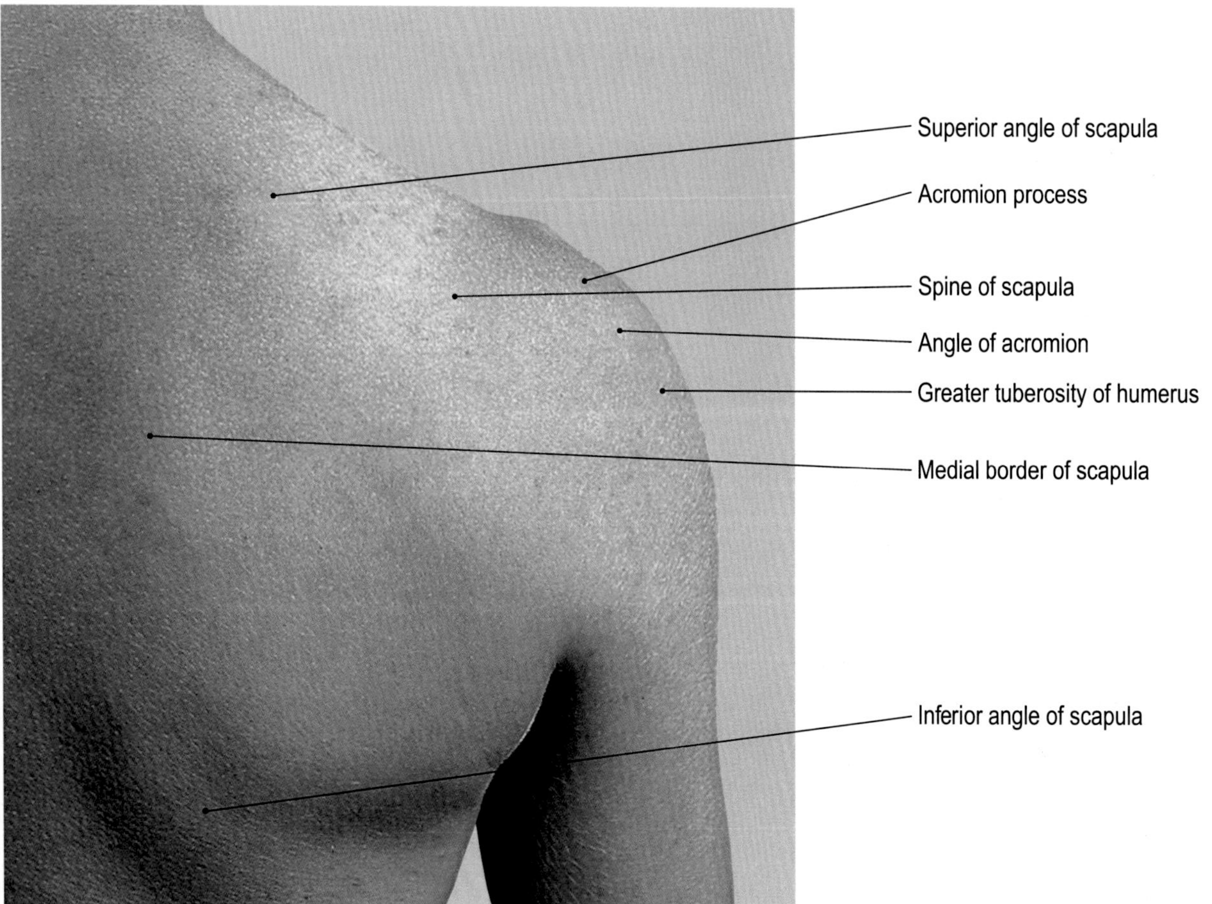

Fig. 2.8 (e) The right shoulder joint (posterior view)

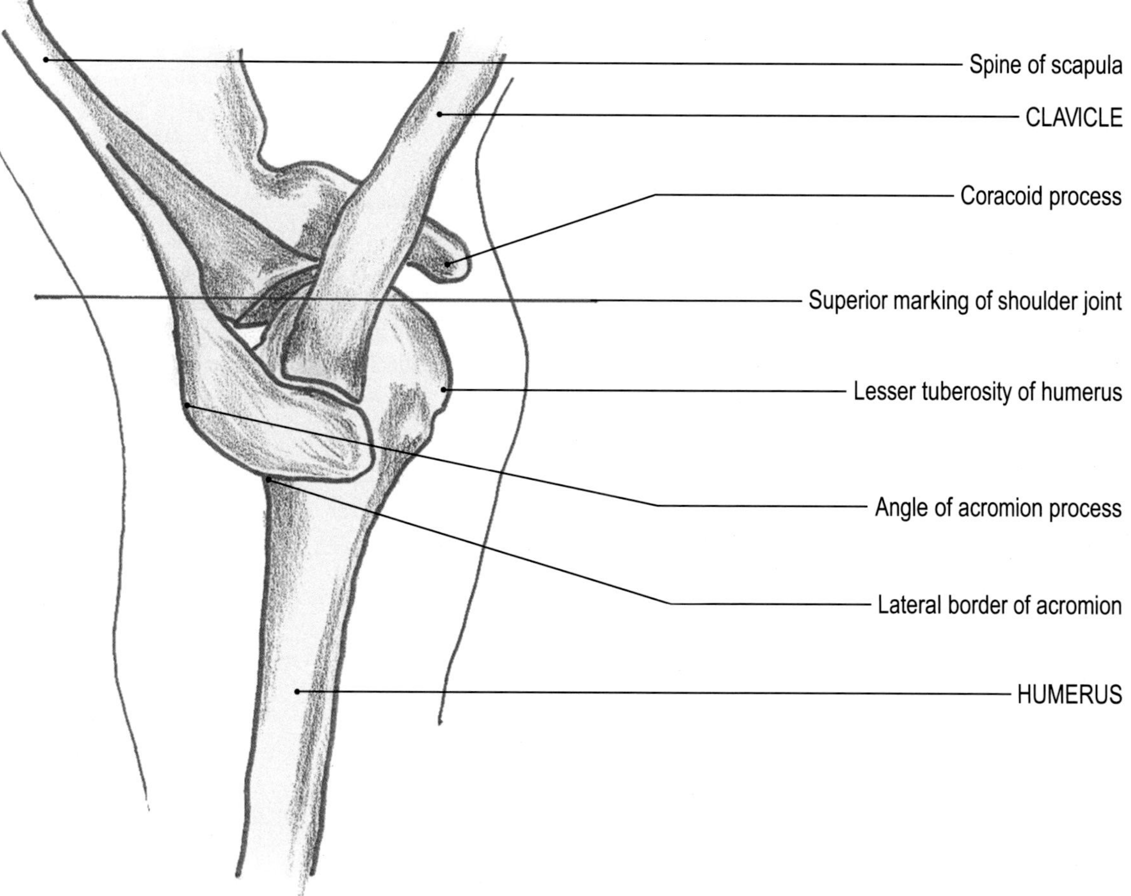

Fig. 2.8 (d) The right shoulder joint (upper lateral view)

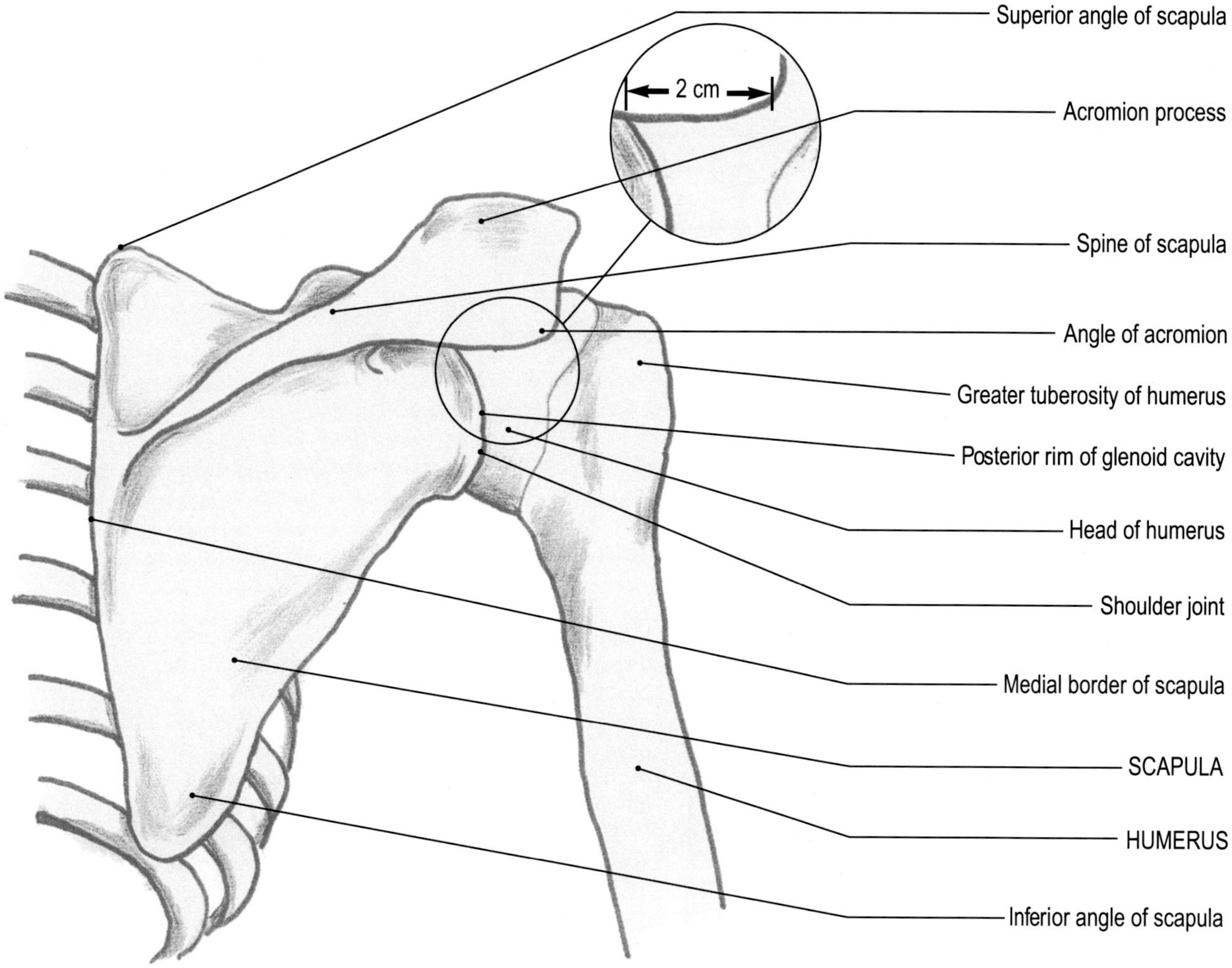

Fig. 2.8 (f) The right shoulder joint (posterior view)

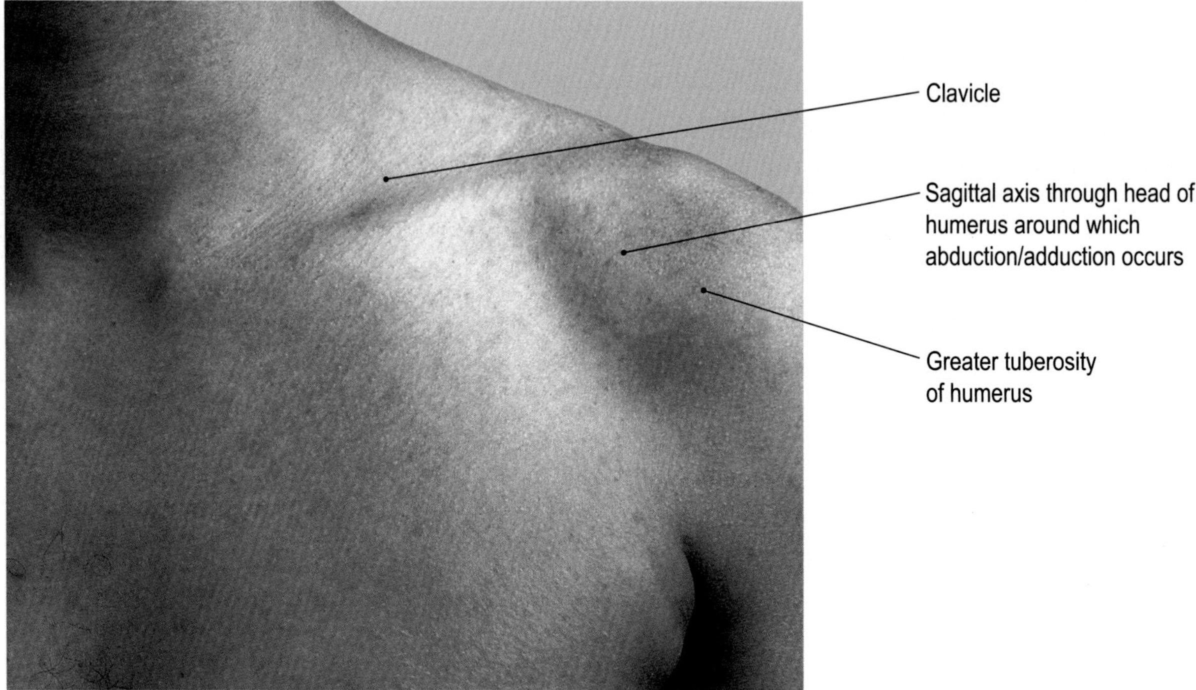

Fig. 2.9 (a) Movements of the head of the humerus (anterior view)

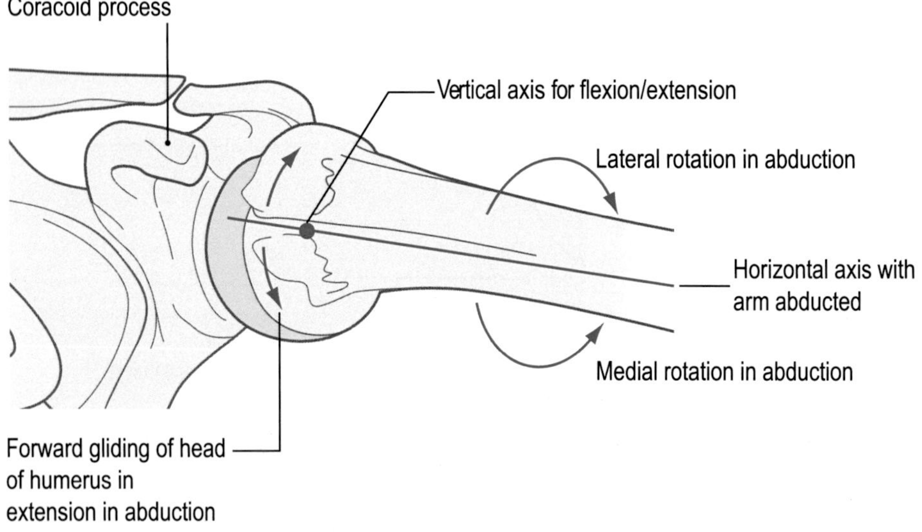

Fig. 2.9 (c) Left humerus in 90° abduction (superior view)

Movements of the head of the humerus

As the axis of movement of the shoulder joint is through the centre of the head of the humerus (Palastanga et al 2002), movements of the distal end of the humerus produce an opposite gliding of the head against the glenoid fossa. Thus, abduction causes a downward gliding and an upward rolling of the head of the humerus on the glenoid cavity around a sagittal axis (Fig. 2.9a, b). Flexion and extension (Fig. 2.9d), however, produce rotation or spin of the head around a frontal axis within the glenoid fossa, similar to that produced by rotating the limb in abduction (Fig. 2.9c). Rotation, with the arm by the side, however, produces a gliding forwards and rolling backwards of the head on lateral rotation and a gliding backwards and rolling forwards on medial rotation around a vertical axis. The combination of rolling in one direction and gliding in the other maintains the position of the centre of axis of the head (Fig. 2.9e). With the subject performing one movement at a time and with your fingers placed over the head of the humerus, these movements can be observed. It becomes even clearer if palpation is performed with one hand and the humerus is carefully taken through the movement passively.

The shoulder joint has a loose joint capsule and relatively weak associated ligaments. It relies to a large extent on muscular activity, especially by the 'rotator cuff' muscles (supraspinatus, infraspinatus, teres minor and subscapularis), for joint stability. It has an extensive range of movement together with a complementary range of accessory movements.

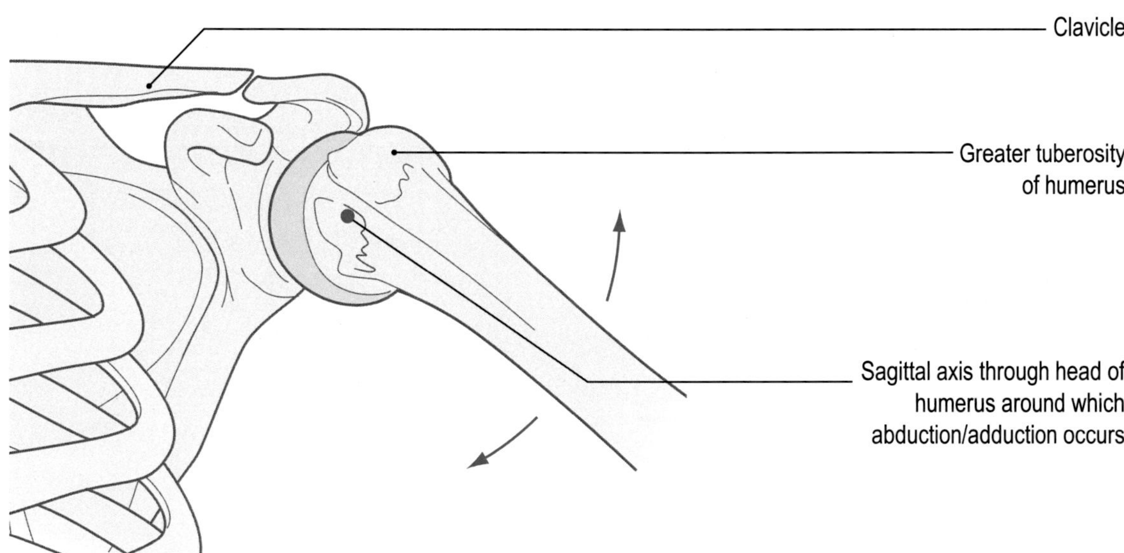

Fig. 2.9 (b) Movements of the head of the humerus (anterior view)

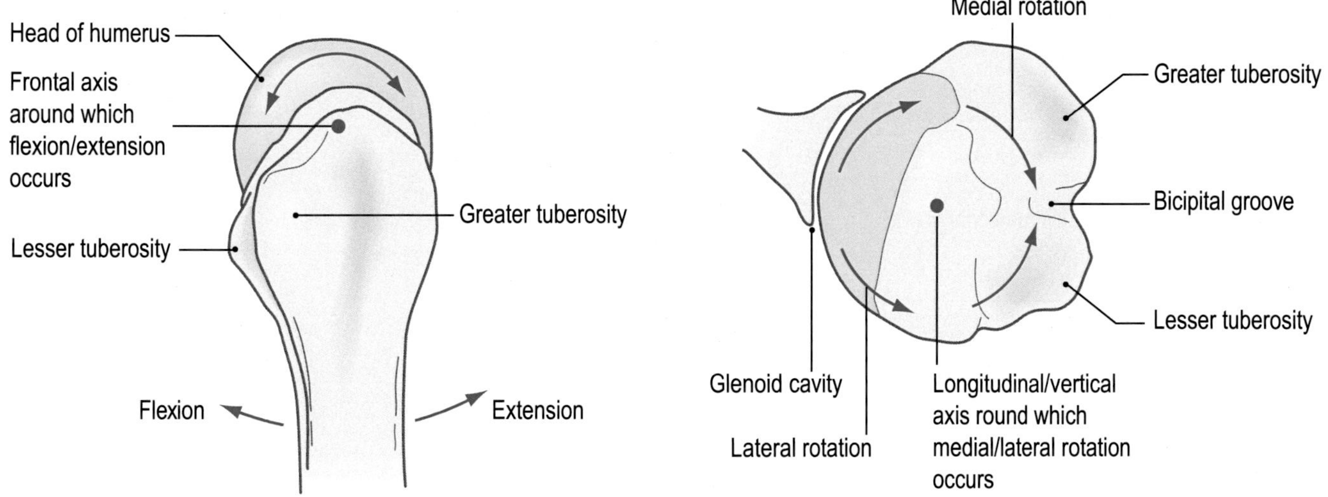

Fig. 2.9 (d) Left humerus (lateral view)

Fig. 2.9 (e) Left humerus (superior view)

Accessory movements

If the accessory movements are reduced, or lost, normal movement becomes reduced or occasionally eliminated.

Palpation

For palpation in this region, the model should be in supine lying or in side lying. Where necessary, the arm should be supported on a pillow.

- Lateral distraction of the humeral head. For this technique to be successfully produced, the muscles of the upper limb need to be completely relaxed. The head of the humerus can now be drawn laterally away from the glenoid fossa for approximately 1–2 cm. The technique is usually possible when the humerus is between 0° and 90° of abduction. You will find it easier to palpate the movement if you ask a colleague to perform the technique. Place your fingers on the anterior aspect of the joint and palpate the head and anterior rim of the glenoid fossa.
- Gliding of the head of the humerus. Gliding of the humeral head can be in either a downwards or an upwards direction. This is achieved by pulling down or pushing up along the line of the humeral shaft. The humeral head can also glide in a forwards or backwards direction within the glenoid fossa. This is achieved by applying direct pressure on the upper end of the humerus. Again, you will find that it is easier to palpate the movement if you ask a colleague to perform the techniques as described above. Using several fingers, you should gently palpate over the area at the front of the joint where the head and glenoid fossa are identifiable.

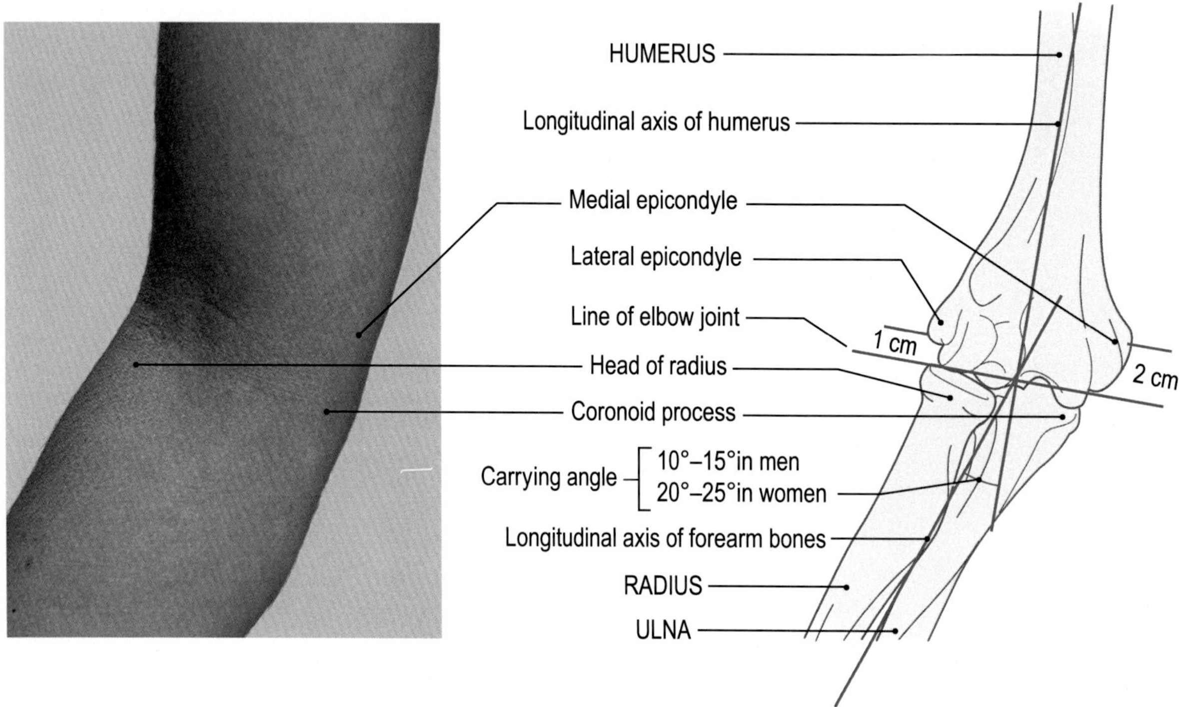

Fig. 2.10 (a, b) The right elbow joint (anterior view)

The elbow joint (Fig. 2.10)

The elbow joint is basically a hinge joint between the **humerus** above and the **ulna** and **radius** below. The articular surfaces are, medially, the trochlea of the humerus above and the trochlear notch of the ulna below, and laterally the capitulum of the humerus above and the upper surface of the **head of radius** below.

The articular surfaces of the trochlea, capitulum, trochlear notch and the head of the radius are all covered with articular cartilage. The joint is surrounded by an extensive capsule which extends up onto the front and back of the humerus above the radial, coronoid and olecranon fossae. It is supported on either side by two strong ligaments. The ulna collateral ligament is triangular and joins the medial epicondyle to the medial side of the olecranon and coronoid processes. The lateral ligament is also triangular and joins the lateral epicondyle to the annular ligament surrounding the head of the radius. The capsule is lined with synovial membrane.

Palpation: surface marking

- Draw a line from a point 2 cm below the tip of the **medial epicondyle** to a point 1 cm below the tip of the lateral epicondyle of the humerus (Fig. 2.10, b). The line passes downwards and medially due to the medial margin of the trochlea projecting down further than the lateral margin.
- **Note.** When viewed from the front, this produces an angle at the elbow where the long axis of the ulna deviates laterally from that of the humerus by approximately 10–15° in men and 20–25° in women (Palastanga et al 2002). The angle at the elbow is only apparent on full extension and supination of the forearm and is commonly termed the '**carrying angle**' (Fig. 2.10b).

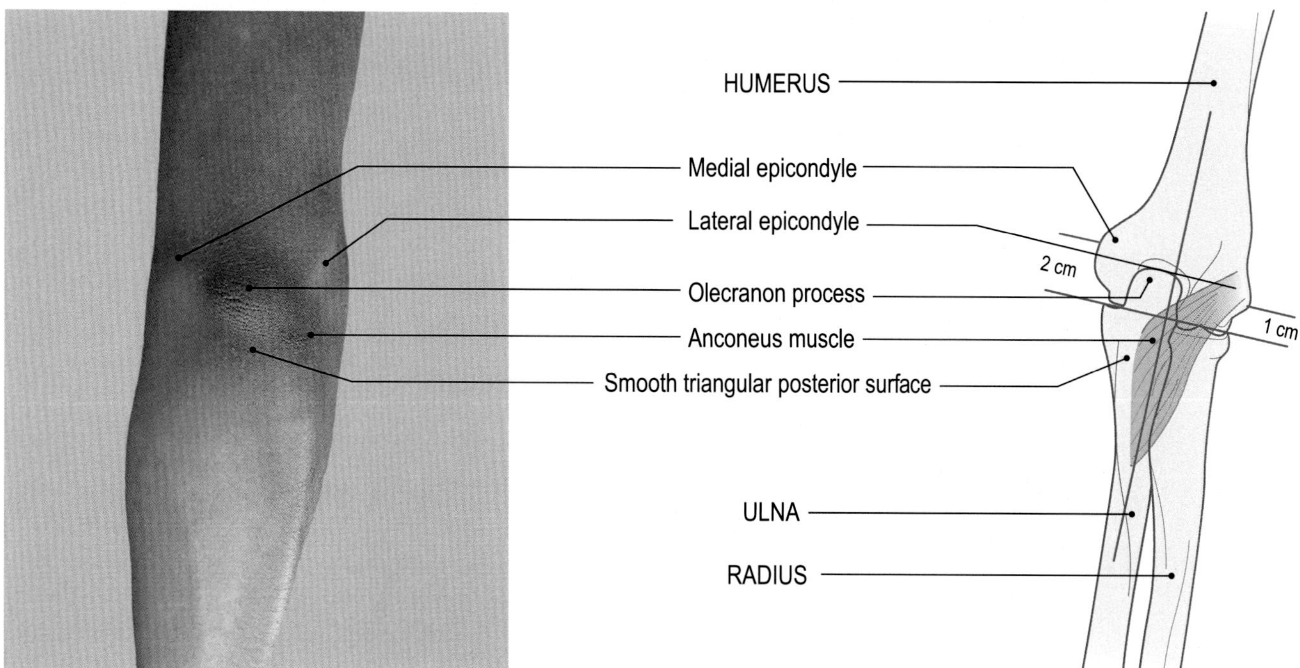

Fig. 2.10 (c, d) The right elbow joint (posterior view)

Palpation

- The lateral aspect of the elbow joint. You will be able to identify the joint easily on the lateral side between the **lateral epicondyle** of the humerus and the lateral side of the head of the radius.
- The anterior aspect of the elbow joint. Anteriorly, the joint is not palpable as it lies deep to muscles: the extensor muscles laterally and the strong flexor muscles anteromedially, with brachialis and biceps between.
- The posterior aspect of the elbow joint. Posteriorly, trace the joint line as far as the radial notch of the ulna at the posterior aspect of the superior radioulnar joint (Fig. 2.10d). Ask the model to flex the elbow joint to 90°. In this position, you can palpate the anterior edge of the **olecranon** which can be traced downwards on either side until it is hidden by **anconeus** laterally and by the medial collateral ligament medially (Fig. 2.10d).

Accessory movements

Palpation

- Rocking. Ask the model to flex the elbow joint to approximately 15°. In this position, the ulna and radius can be rocked from side to side. Stabilize the arm just above the medial and lateral supracondylar ridges with one hand and apply a side-to-side force just above the wrist. The correct angle is critical for the movement to take place which varies from individual to individual.
- Distraction. The model is lying supine or in side lying. Ensure that the muscles are relaxed. Ask the model to flex the elbow joint. Distraction is achieved by applying a considerable force in the direction of the long axis of the humerus. With the elbow at a right angle and the upper arm stabilized, you will be able to move the forearm very slightly in its long axis. This produces a gapping at the anterior and posterior aspect of the joint.
- **Note.** These techniques require practice and are best studied from the mobilization and manipulation literature.

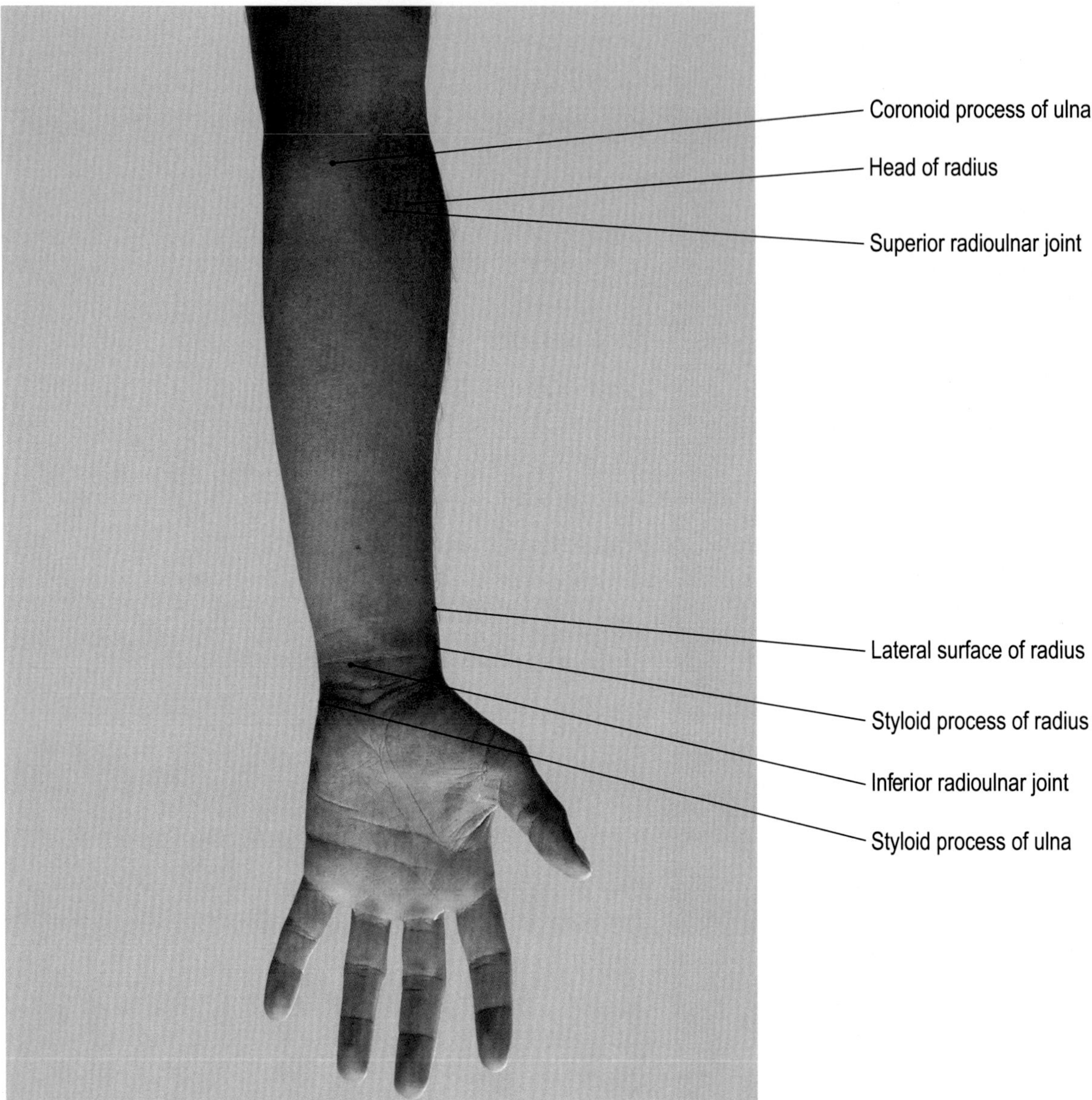

Fig. 2.11 (a) The superior and inferior radioulnar joint of the left arm (anterior view)

The radioulnar union

The movements of pronation and supination occur between the radius and ulna. They involve a type of rotation movement at the superior and inferior radioulnar joint and a twisting movement between the shafts of both bones. This is often referred to as the radioulnar union because the two bones are held together by the interosseous membrane.

The superior radioulnar joint

The superior radioulnar joint is a synovial pivot joint between the medial one-fifth of the head of the radius and the radial notch on the lateral side of the coronoid process of the ulna.

Both surfaces are covered with articular cartilage and are reciprocally curved. The head is surrounded by the annular ligament. This is attached in front and behind the radial notch of the ulna and forms the other four-fifths of the ring and is lined with fibrocartilage. The annular ligament is supported from above by the capsule and the triangular radiocollateral ligament of the elbow joint and from below by the quadrate ligament attaching it to the ulna. The joint is further stabilized by the interosseous membrane which binds the radius and ulna together. Synovial membrane lines the inner surface of the annular ligament in a double fold attaching to the edges of the articular facets of ulna and radius. It emerges just below the annular ligament as a loose fold. It is continuous with that of the elbow joint, although functionally it is a completely separate joint.

Palpation: surface marking

- The superior radioulnar joint. Anteriorly and posteriorly, draw a vertical line 1 cm long downwards from the line of the elbow

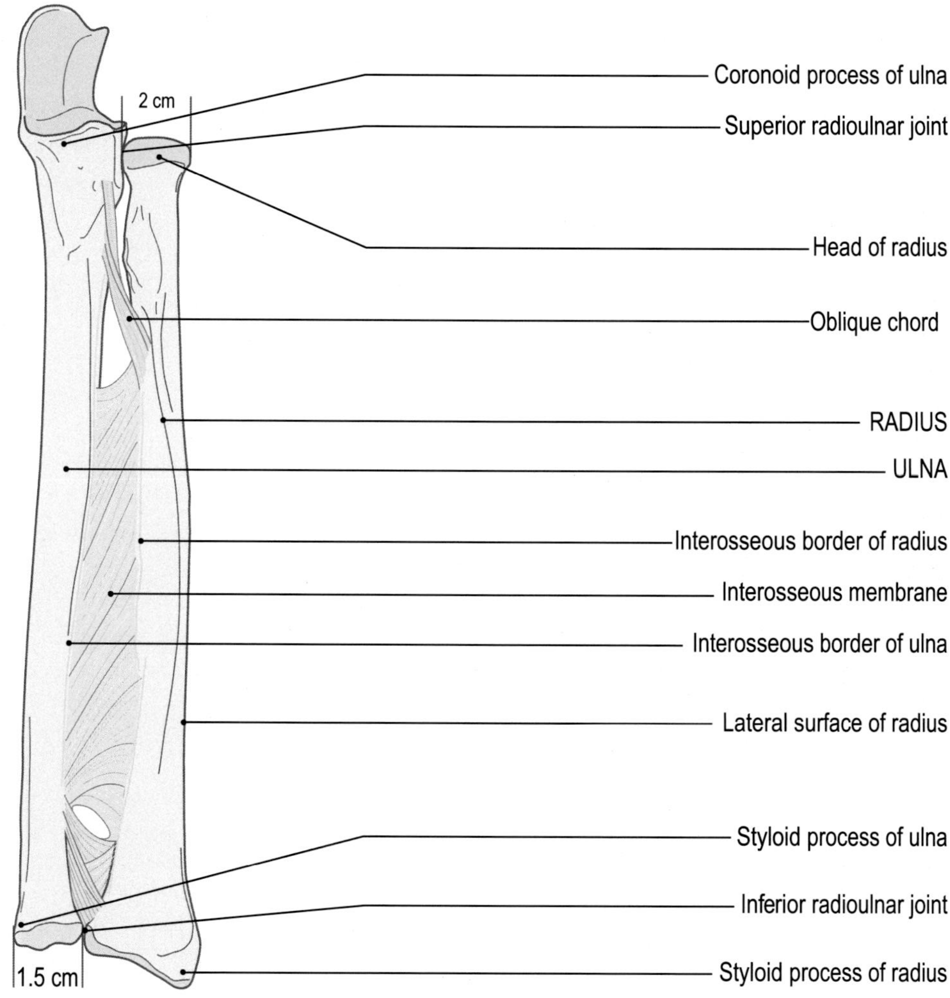

Fig. 2.11 (b) The superior and inferior radioulnar joint of the left arm (anterior view)

joint (see above), 2 cm medial to the lateral edge of the head of the radius (Fig. 2.11).

Palpation on movement

- Pronation and supination. Locate the head of the radius just below the lateral epicondyle of the humerus. Trace backwards around the radial head until the movement is arrested by contact with the lateral side of the ulna. The joint space is usually hidden by anconeus muscle. Anteriorly, the surface marking is covered by muscle and is not palpable. When the forearm is pronated and supinated, you will be able to fcel the head of the radius rotating under your fingers.

Accessory movements

- Gliding of the radial head. The model is in the sitting position. Grip the head of the radius firmly between your fingers and thumb of one hand. Stabilize the upper end of the ulna with your other hand. You will now be able to produce slight backwards and forwards gliding of the head.
- Upwards and downwards gliding of the radial head. If you apply traction on the lower part of the radius, you will produce a slight gliding up and down of the head of the radius against the radial notch of the ulna.
- **Note.** If you apply too much traction to the radius in younger children (as in lifting the child by the forearm) the head of the radius may dislocate out of the annular ring, causing much pain and discomfort.

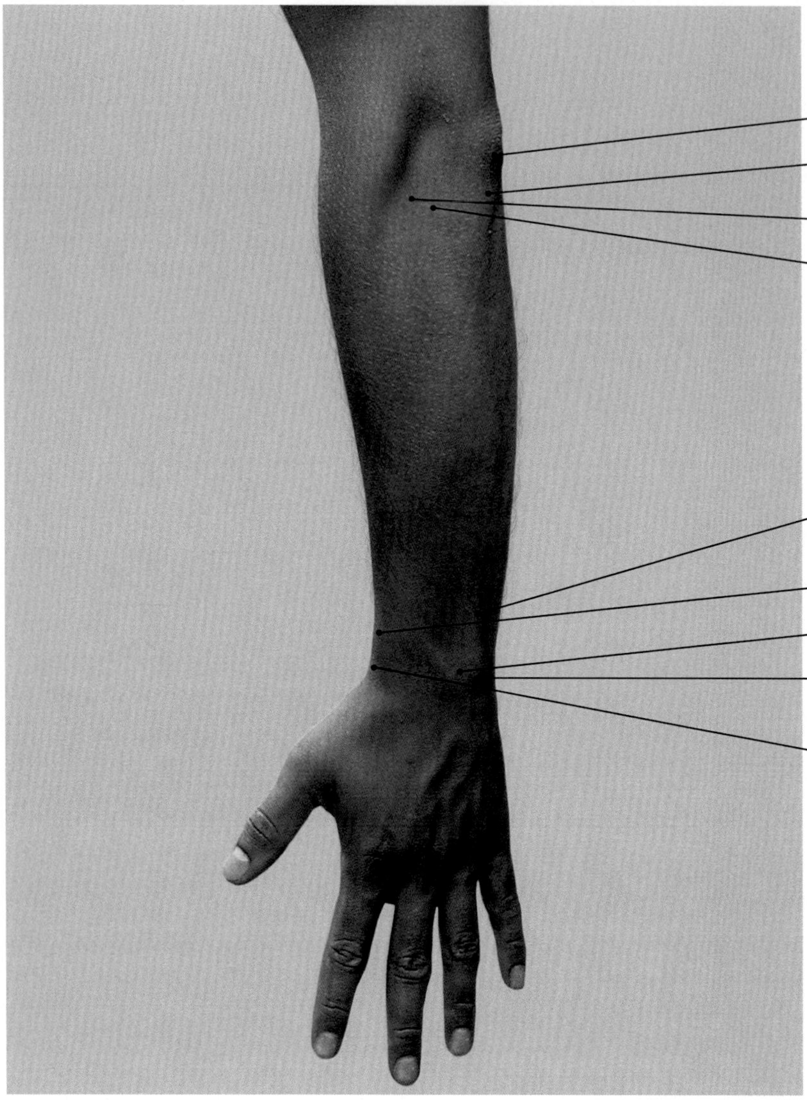

Fig. 2.11 (c) The superior and inferior radioulnar joint of the left arm (posterior view)

The inferior radioulnar joint

This joint is also a synovial pivot joint, being between the ulnar notch on the medial side of the distal end of the radius and the lateral rim of the head of the ulna. Both surfaces are covered with articular cartilage and the joint is surrounded by a capsule which is thicker in front and behind. A triangular interarticular disc is situated between the lower end of the ulna and the carpus. This attaches medially to the base of the **styloid process of ulna** and laterally to the medial edge of the inferior surface of the radius. At this joint, the radius moves around the head of the ulna in conjunction with the rotation of the head of the radius against the ulna at the superior radioulnar joint.

The mid radioulnar union

The **radius** and the **ulna** are joined together for most of their length by the **interosseous membrane**. This attaches to the interosseous borders of both bones, except for a small space at the upper part. This thin collagenous sheet, broader at its middle, is made up of fibres which pass downwards and medially from the radius to the ulna. Its fibres help to bind the two bones together whilst allowing movement between them. It gives support to the **superior** and **inferior radioulnar joints**. Due to the direction of its fibres, it transmits weight from the radius to the ulna.

Palpation

- Specific features of the radius and ulna. Examine both the radius and the ulna. Note that the lower end of the radius is large and takes any force transmitted from the carpus. In contrast, note that the radial head is relatively small and obviously transmits very little, if any, force to the capitulum. Note that, compared with the lower end of the radius, the ulna has a very small head at its lower end. This takes very little force from the carpus. Note also that its upper end is large and obviously transmits most of the force through to the trochlea of the humerus.

There is an **oblique cord** running downwards and laterally which attaches the tubercles at the upper part of the ulna with the radius just below its tuberosity. It is distinct from the interosseous membrane.

The interosseous membrane and oblique cord cannot be palpated.

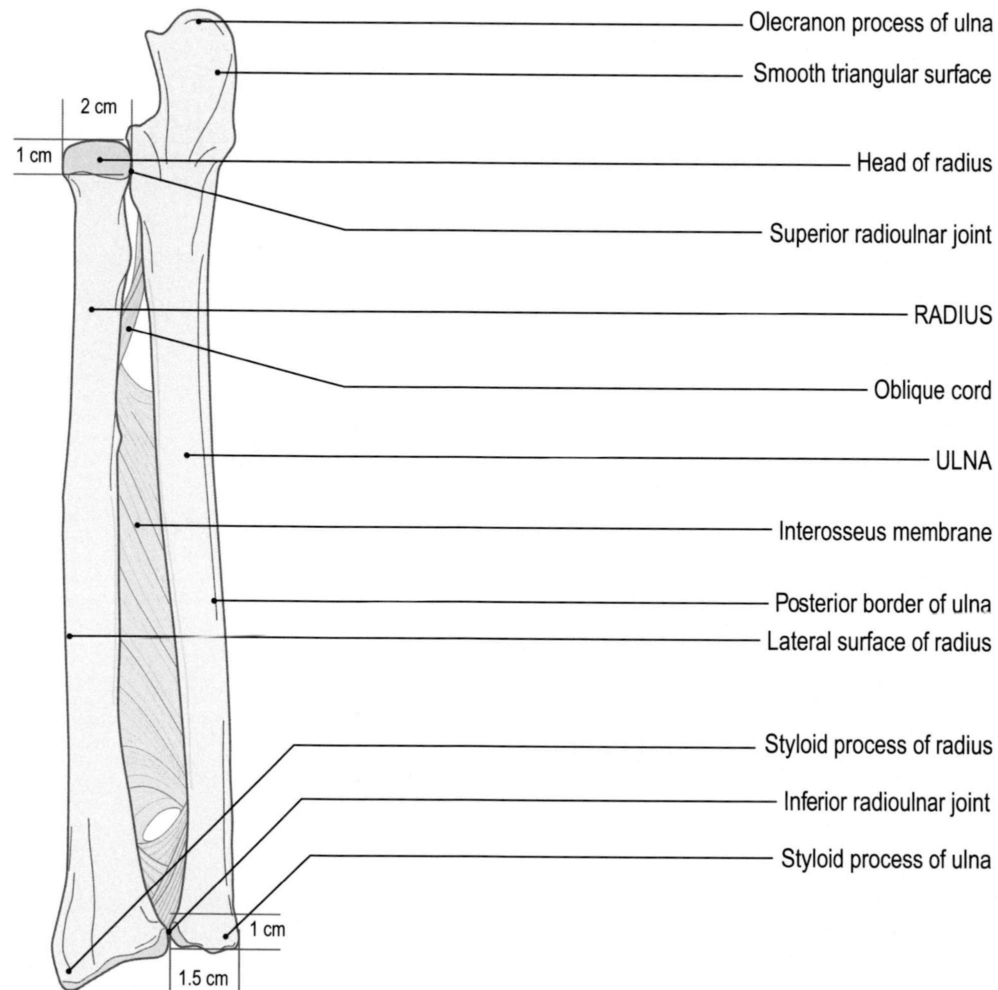

Fig. 2.11 (d) The superior and inferior radioulnar joint of the left arm (posterior view)

Palpation: surface marking

- The inferior radioulnar joint. Palpate the joint line 1.5 cm lateral to the medial rim of the head of the ulna running 1 cm upwards from the line of the wrist joint (Figs 2.11 and 2.12).

Palpation

- The posterior aspect of the inferior radioulnar joint. You will find it easier to palpate the joint line posteriorly where there is a vertical depression for 1 cm immediately above the line of the wrist joint 1.5 cm lateral to the ulnar styloid process (Fig. 2.11). Here, the tendon of extensor digiti minimi crosses the posterior aspect of the joint. Ask the model to extend the little finger and identify the tendon.
- The anterior aspect of the inferior radioulnar joint. Anteriorly the joint is much more difficult to palpate. In order to do so, slip your fingers under the thick tendon of flexor carpi ulnaris from the medial side.
- Pronation and supination. Ask the model to pronate and supinate the forearm. Now feel the radius moving around the lateral side of the head of the ulna. Note that the ulna also moves slightly laterally on pronation and medially on supination.

Accessory movements

Palpation

- Forwards and backwards gliding of the head of the ulna. Grip the head of the ulna firmly between your fingers and thumb of one hand. Now stabilize the lower end of the radius with the other hand. Now glide the lower end of the ulna forwards and backwards.
- Pronation and supination. Ask the model to flex the elbow joint. Hold the model's forearm in your hand. Ask the model to pronate and supinate the forearm. In pronation, note the radius as it rotates around the head of the ulna. At the same time the lower end of the ulna moves slightly laterally. In supination the reverse occurs. Loss of this movement will limit the range.
- Lateral movement of the head of the ulna. Ask the model to pronate the forearm fully. Now apply pressure to the anteromedial aspect of the head of the ulna with your thumbs.
- Medial movement of the head of the ulna. Ask the model to supinate the forearm fully. Now apply pressure with your thumbs to the posterolateral side of the head of the ulna.
- **Note.** Both these manoeuvres achieve slight movement of the head of the ulna.

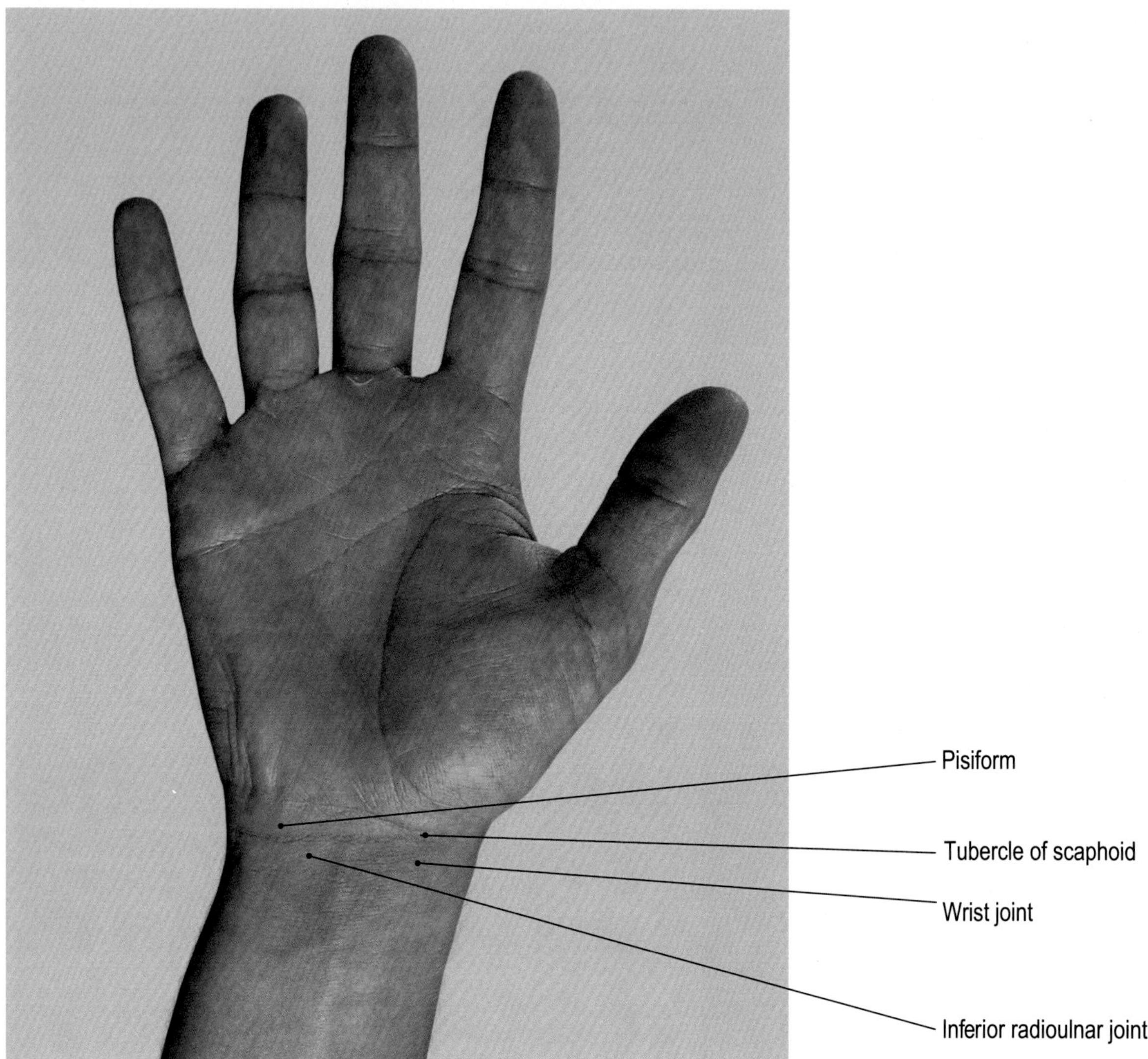

Fig. 2.12 (a) The right wrist joint (radiocarpal joint) (anterior view)

The wrist (radiocarpal) joint (Fig. 2.12)

The wrist joint is formed, superiorly, by the inferior surface of the lower end of the radius and an interarticular disc. Inferiorly, it is formed by the proximal surfaces of the scaphoid, lunate and triquetral bones. These, together with the ulnar and radial styloid processes, form a synovial ellipsoid joint. All joint surfaces are covered with articular cartilage. The joint is surrounded by a capsule, lined with synovial membrane. It is supported by the palmar and dorsal radiocarpal, ulnocarpal, radial and ulnar collateral ligaments. The interarticular disc lies between the inferior surface of the head of the ulna and the triquetral bone.

Palpation: surface marking

- The wrist joint. Draw a line between the tips of the ulnar and radial styloid processes, slightly concave distally. The line becomes increasingly curved as it approaches the styloid processes (Fig. 2.12).

Palpation

For palpation in this area, the model is in the sitting position with the forearm resting on a support.

The joint is covered both anteriorly and posteriorly by tendons running from the forearm into the hand. There are, however, areas, mainly on the medial side, where the joint space of the wrist can be palpated.

- The posteromedial aspect of the wrist joint. Locate the ulnar styloid process on the posteromedial side of the wrist. Trace along both the medial and posterior edges of the head of the ulna. Medially, you will notice a gap just distal to this area. This contains the interarticular disc, the inferior surface of which takes part in the wrist joint articulation.
- The lateral aspect of the wrist joint. Press your fingers between the extensor tendons. Now trace the joint line just distal to the dorsal tubercle of the radius across the back of the wrist as far as the head of the ulna.

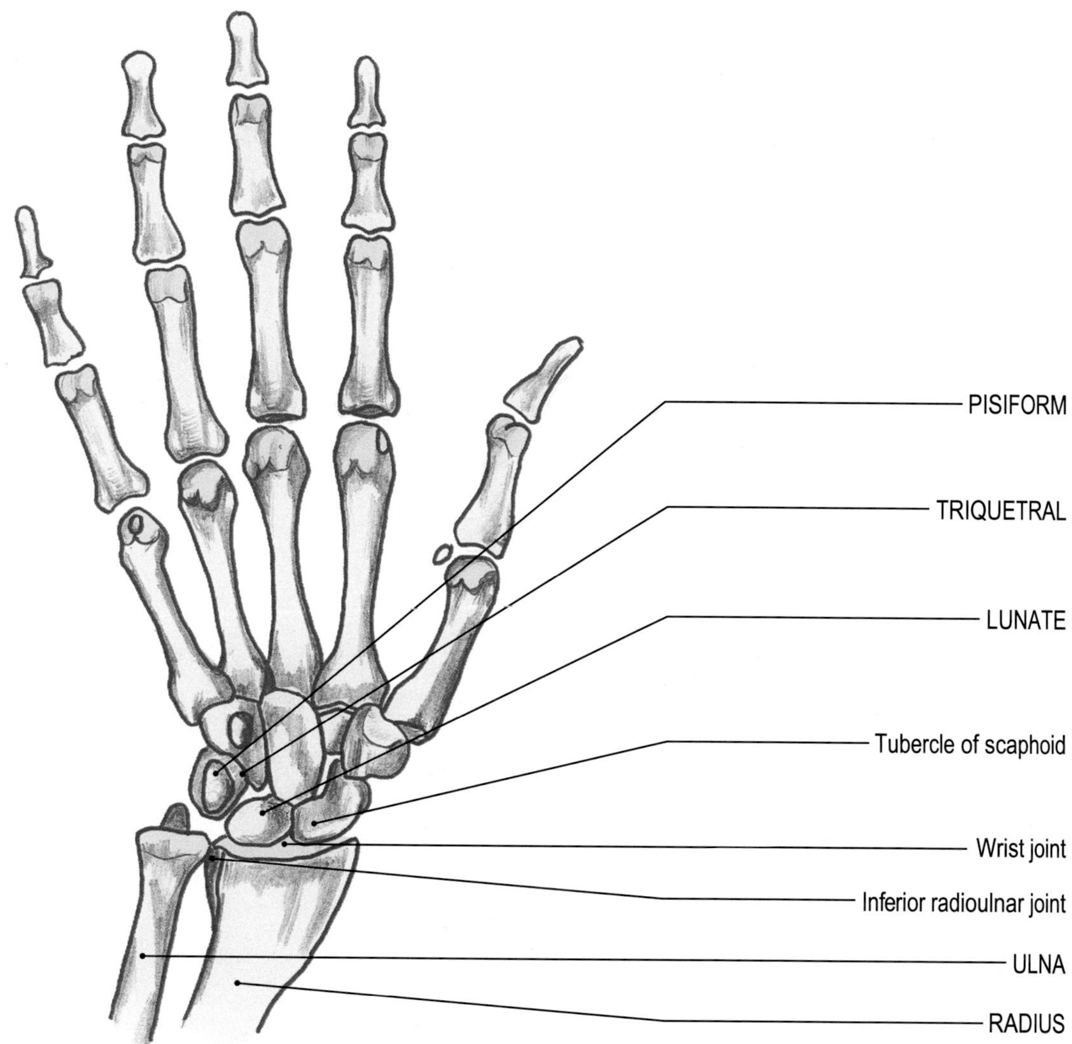

Fig. 2.12 (b) The right wrist joint (radiocarpal joint) (anterior view)

- Note. The joint line cannot be palpated anteriorly. You can draw its line horizontally just proximal to the **tubercle of the scaphoid**.
- The anterior aspect of the wrist joint. Ask the model to flex the wrist slightly. This will facilitate identification of the joint line. Identify the anterior line of the joint by tracing the crease across the anterior aspect of the wrist between the flattened lower end of the forearm and the elevations of the thenar and hypothenar eminences.

Accessory movements

Palpation

- Movements of the carpus. Ask the model to pronate the forearm. Now grip the dorsum of the lower end of the radius and ulna with one hand and the carpal bones with the other, so that the radial sides of your index fingers and thumbs are nearly touching. You can now move the carpus forwards and backwards, from side to side and even rotate it slightly.
- Note. Take care not to flex the wrist joint. The technique is to glide one surface on the other in a transverse plane. It will be difficult to prevent some movement occurring between the bones of the midcarpal joint.
- Distraction. Ask the model to pronate the forearm. Adopt the same hand hold as described above. Draw your two hands apart, taking care to grip the bones tightly. Do not allow too much slide of the skin and fascia.
- Note. Accessory movement at the wrist, if performed correctly, is quite dramatic, producing considerable movement in unusual directions. It must be remembered, however, that some of this movement occurs at the intercarpal and carpometacarpal joints.
- Movement of the carpal bones. With practice, it is possible to move each of the carpal bones individually on each other or on the lower end of the radius and disc. Grip one bone between your finger and thumb of one hand, while stabilizing its neighbour as described above. Alternatively, use the finger and thumb of your other hand. Slight gliding movement between the two bones can be achieved.

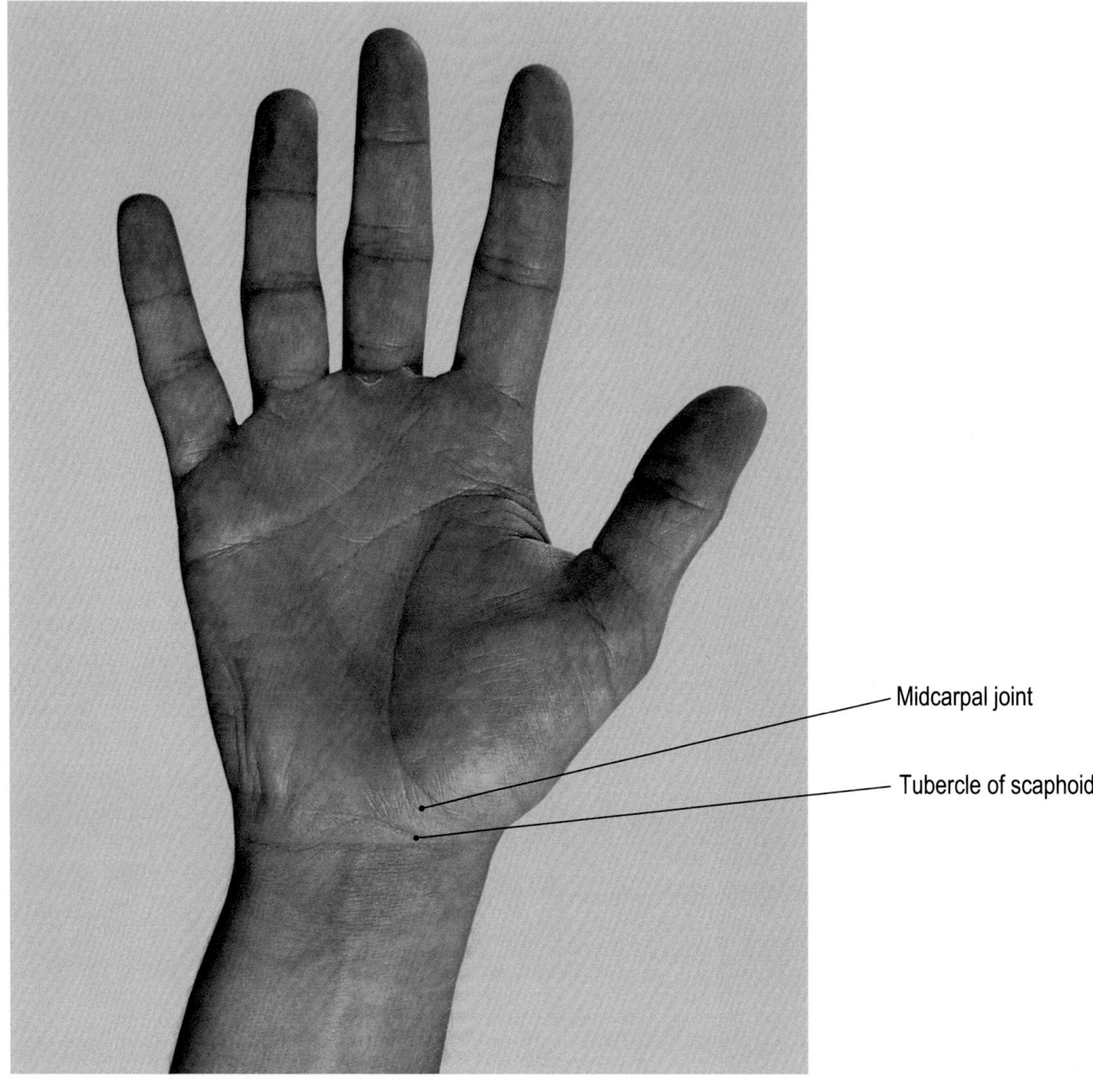

Fig. 2.13 (a) The intercarpal and midcarpal joints of the right hand (anterior view)

The hand

The intercarpal joints (Fig. 2.13)

These are all synovial, plane joints. Their surfaces are covered with articular cartilage and their capsules are lined with synovial membrane. With the exception of the pisotriquetral joint, the capsule is supported by the palmar and dorsal ligaments and radial and ulnar collateral carpal ligaments. There are also some interosseous ligaments between the proximal ends of the proximal row and distal ends of the distal row of carpal bones.

The pisotriquetral joint is also a synovial plane joint, but it has a distinct capsule which is supported by the tendon of flexor carpi ulnaris proximally and pisohamate and pisometacarpal ligaments distally.

Palpation

With the exception of the joint between the pisiform and triquetral, the joints between the carpal bones are very difficult to palpate with any degree of accuracy.

- The posterior aspects of the joints of the carpal bones. These can be identified either by relating their position to the metacarpals or by noting any particular features. You can grip each carpal bone between your finger and thumb and move it against the adjacent bone. The joint line remains elusive to the touch.
- The pisotriquetral joint. The medial aspect of the joint line is the easiest to palpate. Run your fingers dorsally for 1 cm from the anterior point of the **pisiform** on its medial side. Slight movement of the pisiform will emphasize the joint line.
- The midcarpal joint. The joint between the two rows of carpal bones is known as the **midcarpal joint**. It permits gliding forwards, backwards and from side to side, augmenting the movements of flexion, extension, abduction and adduction at the wrist joint.

Palpation: surface marking

- The midcarpal joint. Draw a line across the carpus just below the tips of the radial and ulna styloid processes concave downwards, slightly more concave than that of the wrist joint.

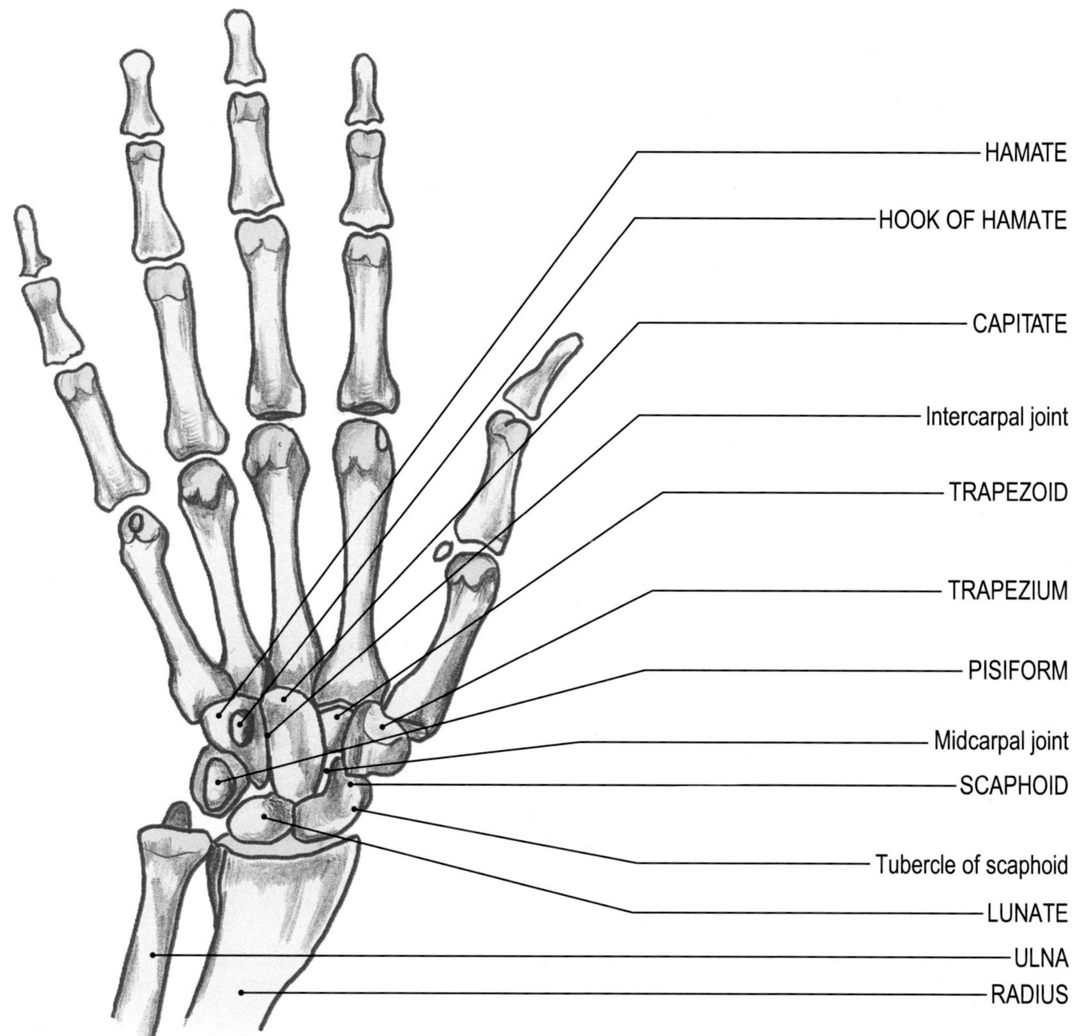

Fig. 2.13 (b) The intercarpal and midcarpal joints of the right hand (anterior view)

Accessory movements

- Side-to-side movement of the pisiform bone. Ask the model to flex the wrist joint slightly and then deviate the joint medially. Ensure that flexor carpi ulnaris is relaxed. The pisiform bone can now be moved from side to side.
- Gliding movement of the carpal bones. Now locate the **capitate** bone which is situated at the base of the third metacarpal bone. Stabilize the capitate bone by gripping it between your index finger anteriorly and your thumb posteriorly. You will be able to glide the surrounding carpal bones anteriorly and posteriorly by using a similar grip with the other hand on each bone in turn.
- Side-to-side and anterior and posterior movement of the trapezium bone. Palpate the **trapezium** at the lateral side of the distal row of carpal bones. Use the same hold as described above and stabilize the rest of the carpus. The trapezium can also be moved anteriorly and posteriorly.
- **Note.** A good knowledge of the anatomy of the carpal bones is essential and should be combined with practise of this type of movement. Consult the literature on mobilization and manipulations for therapeutic techniques.
- Passive movement between the two rows of carpal bones (the midcarpal joint). Use a similar hold to that described for producing accessory movements of the wrist joint. In this case, stabilize the proximal row of bones with one hand and move the distal row with the other. You should grip the proximal row of carpal bones with the index finger and thumb of your stabilizing hand just distal to the radial and ulnar styloid processes.
- **Note.** During the anterior, posterior, lateral and medial gliding, however, it is impossible to prevent some movement occurring in the neighbouring joints.

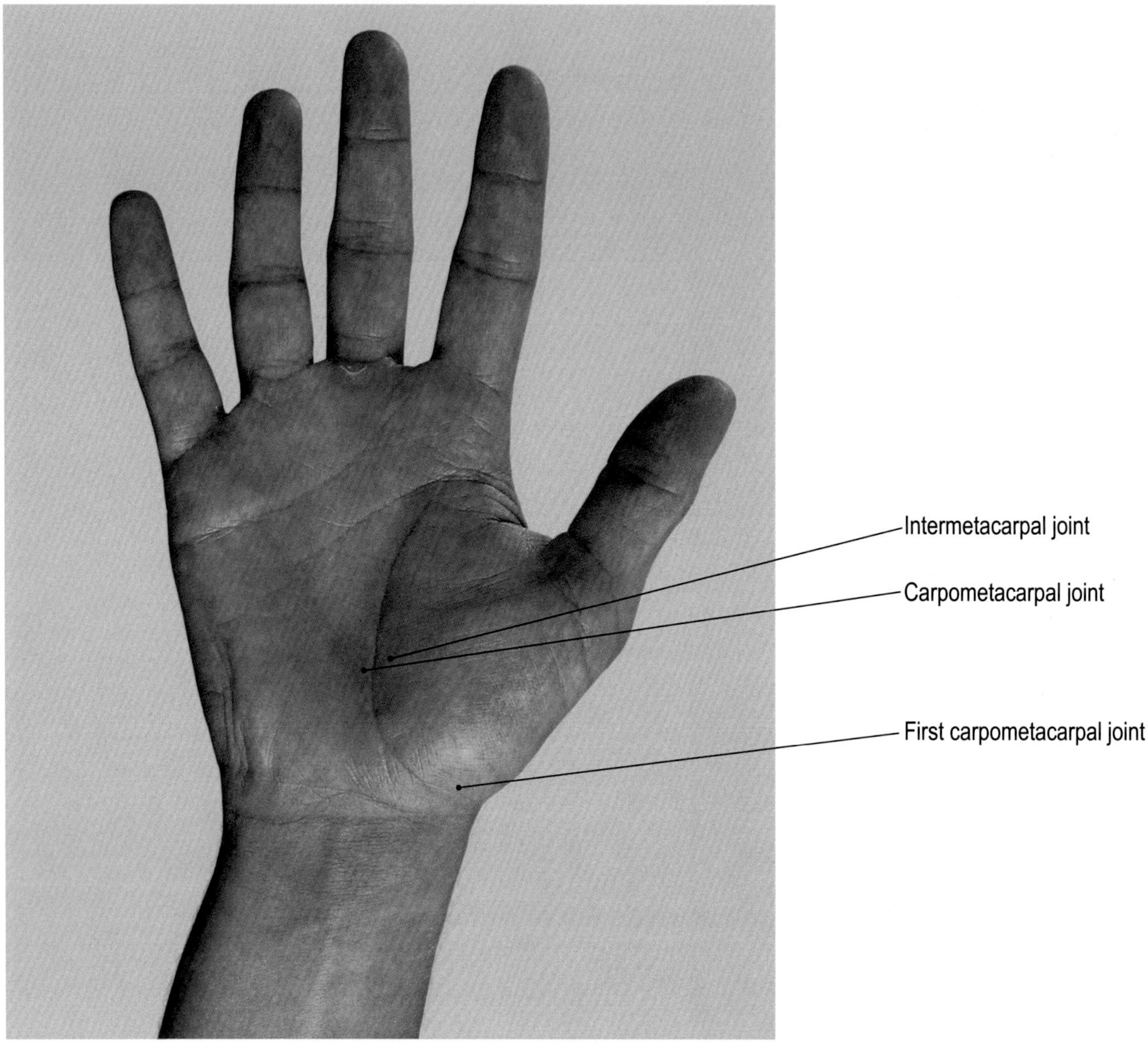

Fig. 2.14 (a) Carpometacarpal and intermetacarpal joints of the right hand (anterior view)

The carpometacarpal joints (Fig. 2.14)

The first metacarpal articulates with the trapezium by means of a synovial saddle (sellar) joint and is separate from the remaining carpometacarpal joints. It is surrounded by a capsule which is lined with synovial membrane and supported by the radial carpometacarpal, anterior and posterior oblique ligaments. The second metacarpal articulates mainly with the trapezoid, having small facets on either side for the trapezium laterally and the capitate medially. The third metacarpal articulates only with the capitate, while the fourth and fifth articulate with the hamate. Except for that of the thumb, they are all plane synovial joints. They have a capsule lined with synovial membrane and are supported by palmar and dorsal ligaments. There is normally an interosseous ligament between the distal ends of the hamate, capitate and trapezoid bones.

Palpation

These joints are only palpable from the posterior aspect.

- The carpometacarpal joints. Trace proximally along the back of the first metacarpal to its enlarged base, beyond which is a depression. At this point, palpate the joint line on either side of the tendon of extensor pollicis longus.
- The common carpometacarpal joint. Dorsally, just proximal to the bases of the second, third, fourth and fifth metacarpals, 2 cm distal to the line of the wrist joint, is a line of depressions between the extensor tendons. These represent the surface marking of the common carpometacarpal joint.
- Movements of the carpometacarpal joint of the thumb. Ask the model to flex, extend, abduct and adduct the thumb. Now feel the base of the first metacarpal moving on the trapezium.
- Note. There is little movement at the common carpometacarpal joint, except a slight gliding of the surfaces against each other accompanying movements of the hand.

Accessory movements

Palpation

- Movements of the carpometacarpal joint of the thumb. Ask the model to flex the elbow joint. Stabilize the trapezium with your finger and thumb of one hand. Grip the first metacarpal bone with your other hand. Now you can produce anterior, posterior, medial and lateral gliding of the metacarpal base against the trapezium. You can also produce a limited amount of rotation

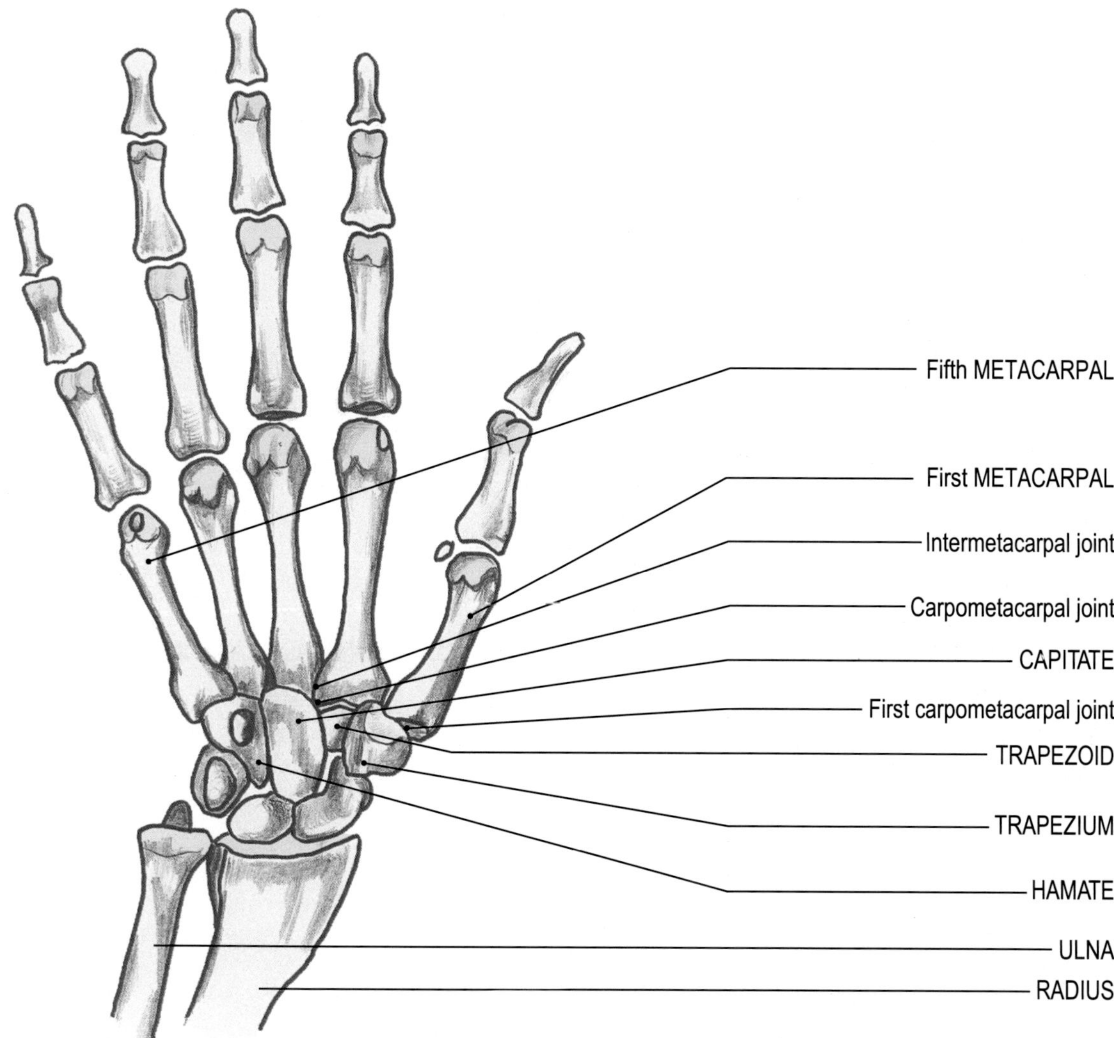

Fig. 2.14 (b) Carpometacarpal and intermetacarpal joints of the right hand (anterior view)

(i.e. rotation of the metacarpal about its long axis). Slight distraction of the joint is also possible.

- Distraction of the metacarpal bones. Stabilize the remaining carpus with one hand. In turn, grip each metacarpal between your fingers and thumb of the other hand. You can now move each metacarpal base slightly forwards and backwards.

The intermetacarpal joints (Fig. 2.14)

Between the bases of the second to fifth metacarpals are small plane synovial joints surrounded by a capsule lined with synovial membrane and supported by palmar, dorsal and interosseous ligaments. These ligaments allow the joints to be moved individually, giving the hand more mobility and thus more dexterity.

Palpation: surface marking

- The intermetacarpal joints. On the posterior aspect of the hand, trace proximally up the spaces between the second and third, third and fourth, and fourth and fifth, metacarpal bones until you feel the two bones touching. Palpate the joint line running vertically for approximately 1 cm from the line of the carpometacarpal joint (see above).

Accessory movements

Palpation

It is extremely difficult to move the base of one metacarpal against another, except when they are used as levers.

- Upwards and downwards movement of the metacarpal bones. Ask the model to pronate the forearm. Now grip one metacarpal head between your index finger and thumb of one hand and its neighbour similarly in the other. Move the bones up and down against each other.
- Note. There may be up to a centimetre of movement at the level of the heads, with a much smaller twisting movement of one base against its neighbour.

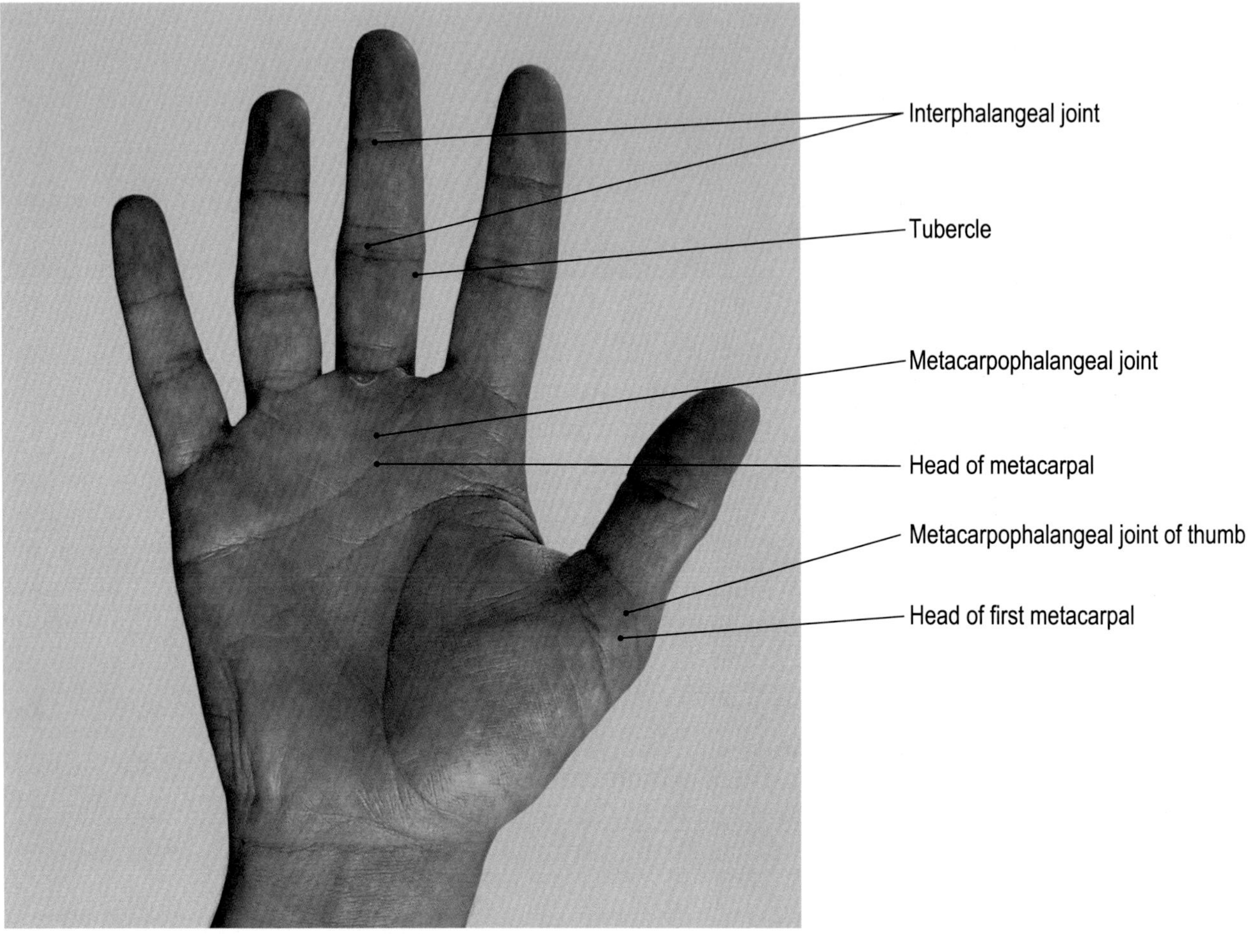

Fig. 2.15 (a) The metacarpophalangeal joints and interphalangeal joints of the right hand (anterior view)

The metacarpophalangeal joints

Metacarpophalangeal joints are synovial ellipsoid joints between the head of each metacarpal and the proximal end of each associated proximal phalanx. Each joint is surrounded by a fibrous capsule enclosing the head of the metacarpal and the proximal surface of the phalanx.

The capsule is lined with synovial membrane and is supported by strong, cord-like collateral ligaments and a dense palmar ligament. The posterior aspect of the joint is protected by the dorsal expansion of extensor digitorum longus tendon. The palmar ligaments of the second to fifth metacarpophalangeal joints are linked by the deep transverse metacarpal ligament.

- Note 1. Flexion of the metacarpophalangeal joint of the thumb is only 45°, whereas that of the fingers is 90°.
- Note 2. This movement occurs at right angles to that in the other metacarpal joints taking the thumb across the palm.

Palpation

- The metacarpophalangeal joints. The joints of each finger can be palpated just distal to the head of the metacarpal. Ask the model to flex the finger to 90°. Palpate the joint line which appears to be beyond the knuckles, on the anterior surface of the head of the metacarpal (Fig. 2.15). It is easily palpable dorsally on either side of extensor digitorum longus tendons.
- The metacarpophalangeal joint of the thumb. Palpate this joint posteriorly, just beyond the metacarpal head.

Accessory movements

Palpation

- Movements of the proximal phalanges. Stabilize the metacarpal with one hand and grip the digit with your other hand. Now move the base of the proximal phalanx forwards, backwards and from side to side. You can also rotate the digit about its long axis, producing spin between the two surfaces. If

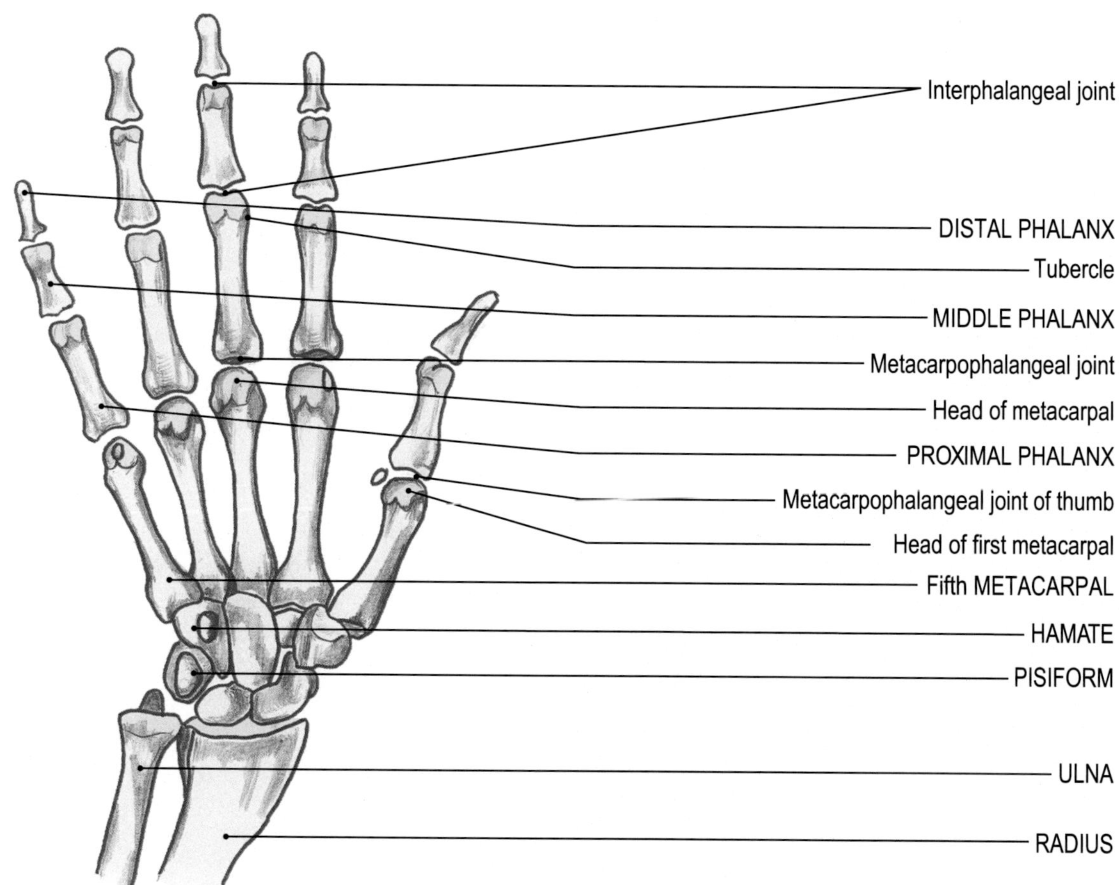

Fig. 2.15 (b) The metacarpophalangeal joints and interphalangeal joints of the right hand (anterior view)

sufficient distraction is applied, you will produce the characteristic 'pop'.

- Note. This is not normally possible at the metacarpophalangeal joint of the thumb.

The interphalangeal joints

Each finger has two **interphalangeal joints**, whereas the thumb has only one. They are synovial hinge joints between the head of the more proximal phalanx and the base of the more **distal phalanx**. These joints are surrounded by a capsule which is lined with synovial membrane and supported by collateral and palmar ligaments.

Palpation

- The interphalangeal joints. The joints are easier to palpate posteriorly. Ask the model to flex the joint to 90°. Now trace distally down the back of each phalanx. Palpate the joint line just beyond the slightly expanded head. It is covered centrally by the expansion of extensor digitorum (dorsal digital expansion).

Accessory movements

Palpation

- Rocking. Ask the model to pronate the forearm and to flex the interphalangeal joint to approximately 30°. Stabilize the more proximal phalanx with one hand and grip the more distal phalanx between fingers and thumb of your other hand. You can now rock the base of the more distal phalanx from side to side. This movement often causes a 'cracking' sound.
- Forwards and backwards gliding. It is possible, but not easy, to produce a slight forwards and backwards gliding of the base on the head.
- Distraction. This movement is limited by the tight collateral ligaments. The space gained between the articular surfaces is only a fraction of that gained at the metacarpophalangeal joints.

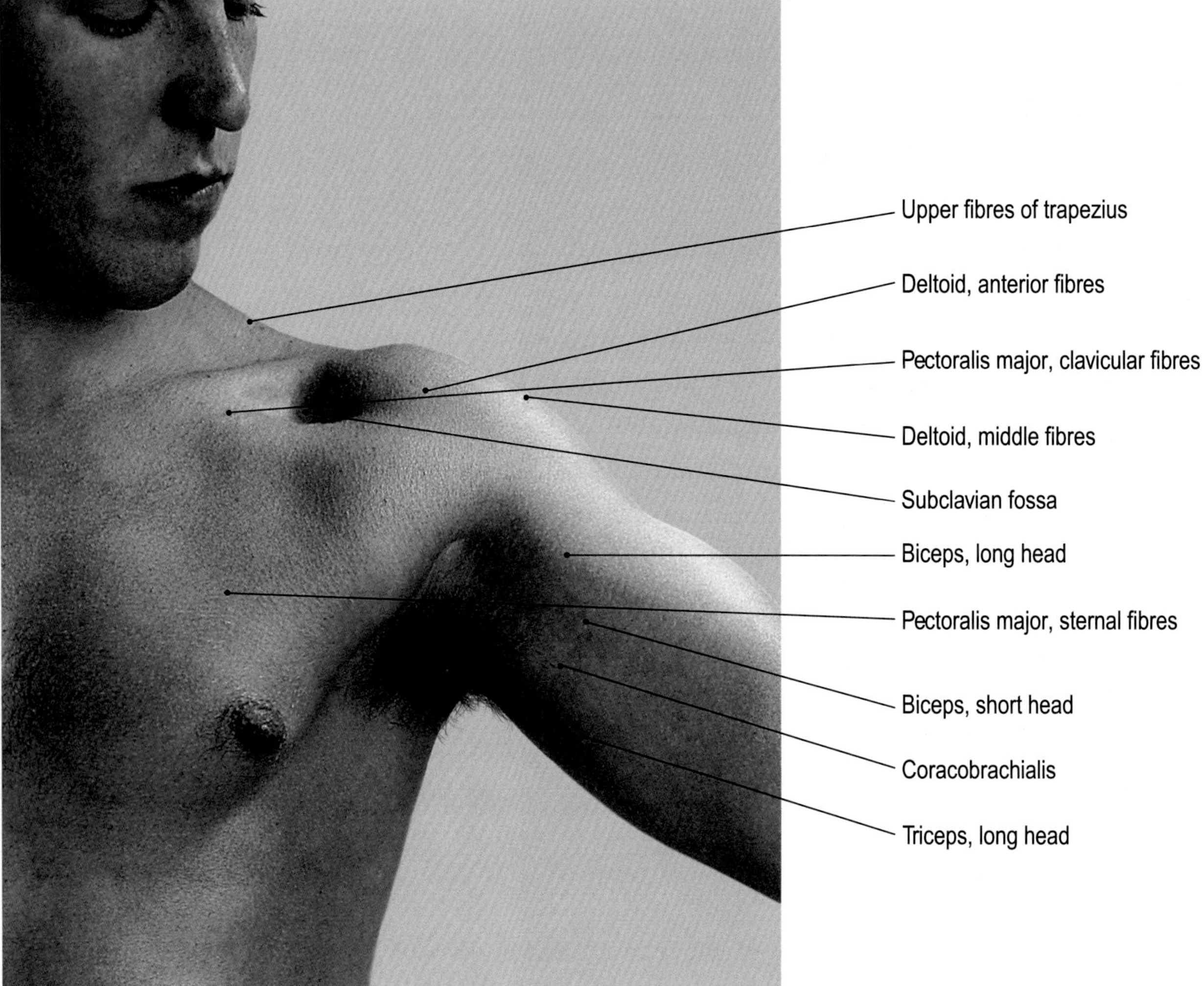

Fig. 2.16 (a) Muscles on the anterior of the left chest, shoulder and arm

MUSCLES

The muscles that move the arm

Deltoid (Figs 2.16 and 2.17)

The deltoid is a triangular or delta-shaped muscle situated on the lateral aspect of the shoulder joint. It comprises anterior, middle and posterior sections. These fibres arise above from the lateral end of the anterior border of the clavicle, anterior, lateral and posterior borders of the acromion process, and the lower lip of the spine of the scapula, respectively. They all unite below to attach to the deltoid tubercle on the lateral side of the humerus.

Below the pectoral girdle, the anterior fibres of deltoid can be seen some 3 cm below the lateral lip of the acromion, level with the greater tuberosity of the humerus. This delta-shaped muscle also covers the anterior and posterior aspects of the shoulder joint and feels thick and well developed.

Palpation

For palpation in this region, the model should be in the standing or sitting positions.

- Deltoid: general features. Palpate the anterior and posterior fibres which feel smooth and strap-like. Now palpate the middle fibres which feel coarse with stringy fibrous bands running vertically. This is because the middle section of deltoid is composed of multipennate muscle fibres, which pass obliquely from one vertical tendinous intersection to another. Palpate these coarse strips of muscle as they pass vertically from the lateral border of the acromion downwards to the final common tendon of all three sections halfway down the lateral aspect of the humerus. Ask the model to abduct the shoulder joint. Palpate the anterior and posterior fibres as triangular sections with facial septa separating them from the central fibres.

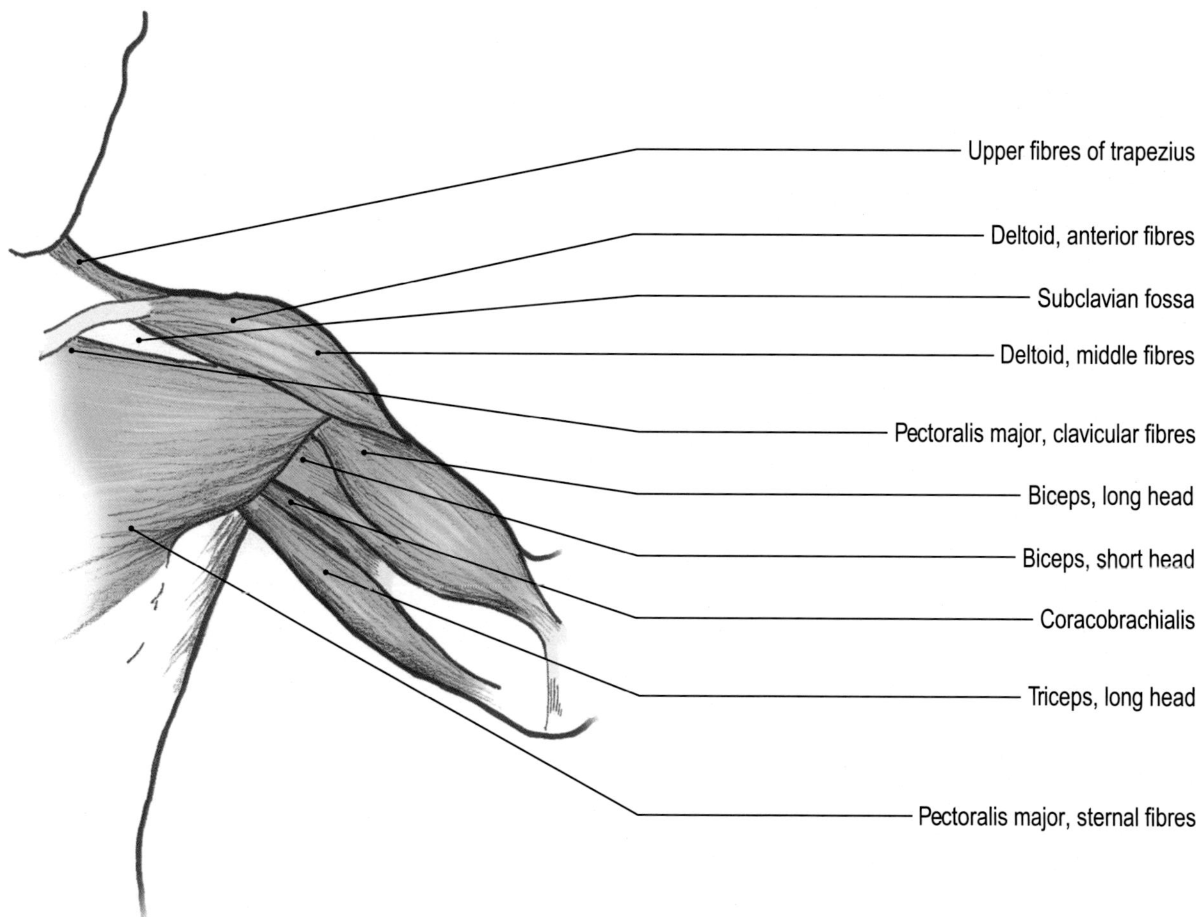

Fig. 2.16 (b) Muscles on the anterior of the left chest, shoulder and arm

- The anterior fibres of deltoid. Ask the model to flex and/or medially rotate the shoulder joint. Now trace the clearly visible anterior fibres from the clavicle above to humerus below.
- The posterior fibres of deltoid. Ask the model to extend and/or laterally rotate the shoulder joint. Now trace the clearly visible posterior fibres from the lower lip of the spine of the scapula above to the humerus below.
- The middle fibres of deltoid. Ask the model to abduct the shoulder joint to 90°. Palpate the middle fibres of deltoid between its anterior and posterior sections.

Pectoralis major (Fig. 2.16)

Pectoralis major is a thick, strong, triangular muscle which covers the upper anterior chest wall. It has its tendinous apex laterally. It comprises two functionally distinct groups of fibres: **clavicular** and **sternal**. The clavicular section attaches medially to the anterior surface of the medial half of the clavicle. The sternal fibres have an extensive attachment medially to the manubrium sterni, body of the sternum, anterior surfaces of the upper six costal cartilages and ribs and the upper part of the aponeurosis of the external oblique muscle. Laterally, the muscle forms a broad tendon which attaches to the lateral lip of the bicipital groove of the humerus. The lower border of the muscle appears thickened. This is due to its lower fibres being folded up behind its upper fibres and forming a bilaminal tendon at its insertion.

Palpation

- Pectoralis major: general features. Trace this muscle laterally as it passes across, and forms the anterior wall of the axilla.
- The clavicular fibres of pectoralis major. Ask the model to flex the shoulder joint. Palpate the clavicular fibres as a thick muscular column passing from the medial end of the clavicle to the humerus.
- The sternal fibres of pectoralis major. Ask the model to extend the shoulder joint from the flexed position. Apply resistance to the movement. Palpate the sternal fibres passing from the lower ribs and sternum to the same insertion.
- **Note.** In women, much of the muscular section is covered by the breast but contraction of the muscle is evident to see or palpate. In men, the whole of the muscle is clearly palpable and becomes hard and tense on adduction and medial rotation of the shoulder joint. Laterally, a groove can be palpated between its upper border and the lower border of deltoid.

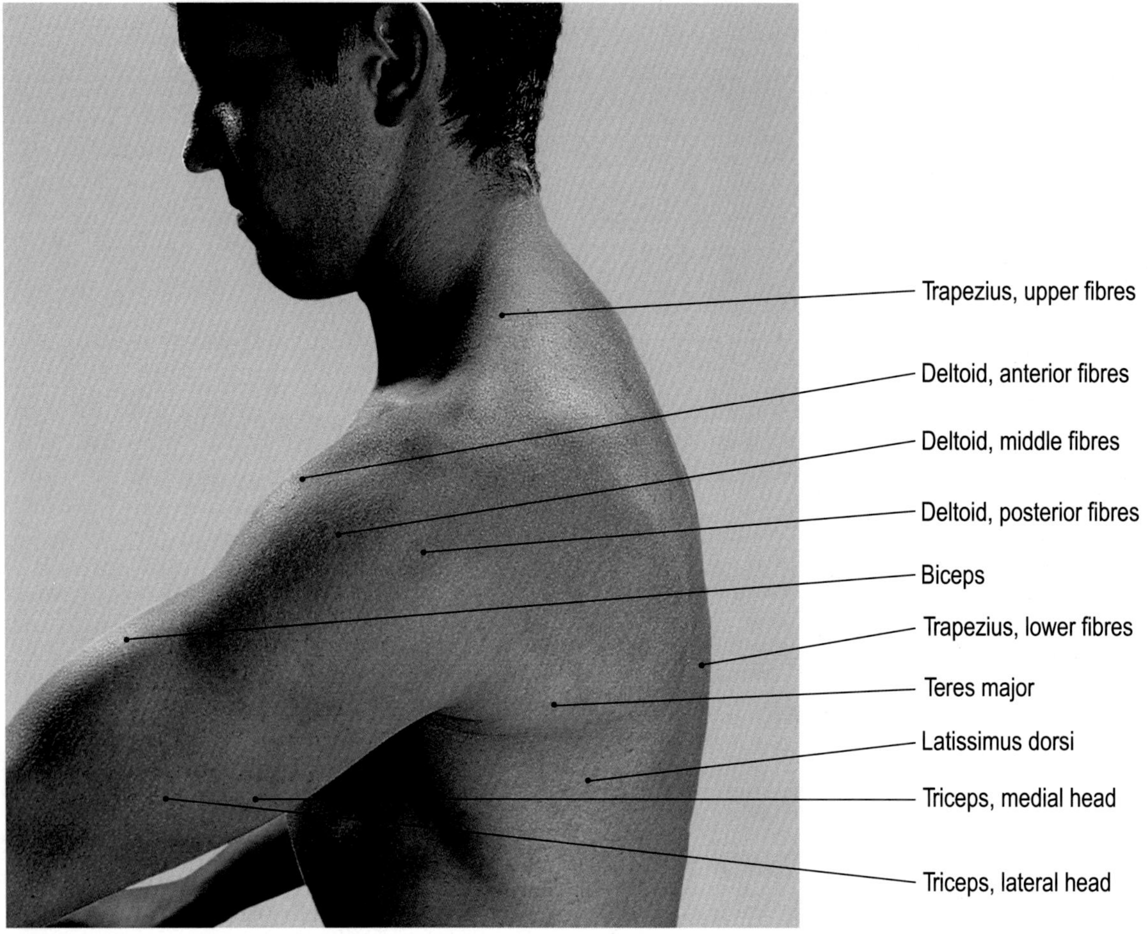

Fig. 2.17 (a) Muscles that move the arm and forearm (lateral view of left arm)

Biceps brachii (Figs 2.16–2.18)

Biceps brachii is fusiform in shape, situated on the anterior aspect of the upper arm. Its upper end attaches by two heads, as its name implies. One attachment is from the supraglenoid tubercle, the other from the tip of the coracoid process of the scapula. Below, it attaches by a strong tendon to the posterior aspect of the radial tubercle on the upper medial aspect of the radius and by an expansion from its medial aspect which blends with the fascia on the medial side of the forearm.

Palpation

- Biceps brachii: general features. The fusiform shape of biceps brachii can be seen and palpated covering the front of the arm. Trace the muscle upwards as it runs deep to pectoralis major and splits into two parts.
- The long head of biceps brachii. Palpate the long head passing as a tendon in the intertubercular groove of the humerus. Trace the tendon up the bicipital (intertubercular) groove and passing over the head of the humerus to the supraglenoid tubercle of the scapula.
- The short head of biceps brachii. Palpate the short head passing medially to the coracoid process of the scapula.
- The common tendon of biceps brachii. Below, palpate the muscle as it forms a well-defined tendon which passes through the cubital fossa giving off an expansion (the bicipital aponeurosis). This blends with the fascia on the medial side of the forearm, reaching as far as the posterior border of the ulna, forming a sickle-shaped edge.
- The bicipital apponeurosis. Ask the model to supinate the flexed forearm. Apply resistance to the movement. You will now find it easier to palpate the shape and tendons of biceps. You will also be able to palpate the aponeurosis spreading medially from the tendon.
- **Note.** In a well-developed subject, you can slip the tips of your fingers under the posterior border of the bicipital aponeurosis approximately 2 cm anteroinferior to the medial epicondyle of the humerus (Fig. 2.18).

Brachialis

Brachialis is a thick, triangular muscle situated deep to the lower part of the biceps. It attaches above to the lower half of the anterolateral and anteromedial surfaces of the humerus, crosses the front of the elbow joint and attaches below to the anterior surface of the coronoid process of the ulna.

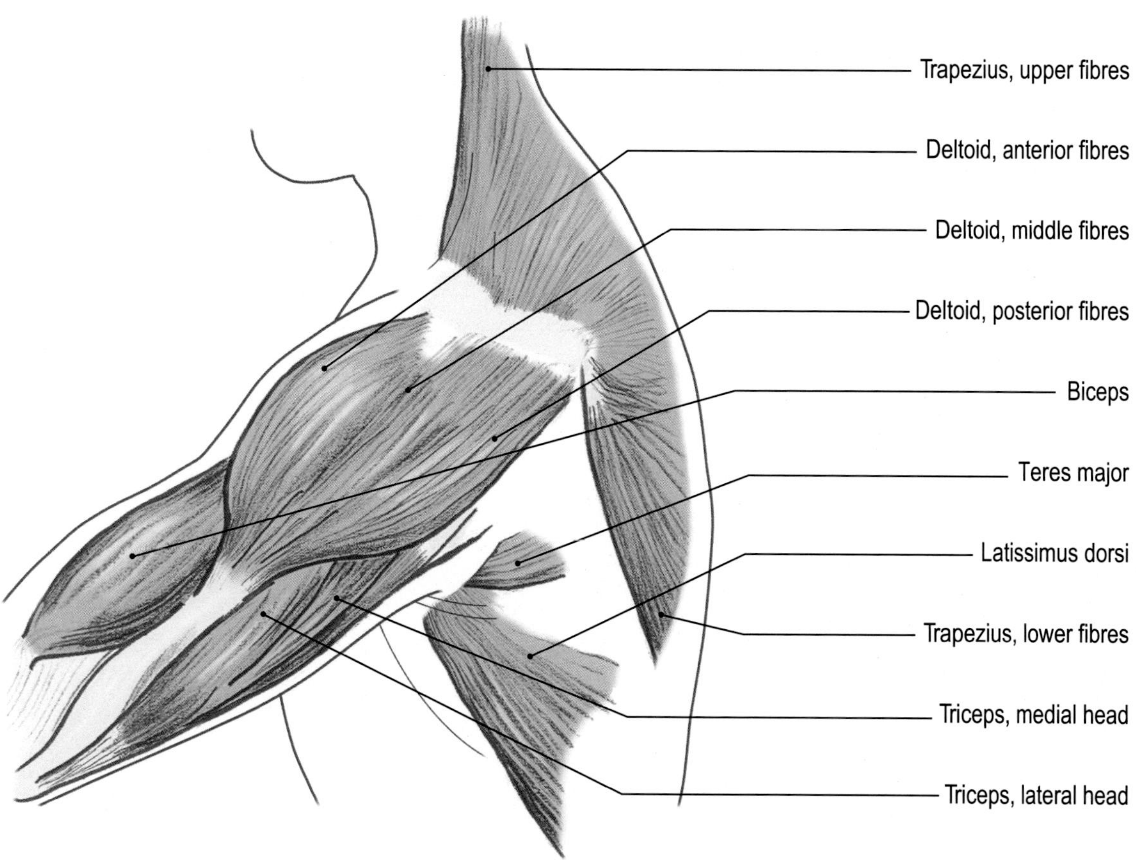

Fig. 2.17 (b) Muscles that move the arm and forearm (lateral view of left arm)

Palpation

Because it is deeply situated this muscle is difficult to palpate.

- Brachialis. Ask the model to flex and extend the elbow joint gently. Locate the tendon of biceps brachii. Now deeply palpate the area. On either side of this tendon, you will be able to feel the contraction and relaxation of brachialis during this movement.

Triceps (Figs 2.16a, b and 2.17a, b)

Triceps is a thick muscular mass situated on the posterior aspect of the arm. As its name implies, it arises from three heads.

1. The long head. This is tendinous and passes upwards, below the shoulder joint to attach to the infraglenoid tubercle of the scapula.
2. The lateral head. This attaches to the upper lateral part of the posterior surface of the humerus above and lateral to the radial groove.
3. The medial head. This attaches to the lower medial part of the posterior surface of the humerus below and medial to the radial groove.

All three heads attach to the posterior part of the superior surface of the olecranon via the triceps tendon.

Palpation

- The long head of triceps. Medially, trace the long head of triceps upwards as a tendon on the medial aspect of the arm. It passes up, under the posterior fibres of deltoid, infraspinatus, teres major and minor, to lie in front of the posterior wall of the axilla.
- The medial and lateral heads of triceps. Palpate these heads as they form a much more fleshy mass down the posterior aspect of the whole of the arm.
- The common tendon of triceps. Just above the elbow joint, palpate the three heads as they form a strong, thick tendon which attaches to the upper surface of the olecranon process.
- Note. You will find it easier to palpate the muscle and its tendon by applying resistance to extension of the elbow joint. On palpation, you will note that the lateral head lies slightly higher and lateral in relation to the medial head. (Fig. 2.17).

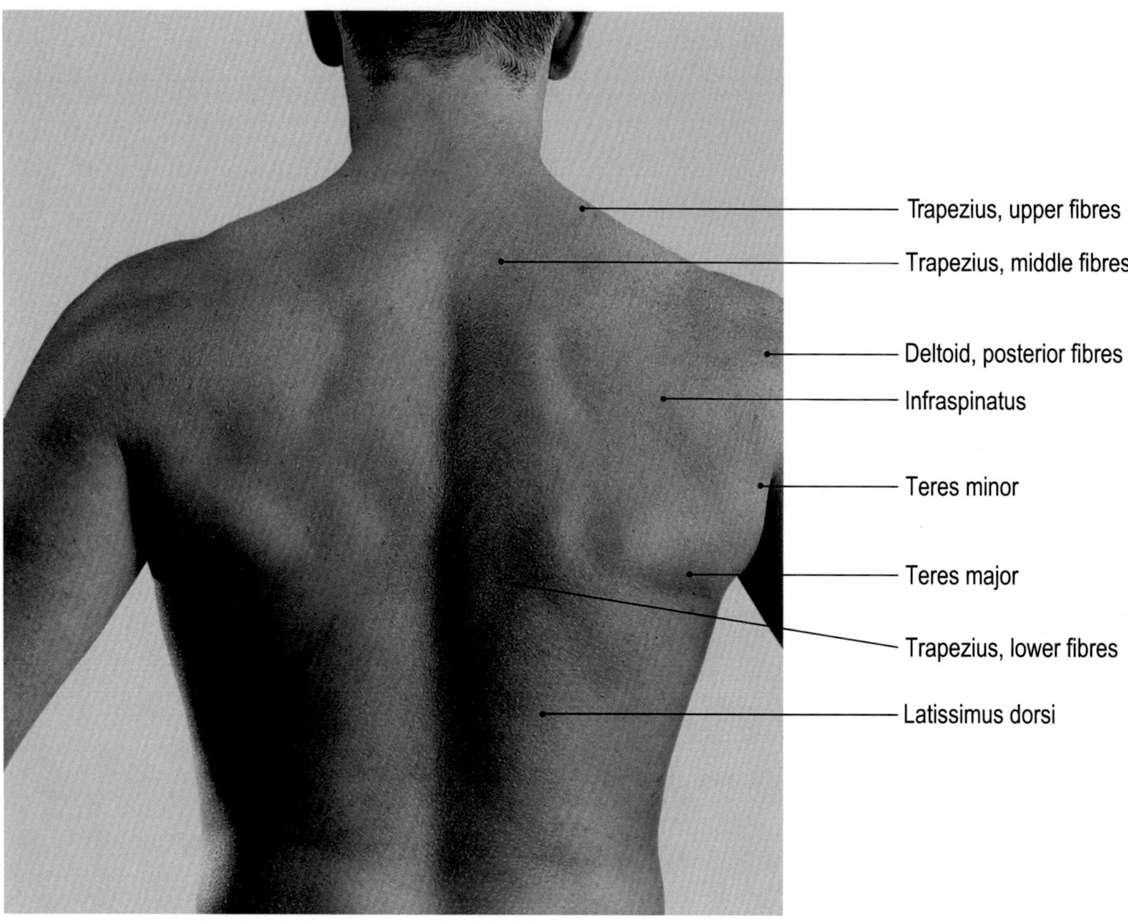

Fig. 2.17 (c) Muscles that move the arm (posterior view)

Latissimus dorsi (Fig. 2.17)

Latissimus dorsi is a large triangular muscle situated on the lower posterior part of the trunk. It passes upwards and laterally to attach to the upper part of the humerus.

This muscle has an extensive origin. It arises from the lower part of the thoracolumbar fascia, the spines of the lower six thoracic, all the lumbar and sacral vertebrae, the supraspinous and interspinous ligaments which lie between the thoracic and lumbar vertebrae and from the outer lip of the posterior sixth of the crest of the iliac crest. As it passes upwards it also attaches to the lower three ribs and the posterior aspect of the inferior angle of the scapula. It attaches above by a flattened tendon, which twists under the axilla and attaches to the floor of the intertubercular groove of the humerus.

Palpation

For palpation in this region the model should be in the standing position.

- The tendon of latissimus dorsi. Palpate the tendon as it passes under teres major, forming the posterior wall of the axilla. Ask the model to extend and medial rotate the arm. Apply resistance to the movement. Now trace the tendon along the medial side of the humerus towards its insertion into the floor of the intertubercular groove.
- The muscle fibres of latissimus dorsi. To facilitate palpation, ask the model to pull down on a fixed beam above the head (beam heaves) and/or to cough. Now palpate the muscle fibres on the posterolateral area of the chest wall.

Coracobrachialis (Fig. 2.16a, b)

Coracobrachialis is a long thin fusiform muscle situated on the upper medial area of the arm. It attaches above to the tip of the coracoid process of the scapula by a tendon common to it and biceps brachii. Below it attaches by a short tendon to a point halfway down the medial side of the humerus.

Palpation

- The tendon of coracobrachialis. Palpation is facilitated by abducting the upper limb. Ask the model to place the hand on the hip and then to adduct the arm forcefully. Now trace the tendon to the posterior aspect of the short head of biceps. It can be identified blending with this tendon.

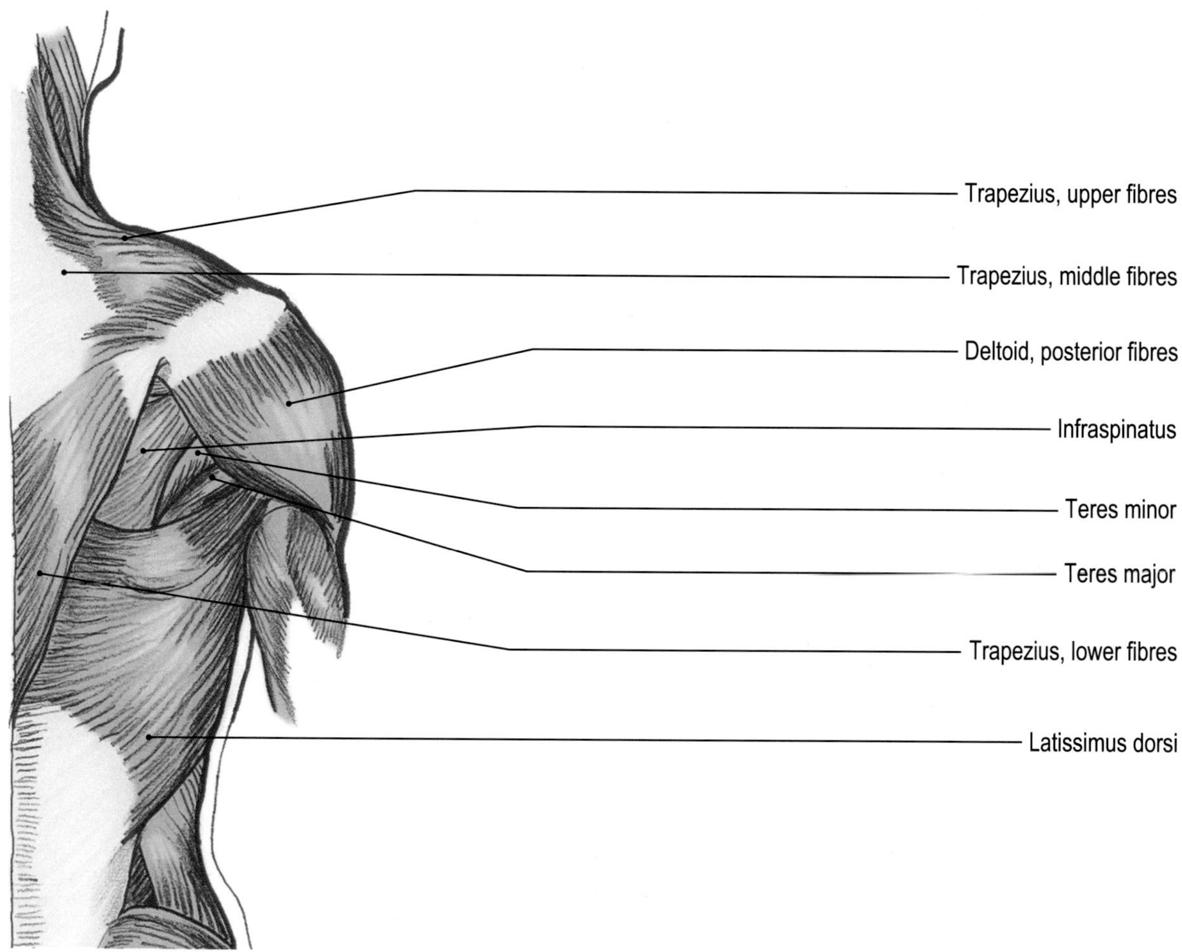

Fig. 2.17 (d) Muscles that move the arm (posterior view)

- The belly of coracobrachialis. Palpate the belly of coracobrachialis (see Fig. 2.16a, b) high up on the medial side of the arm, passing upwards and forwards towards the coracoid process.
- Note. Care must be taken when palpating this area as it contains numerous branches of the brachial plexus and major blood vessels.

The posterior aspect of the scapula (Fig. 2.17c, d)

- Supraspinatus. Supraspinatus arises from the supraspinus fossa on the posterior aspect of the scapula. It attaches laterally to the upper facet on the greater tuberosity of the humerus.
- Infraspinatus arises from the infraspinus fossa on the posterior aspect of the scapula. It passes upwards and laterally to attach to the posterior aspect of the greater tuberosity of the humerus.
- Teres minor arises from the lateral border of the scapula. It passes upwards and laterally to insert into the posterior aspect of the greater tuberosity of the humerus.
- Teres major arises from the lateral border and the inferior angle of the scapula. It inserts into the medial border of the bicipital groove of the humerus.

Palpation

- The muscle belly of supraspinatus. Ask the model to begin to abduct the arm. Now palpate the muscle belly above the spine of the scapula.
- The muscle belly of infraspinatus. Ask the model to laterally rotate the arm. Apply resistance to the movement. Now palpate the muscle belly below the scapula spine as it passes upwards and laterally to the humerus.
- Teres major and the upper part of latissimus dorsi. Ask the model to adduct the arm. Apply resistance to the movement. Palpate these muscles which form the large bulk of muscle covering the lateral border of the scapula.
- Teres minor. Ask the model to rotate the arm laterally. Apply resistance to the movement. Palpate the teres minor.
- Teres major and latissimus dorsi. Ask the model to rotate the arm medially. Apply resistance to the movement. Palpate the teres major and latissimus dorsi.

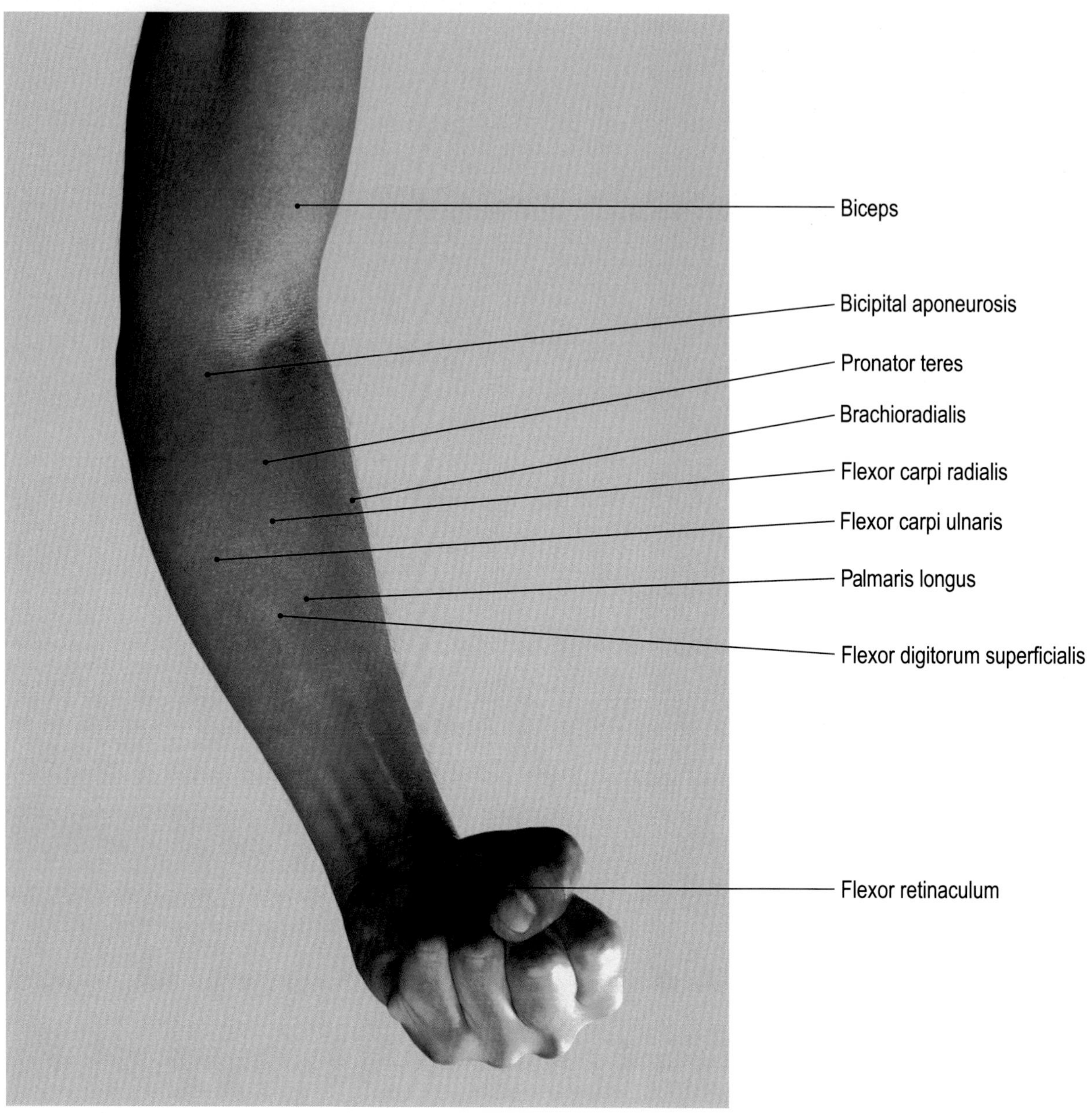

Fig. 2.18 (a) The left forearm (anterior view)

The anterior aspect of the forearm and wrist

Because of their close proximity, palpation of individual forearm muscles is difficult. The point at which they are most easily identifiable is where their tendons cross the wrist joint. For purposes of palpation, therefore, most muscles will be identified at this point and then traced proximally and distally.

Generally the forearm is greater in circumference in its upper half than in its lower half owing to the presence of the muscle bellies, whereas lower down the muscles give way to tendons (Fig. 2.18).

Palpation

For palpation in this region, the model is in the sitting position.

- **Brachioradialis**. Palpate this muscle which is situated most laterally and which gives shape to the upper part of the forearm. Note its strap-like shape, being thicker near the elbow and narrowing to a broad tendon towards the lateral surface of the radius. Ask the model to flex the elbow in the mid-prone position. Apply resistance to the movement. Palpate the muscle from its origin at the supracondylar ridge of the humerus (Fig. 2.18).
- Flexor carpi radalis. Palpate the tendon of **flexor carpi radialis** on the anterior aspect of the wrist, approximately 1 cm medial to the styloid process of the radius. Distally, it passes in front of the scaphoid, being lost in the groove on the front of the trapezium. Now trace the tendon halfway up the front of the forearm. Note that it becomes muscular in the upper part which attaches to the medial epicondyle of the humerus (Fig. 2.18).
- The tendon of **palmaris longus**. Ask the model to flex the wrist slightly and to draw the base of the thumb and the little finger together. Now palpate the slim tendon of palmaris longus medial to the tendon of flexor carpi radialis. Trace the tendon distally and note that it blends with the palmar aponeurosis.
- The belly of palmaris longus. Trace the tendon proximally. Now palpate the narrow belly of palmaris longus on the medial side of flexor carpi radialis muscle.

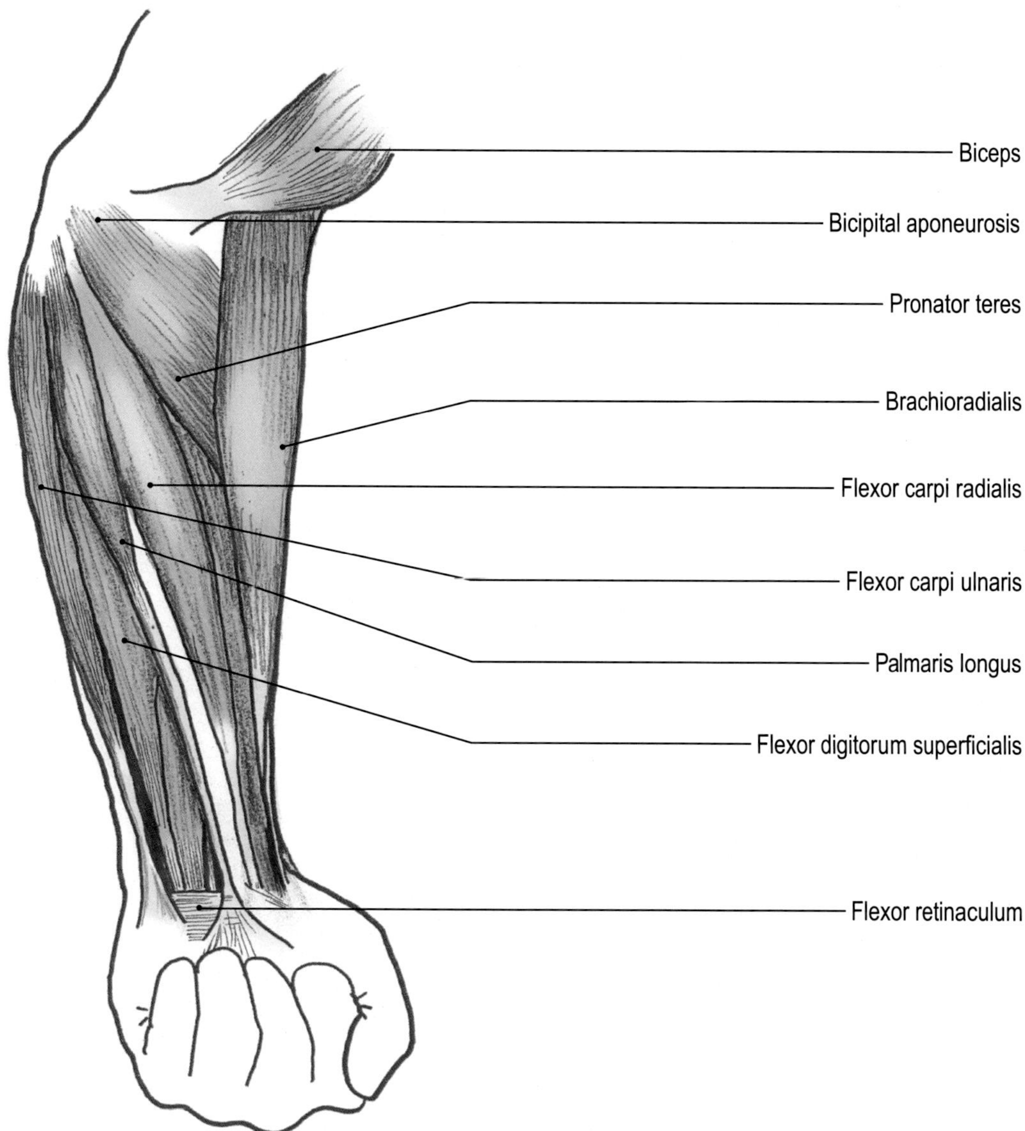

Fig. 2.18 (b) Muscles of the left forearm (anterior view)

- **Note.** Palmaris longus may not be present in all subjects.
- **Flexor carpi ulnaris.** Palpate the stout tendon of flexor carpi ulnaris on the anteromedial aspect of the wrist. Distally, it blends with the pisiform bone. Proximally, trace the tendon to a point almost halfway up the forearm, approximately 2 cm anterior to the posterior border of the ulna. Now palpate the thick muscle which replaces the tendon lying in front of the posterior border of the ulna.
- The tendons of **flexor digitorum superficialis**. Locate the depressed area between the tendons of palmaris and flexor carpi ulnaris. Ask the model to flex the fingers (particularly the middle and ring fingers). Observe and palpate the tendons of flexor digitorum superficialis in that groove.
- **Note.** The tendons to the index and little fingers, and those of flexor digitorum profundus, lie deeper and are difficult to differentiate.
- The belly of flexor digitorum superficialis. Ask the model to flex the fingers only at the metacarpophalangeal and proximal interphalangeal joints. Now palpate flexor digitorum superficialis immediately medial to the tendon of palmaris longus.
- Flexor digitorum profundus. Ask the model to press the fingertips against the palm of the hand. Palpate flexor digitorum profundus on the medial side of the forearm, deep to flexor carpi ulnaris.
- **Note.** In the palm, the tendons of these muscles are well covered with fascia and are difficult to determine, except for an area just proximal to the metacarpophalangeal joints.

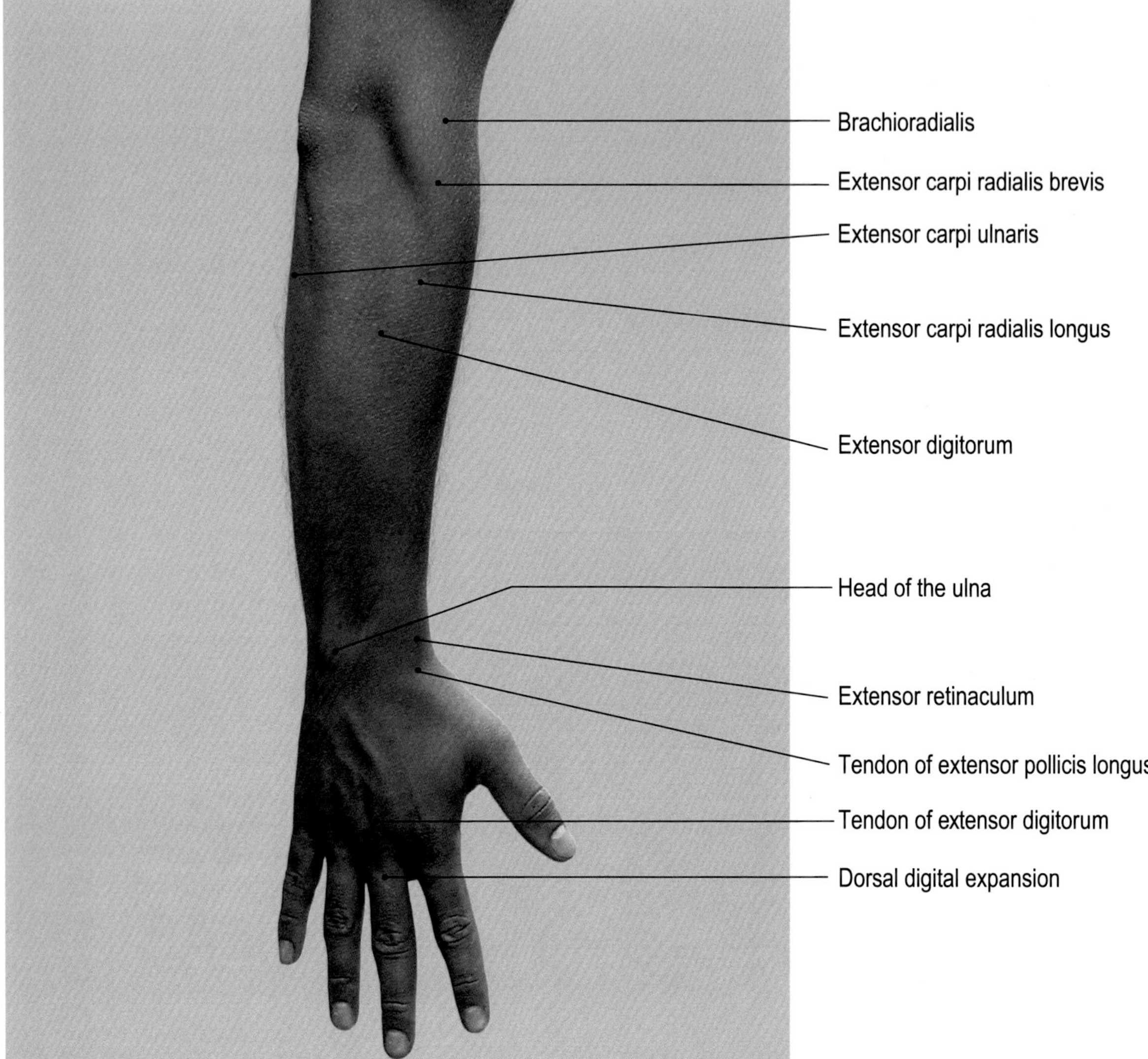

Fig. 2.19 (a) The right forearm (posterior view)

The posterior aspect of the forearm and wrist

Palpation

In order to palpate muscles in this area, you must ensure that the model's forearm is maintained in the anatomical position: i.e. the arm should be hanging loosely by the side with the palms facing forwards.

- **Brachioradialis**. This muscle can be palpated most laterally (see above).
- **Extensor carpi radialis longus** and **brevis**. Locate a point about 1 cm medial to the radial styloid process. Here two tendons cross the wrist. They are so close to each other that they are often mistaken as one. Palpation is facilitated if you ask the model to extend the wrist gently. The most lateral tendon is that of extensor carpi radialis longus. Trace this tendon distally to the base of the second metacarpal. The most medial is the tendon of extensor carpi radialis brevis, which can be traced to its attachment to the base of the third metacarpal distally (see Fig. 2.21a). Proximally, trace both muscles along the medial side of the bulk of brachioradialis to their attachment to, and just above, the lateral epicondyle of the humerus.
- The tendon of **extensor pollicis longus**. Ask the model to extend the thumb. Now palpate this tendon where it passes around the dorsal tubercle of the radius. Follow the tendon to its insertion into the base of the distal phalanx of the thumb. Proximally, the tendon is covered almost immediately by superficial muscles (Figs 2.19 and 2.21).
- **Extensor digitorum**. Ask the model to extend all the fingers. Palpate the tendon of extensor digitorum immediately medial to the tendon of extensor pollicis longus (Fig. 2.19). Note that it is broad and flat, dividing into four separate tendons distally. Trace each tendon over the back of the hand and along the posterior aspect of each finger. Note that each becomes slightly broader over the back of the metacarpophalangeal joint (**dorsal digital expansion**). Distally, trace each tendon to its attachment to the base of the distal phalanx.

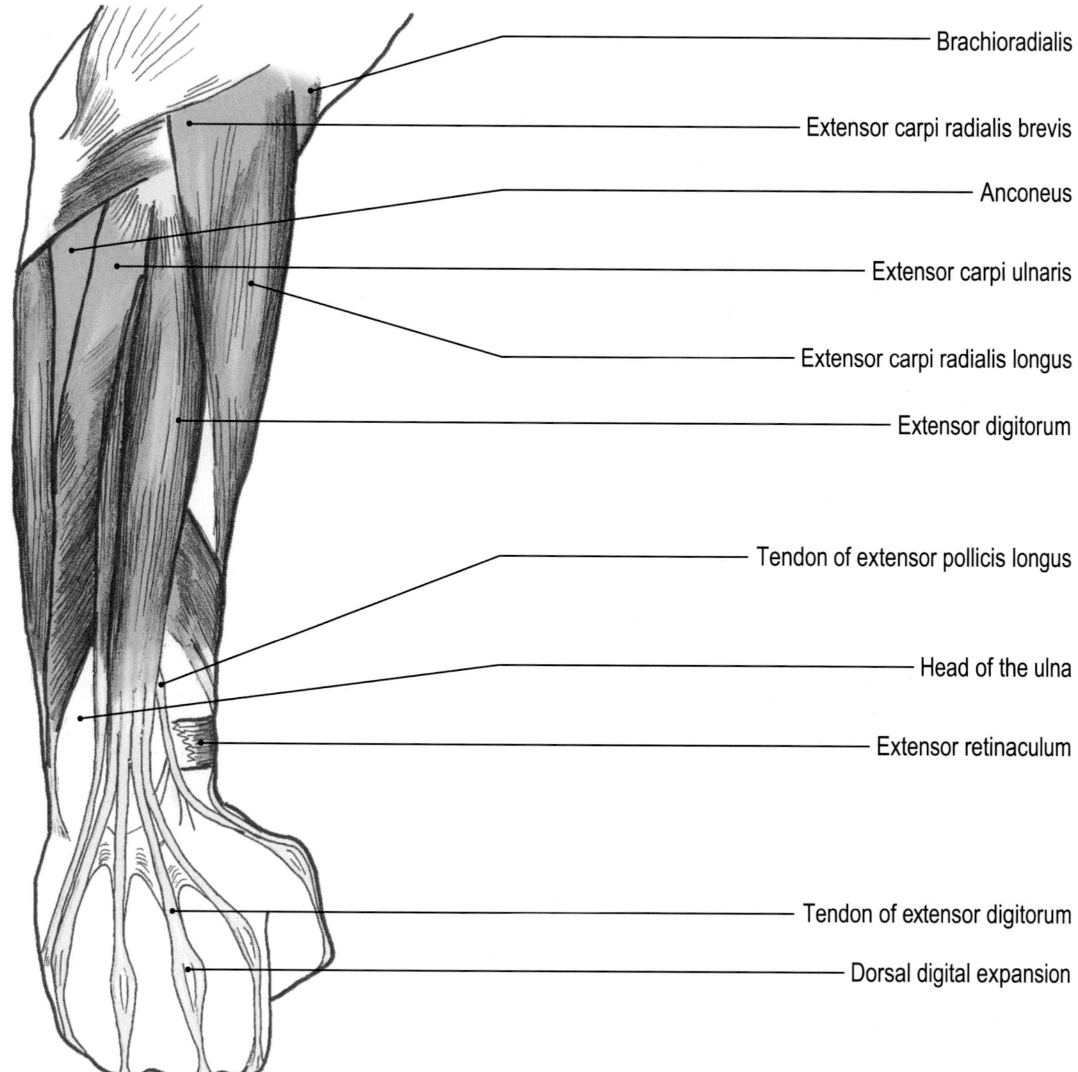

Fig. 2.19 (b) Muscles of the right forearm (posterior view)

- The belly of extensor digitorum. Proximally, trace extensor digitorum up the middle of the forearm medial to extensor carpi radialis longus and brevis to its attachment to the lateral epicondyle of the humerus.
- Note. Often a separate muscle belly can be identified on the lateral side which passes to the index finger only.
- The tendon of extensor indicis. Palpate this tendon as it accompanies extensor digitorum across the back of the wrist. Note that it is more easily identifiable as it joins the ulnar side of the tendon of extensor digitorum to the index finger at the metacarpophalangeal joint.
- The tendon of extensor digiti minimi. Palpation is facilitated if you ask the model to extend and relax the little finger rhythmically. Trace this thin tendon as it passes over the inferior radioulnar joint towards the little finger where it joins the tendon of extensor digitorum at its dorsal digital expansion.
- The belly of extensor digiti minimi. Trace the tendon proximally to a thin fusiform belly which attaches to the lateral epicondyle of the humerus.
- The tendon of extensor carpi ulnaris. Palpation of this tendon is facilitated if you ask the model to extend the wrist. Palpate this thick tendon as it crosses the posteromedial aspect of the wrist, just lateral to the styloid process of the ulna. Trace it distally to the base of the fifth metacarpal and proximally, via its muscle belly, to the lateral epicondyle of the humerus (Fig. 2.19). In the mid-forearm the muscle belly lies lateral to the posterior border of the ulna.

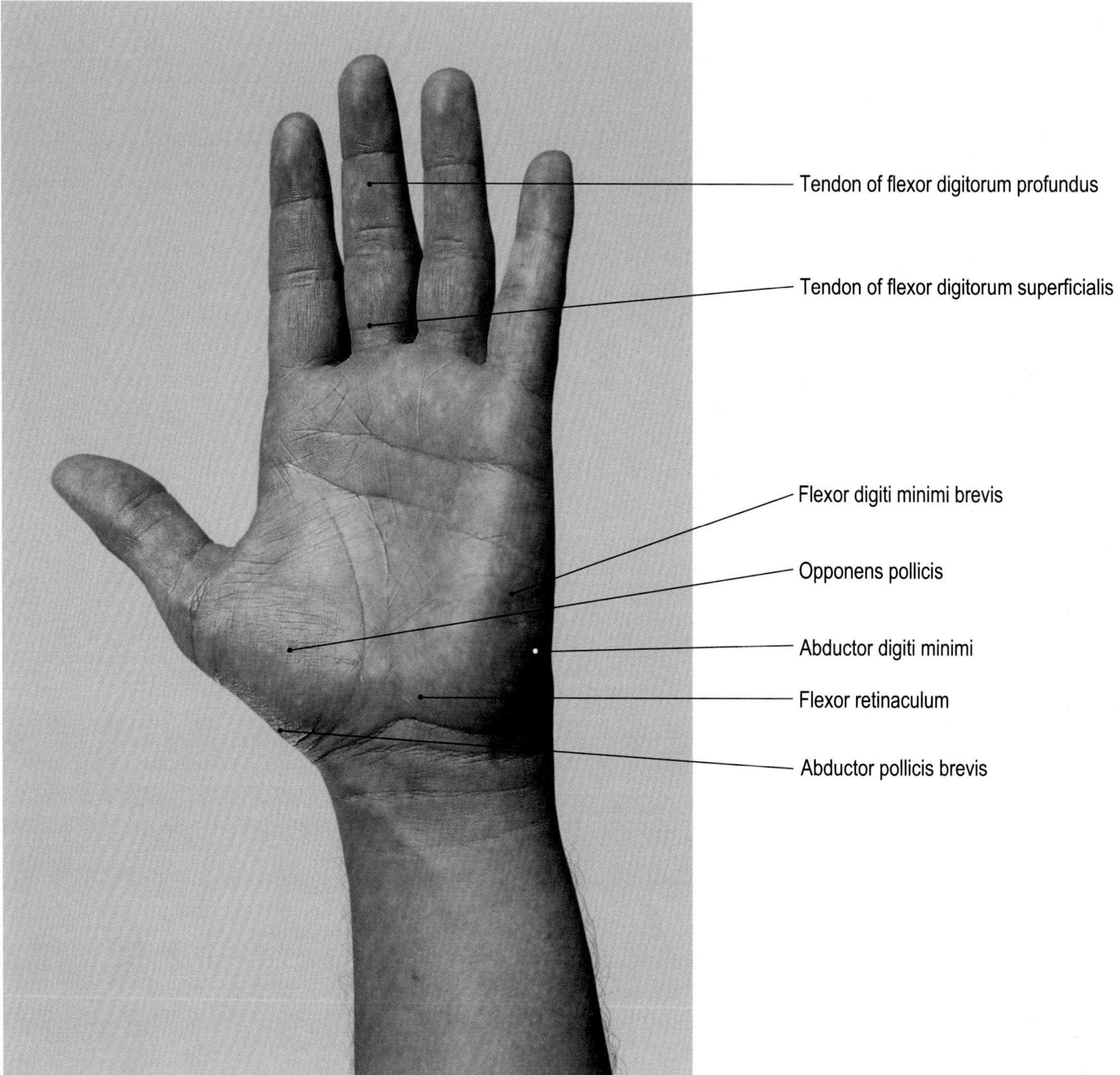

Fig. 2.20 (a) Muscles on the anterior aspect of the left hand (lumbrical muscles cannot be palpated)

The anterior aspect of the hand

The bones and joints of the hand are moved and controlled by two main groups of muscles:

1. The muscles of the forearm: the extrinsic muscles. Their tendons pass over the wrist to attach to particular bony points in the hand and govern the relationships between the forearm and hand.
2. The muscles within the hand: the intrinsic muscles. These change the relationships of the component parts of the hand from within.

The palm appears to have a flattened central portion with muscular masses on either side which are closer together proximally and diverge distally (Fig. 2.20a). The lateral mass, the thenar eminence, is the larger of the two and consists of muscles responsible for producing movements of the thumb. The medial mass, the hypothenar eminence, consists of muscles responsible for producing movements of the little finger.

- **Note.** Movements of the thumb take place in a plane at right angles to the palm of the hand. Consequently, abduction is movement of the thumb anteriorly away from the index finger. Flexion is movement of the thumb medially across the palm of the hand.

Palpation

- The belly of **abductor pollicis brevis**. Ask the model to abduct the thumb. Palpate the belly of abductor pollicis brevis on the lateral side of the thenar eminence.

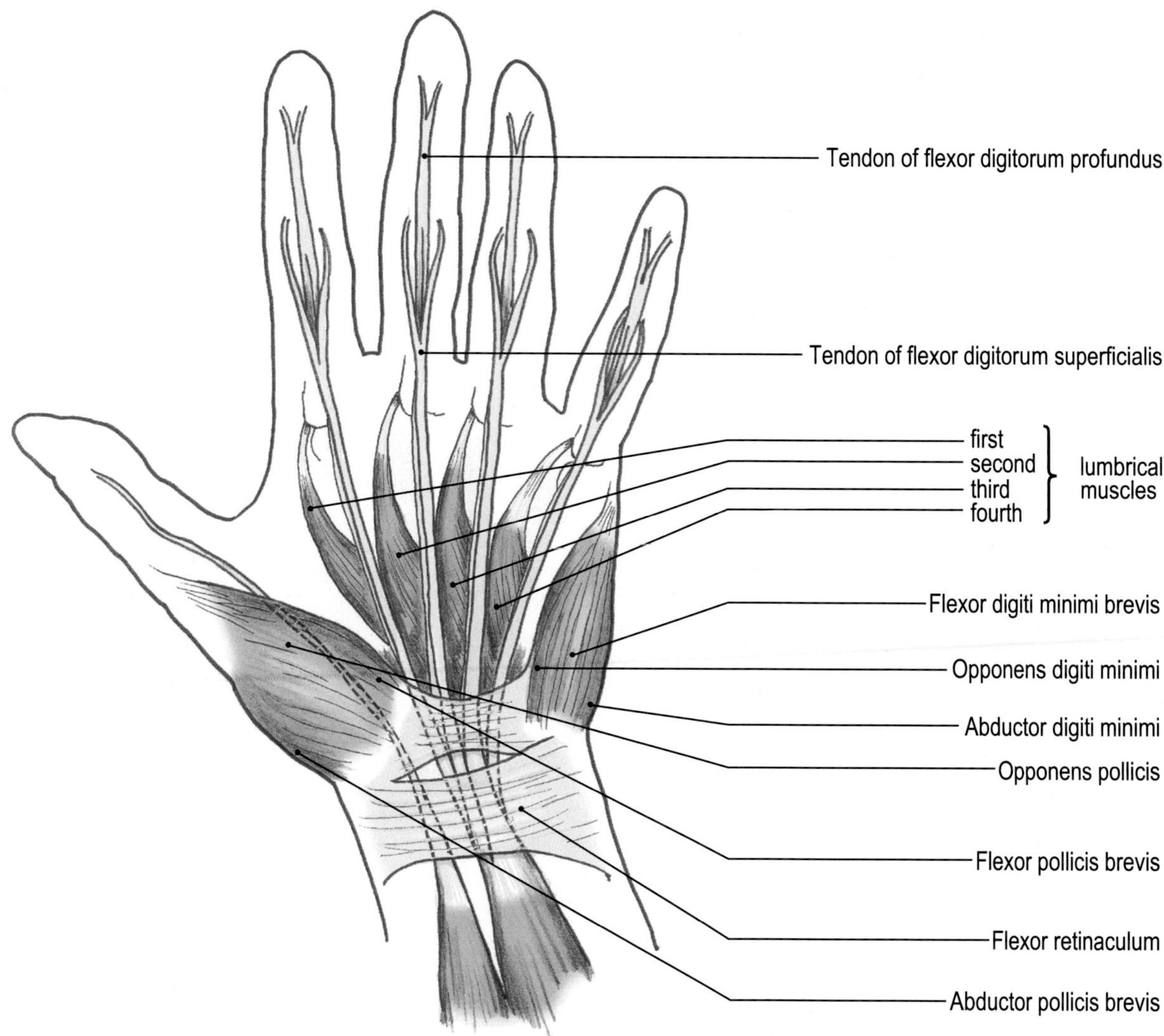

Fig. 2.20 (b) Muscles on the anterior aspect of the left hand (lumbrical muscles cannot be palpated)

- The tendon of abductor pollicis brevis. Palpate this tendon as it passes distally to the lateral side of the proximal phalanx of the thumb (Fig. 2.20).
- **Opponens pollicis**. Ask the model to oppose the pad of the thumb to the pads of the fingers. Palpate opponens pollicis and the resulting contraction of the whole central section of the thenar eminence.
- **Flexor pollicis brevis**. Ask the model to flex the thumb at the metacarpophalangeal joint. Apply resistance to the movement. Palpate flexor pollicis brevis contracting on the medial aspect of the thenar eminence.
- **Abductor digiti minimi**. Ask the model to abduct the little finger (to move it away from the ring finger). Palpate abductor digiti minimi on the medial side of the hypothenar eminence. Trace this via a short tendon to the medial side of the base of the proximal phalanx of the little finger (Fig. 2.20).
- **Opponens digiti minimi**. Ask the model to oppose the little finger to the thumb. Palpate the hard hypothenar eminence caused by the contraction of opponens digiti minimi.
- **Flexor digiti minimi brevis**. Ask the model to flex the little finger. Apply resistance to the movement. You should be able to palpate flexor digiti minimi brevis on the lateral side of opponens digiti minimi (Fig. 2.20).
- **Note.** The central section of the palm of the hand is covered by the strong and thick palmar aponeurosis, making palpation of muscles such as adductor pollicis (transverse head), the palmar interossei or the **lumbrical muscles** impossible.
- The long tendons of **flexor digitorum superficialis** and **profundus**. Palpation is facilitated if you ask the model to flex the fingers and apply resistance to the movement. Whilst it may be difficult, trace these tendons, particularly over the fronts of the metacarpophalangeal joints.

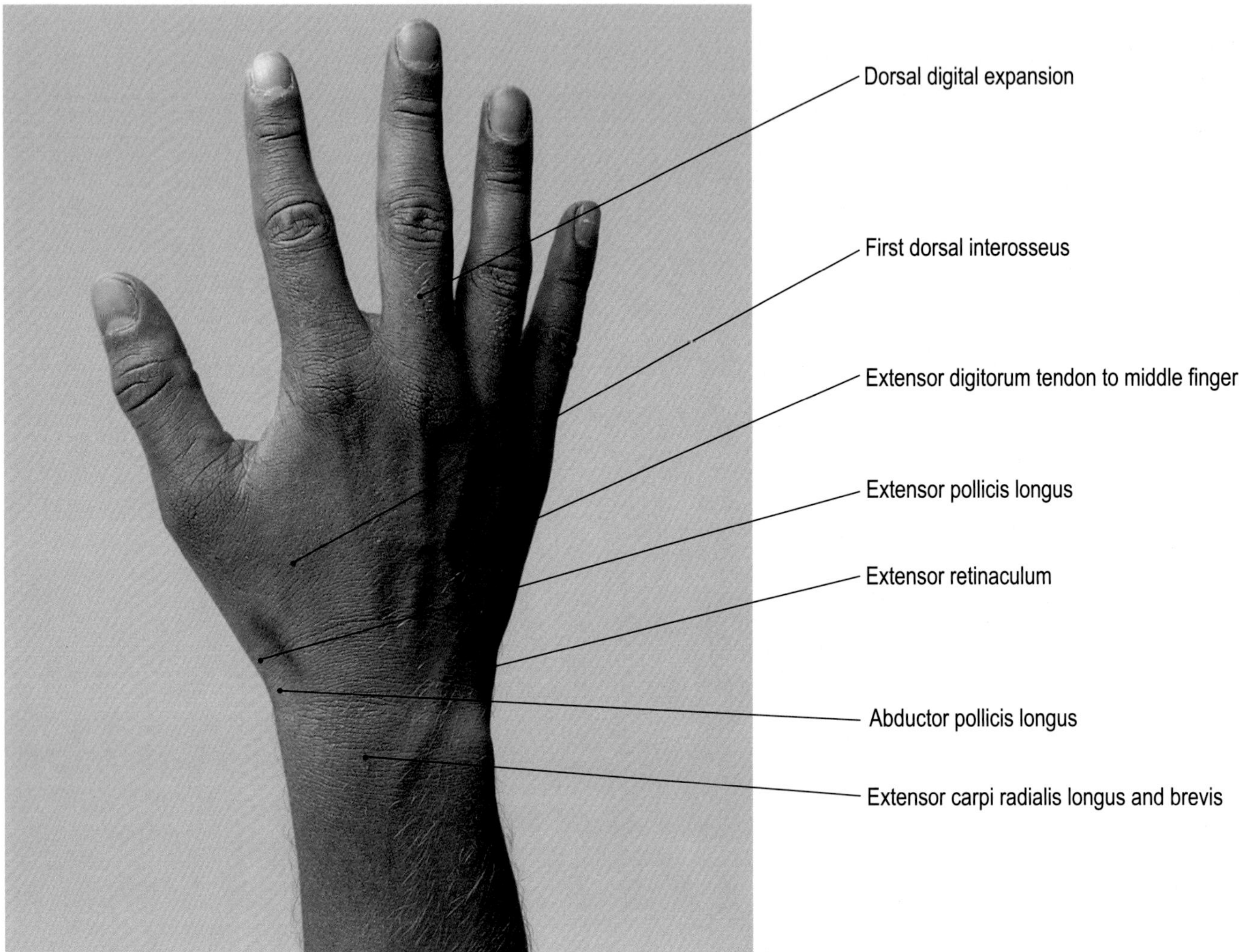

Fig. 2.21 (a) The posterior aspect of the right hand (for clarity only the first dorsal interosseus is identified, but all can be palpated)

The posterior aspect of the hand (Fig. 2.21)

The skin and fascia on the posterior aspect of the hand are thin and relatively loose, giving easy access for palpation of muscles. As the main function of the hand is to manipulate and hold implements and tools, often with great care and precision, most of the muscles are situated anteriorly. Releasing the grip tends to be left to the long extensor muscles whose bellies lie in the forearm, with their connection to the hand being through long tendons which cross the back of the wrist (see muscles on the posterior aspect of the forearm). Nevertheless, there are a few muscles which can be palpated and are worthy of note.

Palpation

- The posterior part of **abductor pollicis brevis**. Palpate the posterior part of this muscle on the lateral side of the thumb, lying just lateral to the tendon of **extensor pollicis longus**.
- The tendon of abductor pollicis brevis. Palpate the short tendon attaching to the lateral side of the proximal phalanx of the thumb. Trace its proximal attachment to the tubercle of the scaphoid.
- Abductor pollicis longus. Ask the model to abduct and extend the thumb. Identify two tendons crossing the wrist joint just in front of the radial styloid. Abductor pollicis longus is the most lateral. Trace this tendon to the base of the metacarpal.
- Extensor pollicis brevis. This lies medial to abductor pollicis longus. Ask the model to extend and abduct the thumb. Trace the tendon to the base of the proximal phalanx.
- **Note.** Proximal to the radial styloid both tendons wrap posteriorly around the lateral surface of the radius and disappear deep between the other muscles.
- The **first dorsal interosseous**. Palpation is facilitated by asking the model to place the fingers on the upper surface of a table with the thumb over the edge running down the vertical section. Ask the model to abduct the index finger (to draw it laterally away from the middle finger). Palpate the contraction of the large muscle mass in the cleft between the thumb and index finger. Trace the muscle belly from its attachment at both the first and second metacarpals to its tendon which attaches

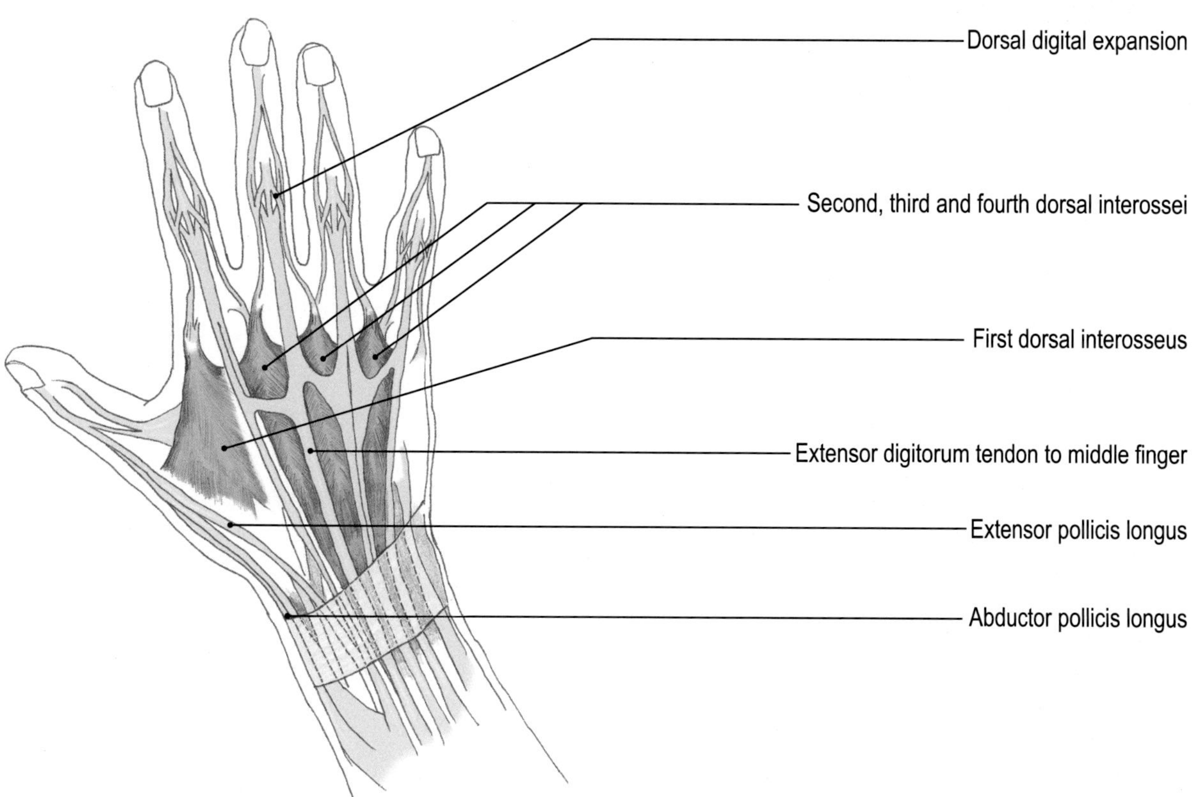

Fig. 2.21 (b) The posterior aspect of the right hand

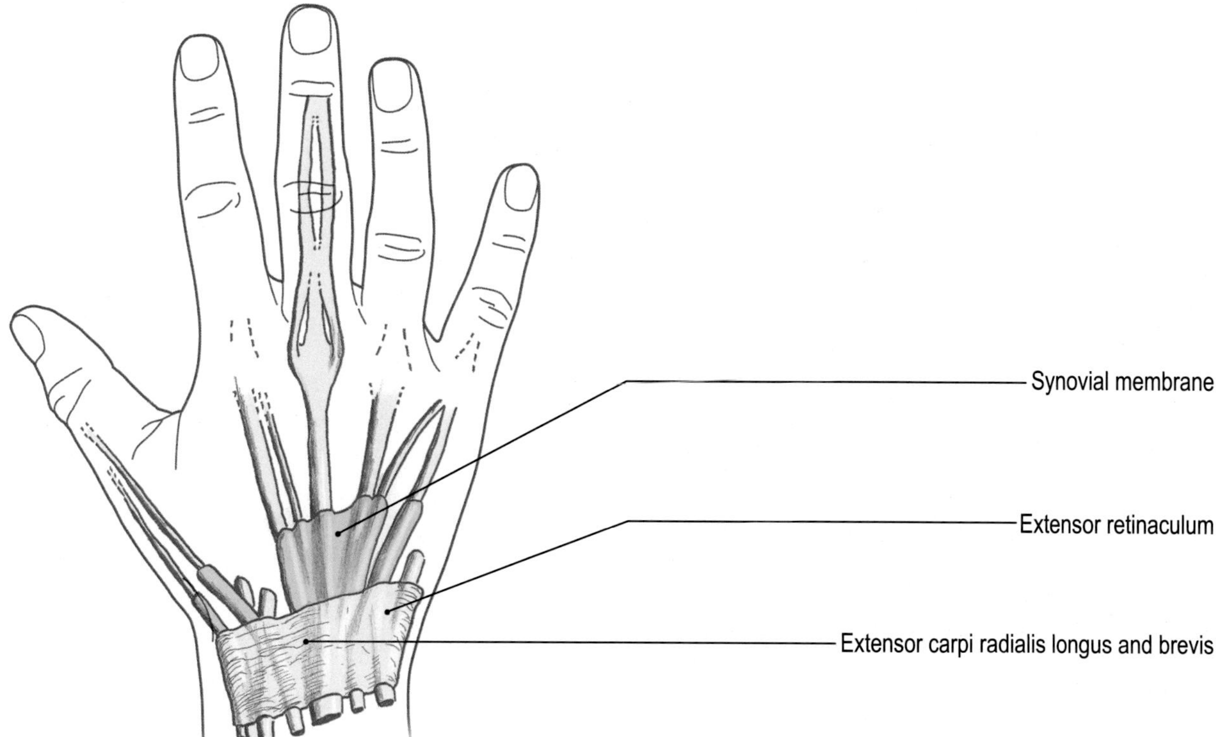

Fig. 2.21 (c) The posterior aspect of the right hand

distally to the lateral side of the base of the proximal phalanx of the index finger (Fig. 2.21a).

- The **second dorsal interosseous**. Ask the model to abduct the middle finger laterally (i.e. towards the index finger). Palpate the muscle fibres bulging between the proximal half of the second and third metacarpals.
- The **third dorsal interosseous**. Ask the model to abduct the middle finger medially (i.e. towards the ring finger). Palpate the muscle between the proximal half of the third and fourth metacarpals (Fig. 2.21d).
- The **fourth dorsal interosseous**. Ask the model to abduct the ring finger. Palpate the muscle between the proximal half of the fourth and fifth metacarpals.
- Abductor digiti minimi. Palpate the muscle on the medial side of the hand (see above).

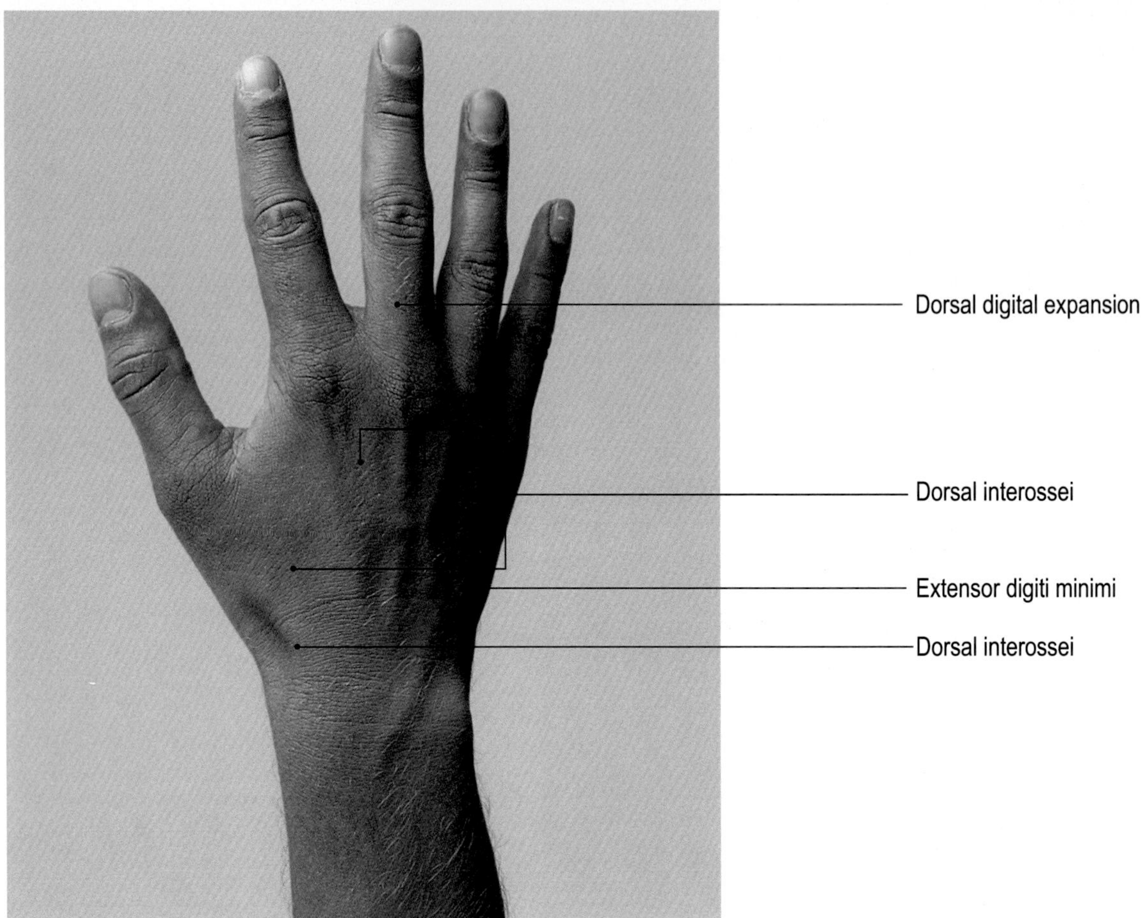

Fig. 2.21 (d) Muscles and tendons of the right hand (posterior aspect)

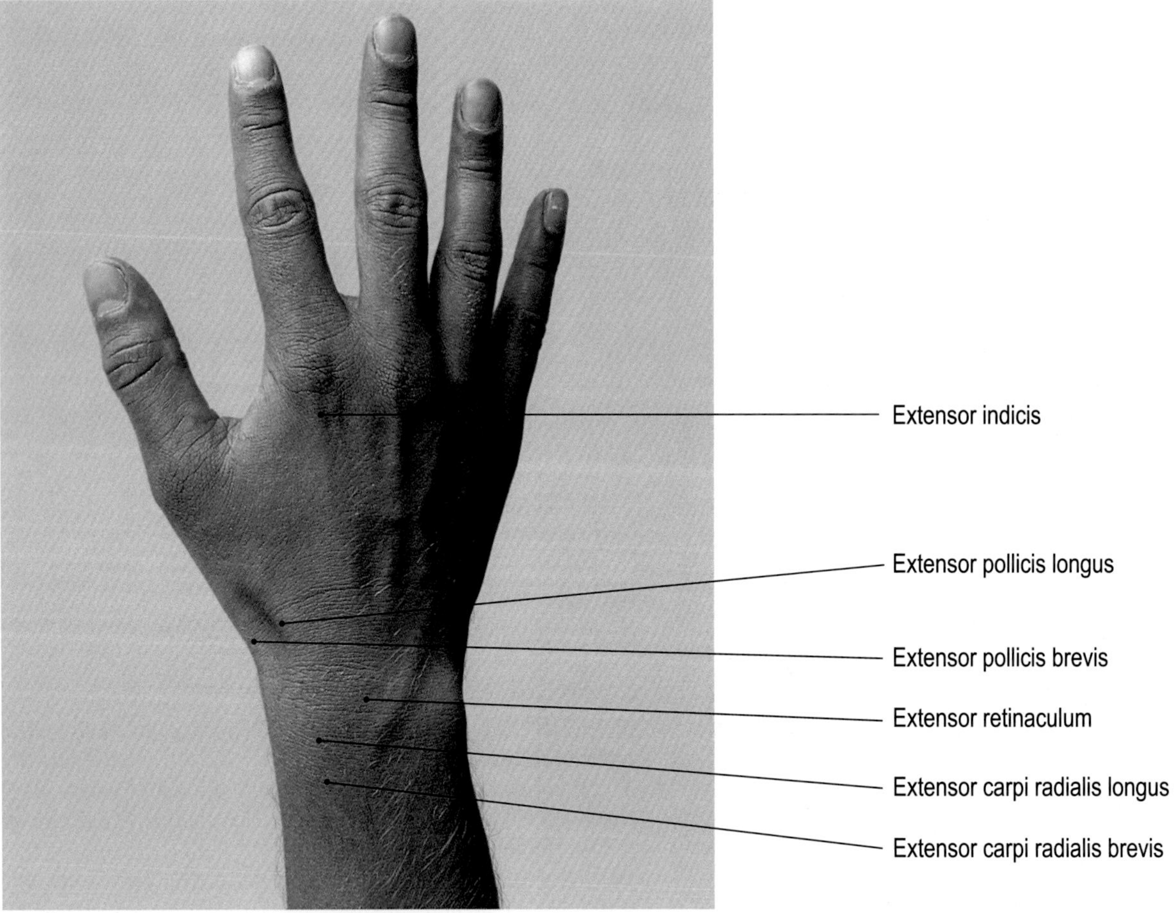

Fig. 2.21 (f) The posterior aspect of the right hand

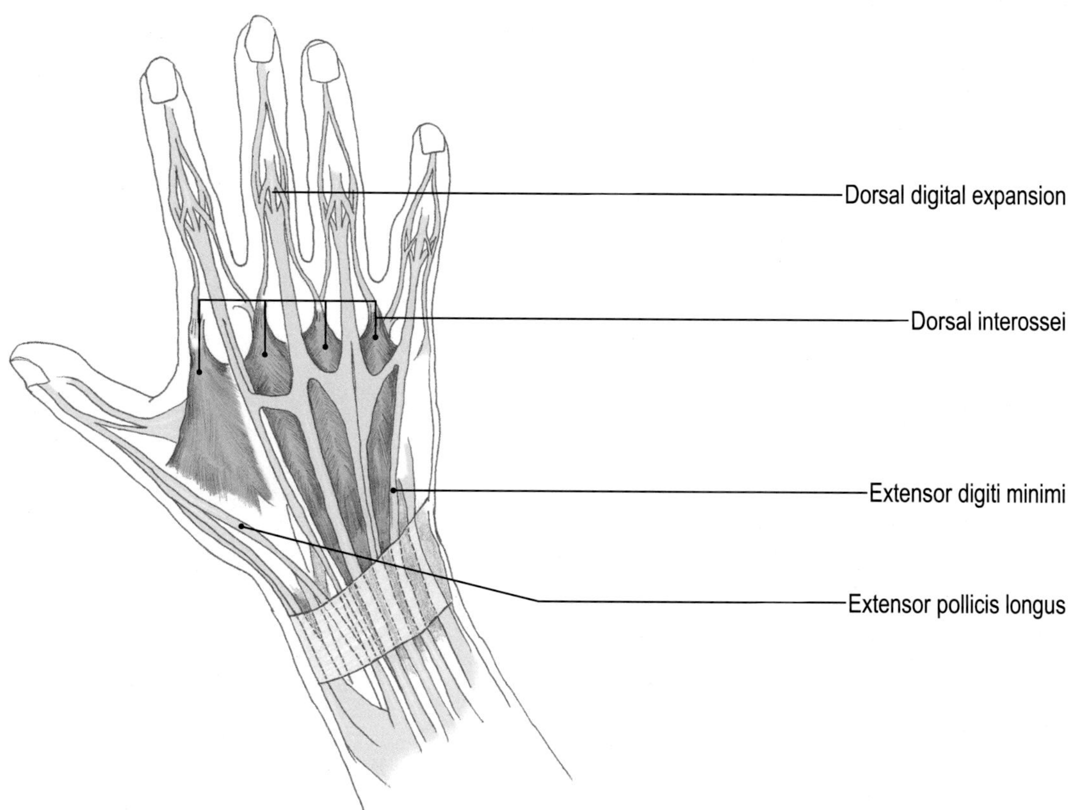

Fig. 2.21 (e) Muscles and tendons of the right hand (posterior aspect)

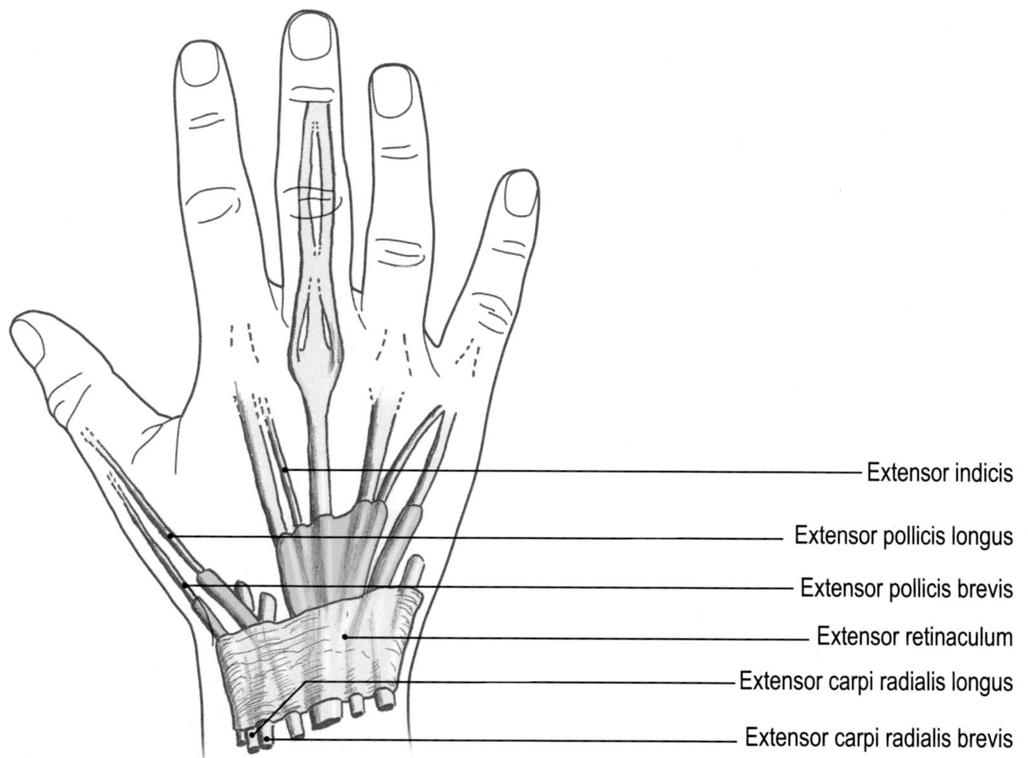

Fig. 2.21 (g) The posterior aspect of the right hand

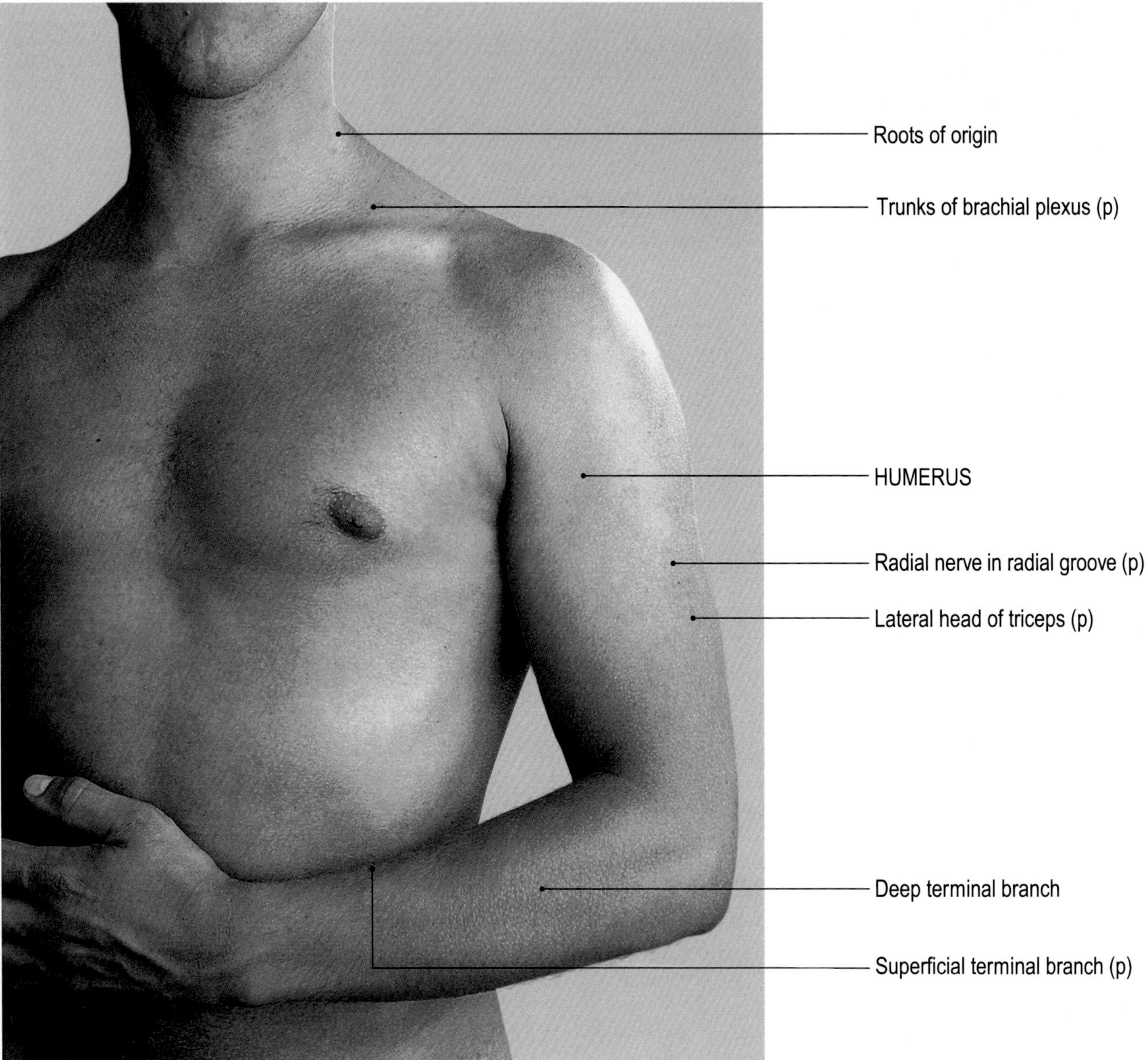

Fig. 2.22 (a) The radial nerve of the left upper limb (p, palpable)

NERVES (FIGS 2.22 AND 2.23)

Most of the upper limb is innervated by nerves via the brachial plexus. The nerve roots contributing to this plexus are C5, C6, 7, C8 and T1. The root of C5 may receive a contribution from C4 (pre-fixed plexus), while the T1 root may receive a contribution from T2 (post-fixed plexus). The roots combine to form three trunks: the upper, middle and lower trunks, each of which split into anterior and posterior divisions. The posterior divisions of all three join together to form the posterior cord. The anterior divisions of the upper and middle form the lateral cord. The anterior division of the lower forms the medial cord of the brachial plexus. It is from these cords that the majority of branches arise to be distributed to the whole of the upper limb. For a more detailed description see Palastanga et al (2002).

Palpation

Palpation of nerves must be performed with care. To the palpator, nerves appear as slippery cord-like structures which only occasionally become superficial, being mostly buried deep to other structures for protection.

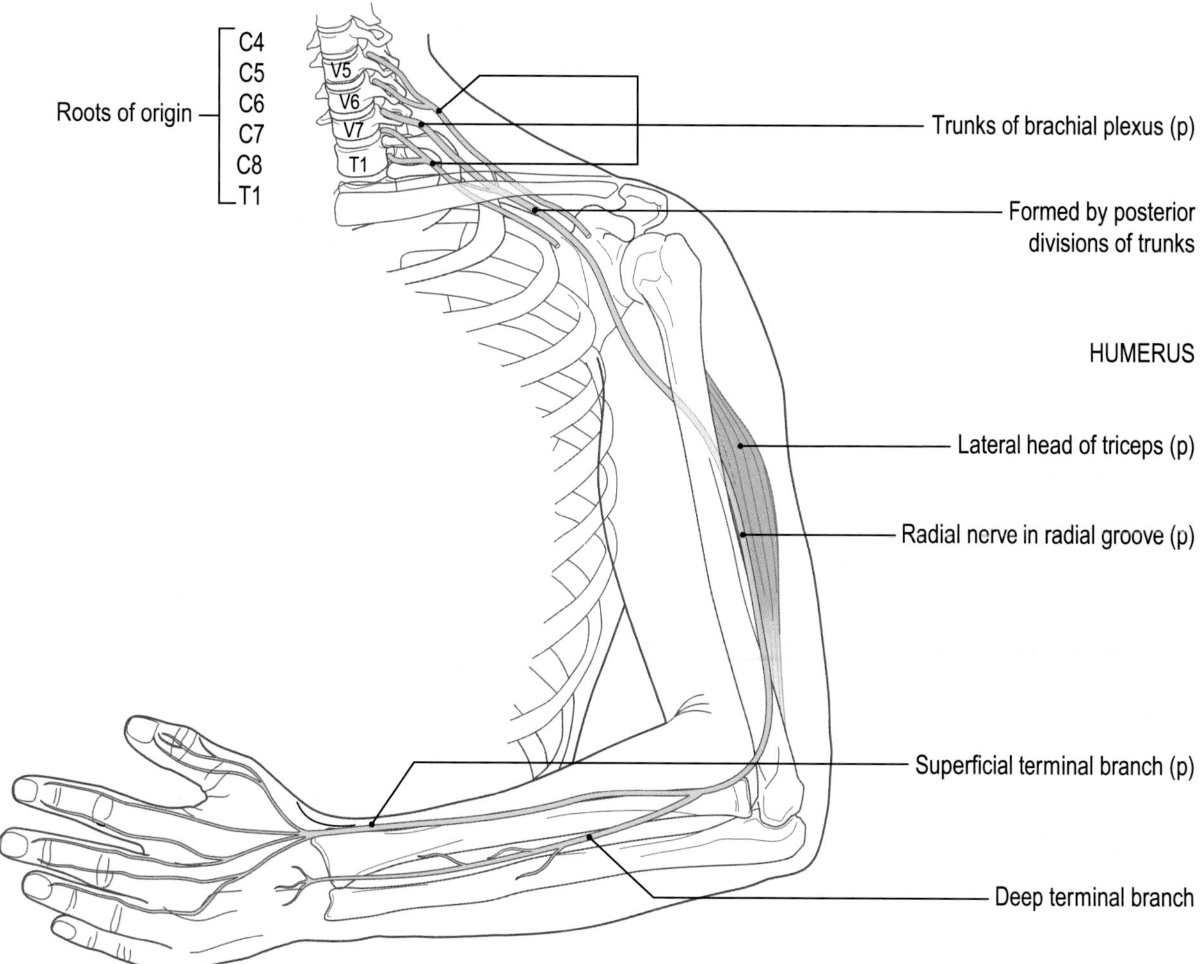

Fig. 2.22 (b) The radial nerve of the left upper limb (p, palpable)

- **Note.** Pressure on a nerve may elicit localized pain. Palpation may also produce a tingling sensation, pain or numbness over the area of its distribution. The accurate location of nerves is important, but over-palpation must be avoided as this may lead to unpleasant sensations.

For palpation in this area, the model should be in the sitting position.

- The trunks of the brachial plexus. Press your fingers into the depression above the medial end of the clavicle, just lateral to sternocleidomastoid. Palpate the trunks of the brachial plexus which appear as a bundle of tense cords running downwards and laterally.
- **Note.** Palpation in this area can be uncomfortable if you apply too much pressure.
- The **radial nerve**. Locate the groove approximately halfway down the lateral side of the arm, below the insertion of deltoid, running downwards and forwards. Palpation of the nerve is facilitated in the area just behind the groove. With care, roll the nerve against the humerus just anterior to the **lateral head of triceps**.
- **Note.** Anteriorly, the nerve enters a muscular groove between brachioradialis and brachialis, passing anterolateral to the elbow joint but too deep to be palpated.
- The superficial branch of the radial nerve. Take the model's right forearm in your left hand with the thumb uppermost. Now glide the radial side of your right thumb up and down the lower end of the radius. You will feel the superficial branch(es) of the radial nerve rolling against the bone. Repeat this at variable points on the lower half of the lateral side of the radius as the nerve passes from under brachioradialis to its distribution on the back of the lateral side of the hand.
- **Note 1.** The nerve may be single or split into five divisions (Fig. 2.22).
- **Note 2.** Even though the superficial branches of the radial nerve lie superficially on the back of the hand, they are still difficult to trace.

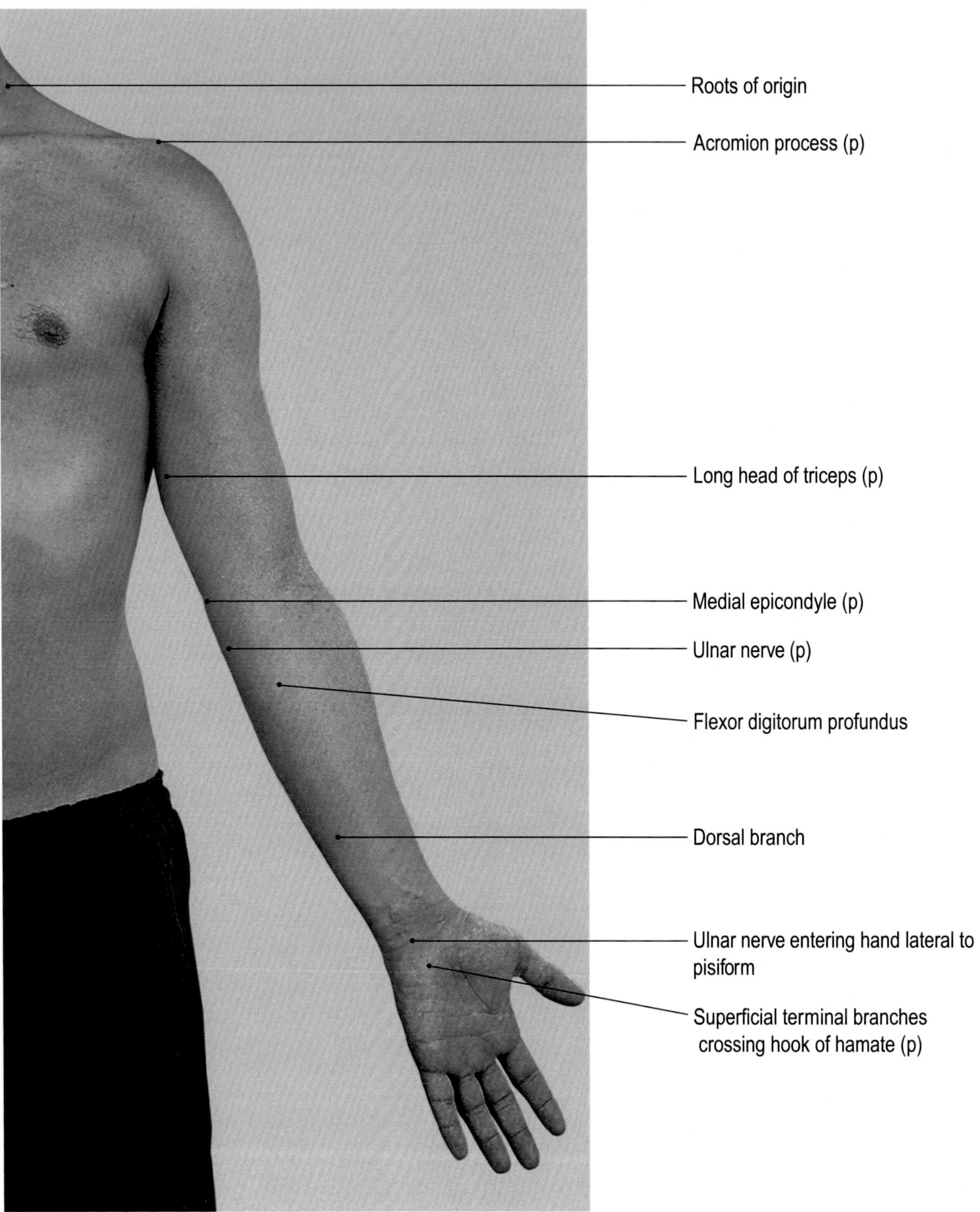

Fig. 2.23 (a) The ulnar nerve of the left upper limb, anterior view (p, palpable)

- Branches of the brachial plexus (including the ulnar and median nerves). Press the pads of your fingers against the lateral wall of the axilla (the upper medial surface of the arm). Palpate the cord-like structures extending down the medial aspect of the arm. You will be able to palpate numerous branches of the brachial plexus surrounding the brachial artery, including the ulnar and median nerves on the medial side of the arm. They are not, however, easily identifiable.
- The upper section of the **ulnar nerve**. Locate the medial supracondylar ridge of the humerus with the **medial epicondyle** projecting medially. Move the tips of your fingers to the posterior aspect of this structure. Palpate the nerve behind the medial epicondyle as it passes from the medial aspect of the arm, over the medial collateral ligament of the elbow joint, to enter the forearm between the two heads of flexor carpi ulnaris.
- **Note.** Careful palpation is essential because the entire medial aspect of the arm is tender.

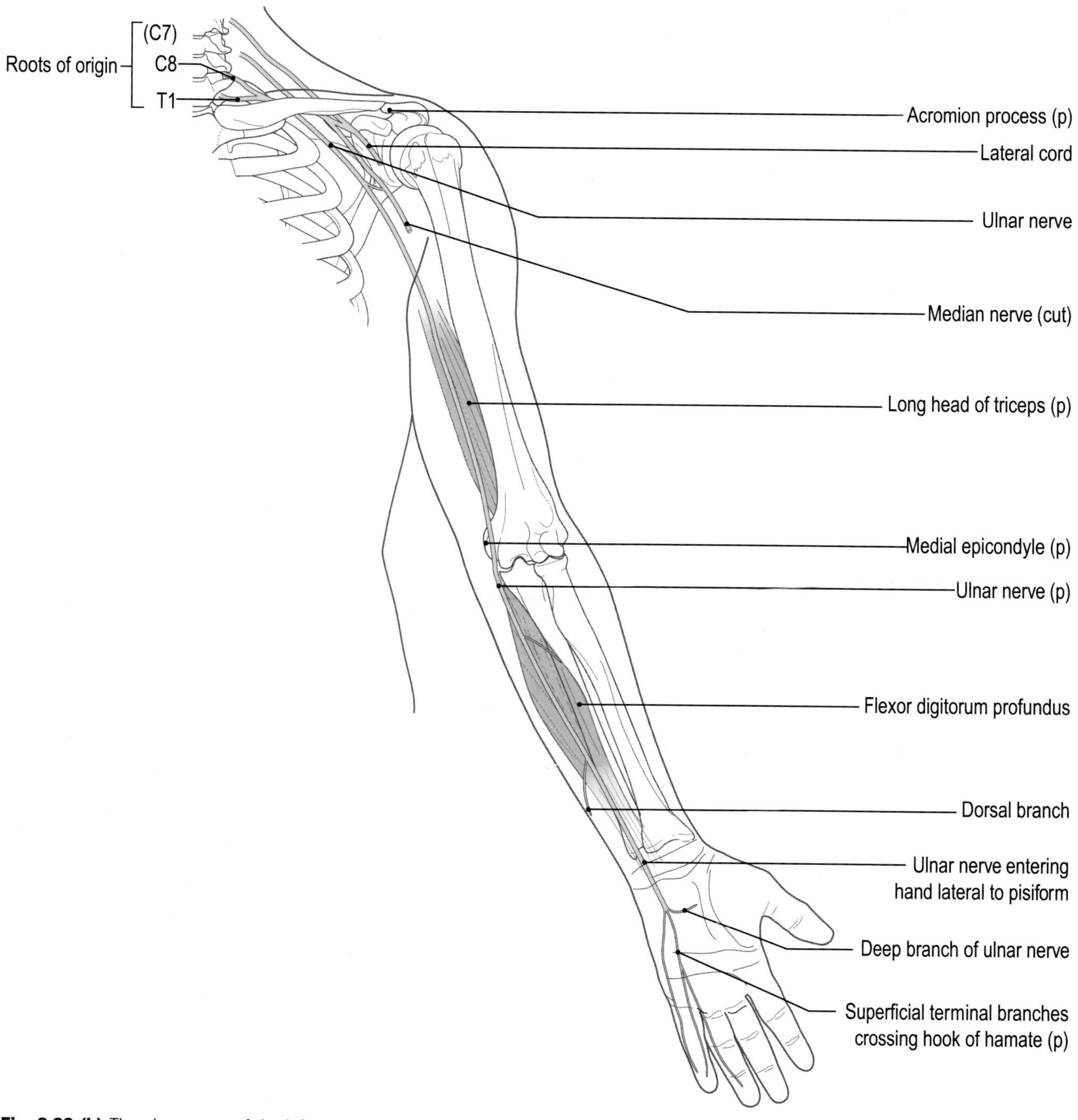

Fig. 2.23 (b) The ulnar nerve of the left upper limb, anterior view (p, palpable)

- The lower section of the ulnar nerve (Fig. 2.23a, b). Trace the nerve from the groove behind the medial epicondyle of the humerus, down the medial aspect of the elbow joint and medial side of the olecranon until it disappears under the fibrous arch of flexor carpi ulnaris. Follow its course down the medial aspect of the forearm deep to this muscle until approximately 7 cm above the wrist. Here it appears on the lateral side of the tendon before passing over the flexor retinaculum to enter the medial side of the hand.
- **Note.** You may find it difficult to palpate the nerve where it lies lateral to the tendon of flexor carpi ulnaris because it is often covered with a layer of fascia.
- The superficial branches of the ulnar nerve. You will be able to roll its **two superficial terminal branches** against the hook of the hamate just distal to the pisiform, deep in the hypothenar eminence.
- **Note.** This procedure will elicit a sensation of tingling over the anterior surface of the medial one-and-a-half digits.

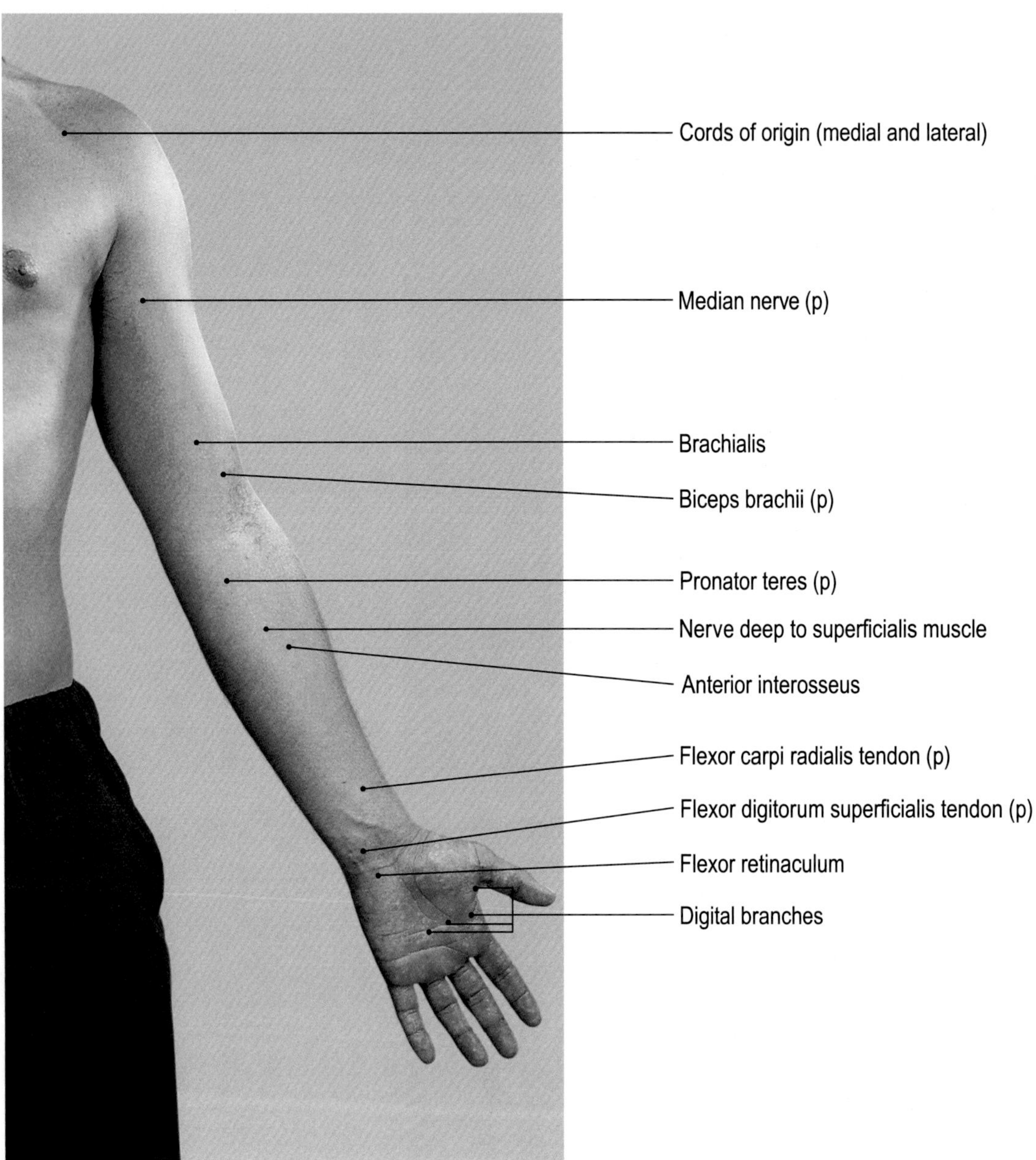

Fig. 2.23 (c) The median nerve of the left upper limb, anterior view (p, palpable)

- The **median nerve**. You will only be able to palpate this nerve in the arm, on the medial side of biceps just before it forms its tendon.
- **Note.** The nerve then passes under biceps tendon and retinaculum to enter the forearm. It is too well covered by **flexor digitorum superficialis** to be palpated in the upper forearm.
- The superficial section of the median nerve. Palpate the nerve where it becomes superficial and emerges from the lateral side of flexor digitorum superficialis to cross the wrist. You will

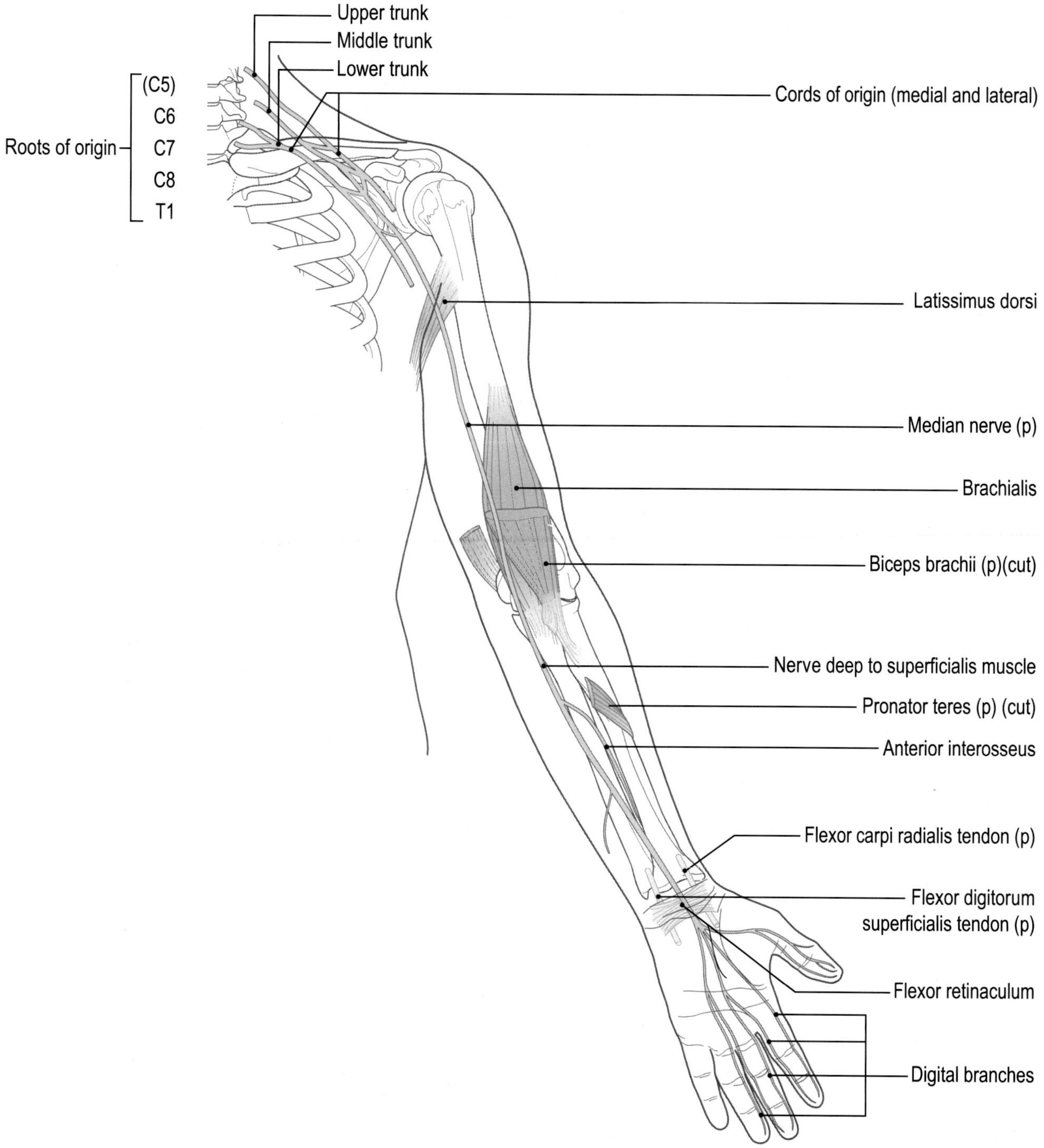

Fig. 2.23 (d) The median nerve of the left upper limb, anterior view (p, palpable)

feel it as a cord-like structure between the tendons of this muscle and those of **flexor carpi radialis**. It then disappears into the thenar muscles on the lateral side of the hand.

- **Note.** Because the median nerve passes through the same compartment as the tendons of flexor digitorum superficialis and profundus it can become compressed. This is commonly due to tightening of the **flexor retinaculum** or swelling of the synovial sheath surrounding the flexor tendons. This condition is referred to as 'carpal tunnel syndrome'.

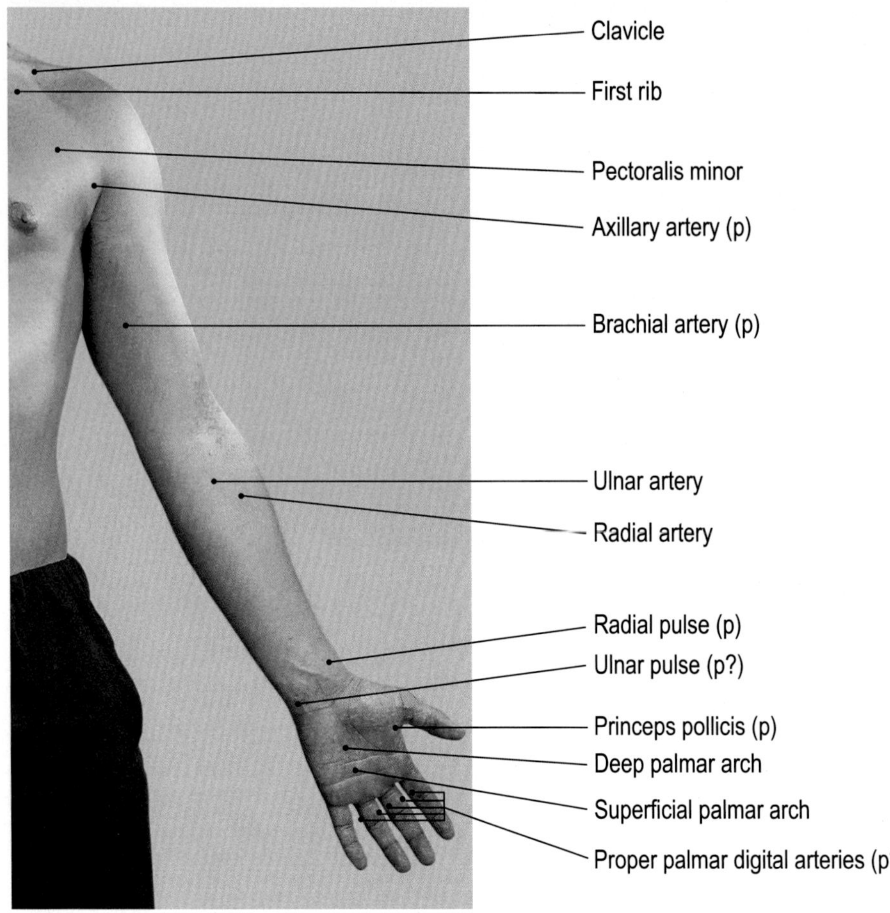

Fig. 2.24 (a) Arteries of the left upper limb, anterior view (p, palpable)

ARTERIES (FIG. 2.24)

Important preliminary notes

A different technique from that described for palpating other structures must be used when palpating arteries. As previously noted, your fingers should remain stationary when the tissue to be palpated is moving. When palpating arteries you should use only your fingertips. Never use your thumb because you could be misled by the pulse in your own thumb. This is due to the presence of the relatively large artery (princeps pollicis) which supplies its pulp. Although the index finger is commonly used, all the fingertips are extremely sensitive. Sometimes the fingers are placed along the line of the artery, as it may be concealed for a short distance by another structure. Very gentle, sensitive touch must be employed because too much pressure may compress the artery and prevent its pulsations.

Palpation

For palpation in this region the model should be in the sitting position.

- Note. Palpation of arteries throughout the limb varies from individual to individual. It is modified by such factors as:
  - the texture of the skin
  - the thickness or tightness of fascial coverings
  - the bulk of muscles
  - the quantity of subcutaneous fat
  - the size of the artery and the patency of its walls, which varies enormously and may be affected by age and disease, particularly of the cardiovascular system.
- Note. The blood supply to the upper limbs is via the left subclavian artery, directly from the arch of the aorta, and the right subclavian, via the brachiocephalic trunk. All of these arteries are too deep to palpate, except where the **subclavian** passes over the **first rib**.
- The subclavian artery. Carefully palpate the pulsations of this artery just posterior to the mid-point of the **clavicle**, behind the insertion of scalenus anterior to the first rib.
- The **axillary artery**. As the subclavian artery passes into the axilla it becomes the axillary artery. Palpate the artery behind the anterior and against the lateral wall of the axilla by pressing gently upwards and laterally with your fingers.
- Note. This may prove uncomfortable for the model because the cords of the brachial plexus may intervene.
- The **brachial artery**. Carefully trace the pulsations of the artery down the medial side of the arm where its upper part lies in a furrow anterior to coracobrachialis, in its upper part, and medial to biceps and its tendon in its lower part.
- Note 1. If you apply too much pressure, discomfort will be experienced throughout the the whole length of the artery. This is because the ulnar nerve lies superficial to the artery in its upper half and the median nerve lies superficial to it in the lower half of its course.
- Note 2. The artery becomes easier to palpate just prior to passing under the bicipital aponeurosis in front of the **elbow joint**, but even here it can remain quite elusive.
- Note 3. It is at this point that the pulsation of the brachial artery is auscultated with a stethoscope when taking blood pressure.
- The brachial artery divides into the **radial** and **ulnar arteries** just below the line of the elbow joint. These are both well covered by muscle and difficult to palpate until they emerge from between the tendons proximal to the wrist.
- The radial artery 1. This is the easiest artery to palpate. Wrap your hand around the back of the model's wrist. Rest your fingertips on the lower end of the anterior border and styloid process of the radius. The artery lies in a groove between flexor carpi radialis and the anterior border of the radius. Now move your fingers gently medially some 0.5 cm. Here, you will be able to identify the pulsation of the artery.

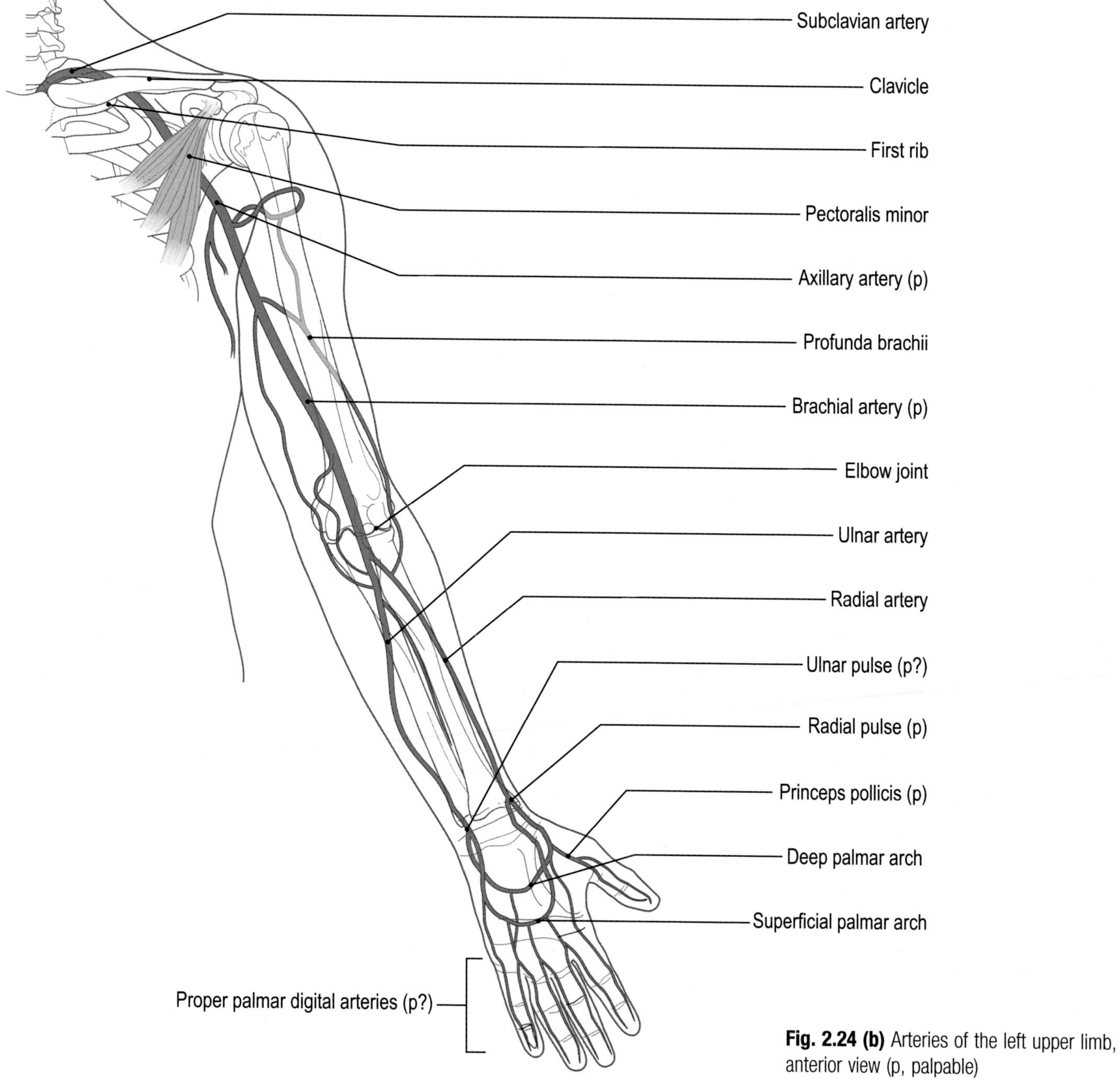

Fig. 2.24 (b) Arteries of the left upper limb, anterior view (p, palpable)

- Note. This technique should be practised regularly because it is the pulse that is most commonly checked during a medical examination.
- The radial artery 2. Palpate the artery on the lateral side of the scaphoid deep in the 'anatomical snuff box', between the tendons of extensor pollicis longus medially, and extensor pollicis brevis and abductor pollicis longus laterally.
- Note. This area is, however, quite tender if too much pressure is applied.

The ulnar artery is much more difficult to palpate in the region of the wrist and hand as it is covered by the palmar aponeurosis. Nevertheless, its pulsations are recognizable just lateral to the pisiform bone. It then passes deep into the palm as the superficial palmar arch, too deep to be palpated.

Branches of the radial and ulnar arteries

Throughout the hand, small branches of the radial and ulnar arteries can be palpated by an experienced practitioner beyond the superficial and deep palmar and carpal arches.

- The posterior metacarpal arteries. Palpation of these arteries is possible between the metacarpal bones, especially at their bases.
- The palmar digital arteries. Palpate the pulsations of the very slender proper palmar digital arteries on each side of the palmar aspect of each finger. These become clearer beyond the cleft of the fingers.
- The dorsal digital arteries. Situated on either side of the dorsum of each finger. These are less obvious.
- The princeps pollicis artery. Palpate the pulsations of this artery in the cleft between the thumb and index finger. Trace this relatively large artery up the anteromedial side of the thumb, particularly opposite the proximal phalanx.
- The radalis indicis artery. Palpate this artery on the lateral side of the metacarpal of the index finger, running up the dorsolateral side of the finger.
- The posterior carpal arch arteries. It is sometimes possible to palpate these arteries as they cross the posterior aspect of the carpus, just below the level of the wrist joint. This will only be possible in those subjects who have good strong pulsations and thin fascia.

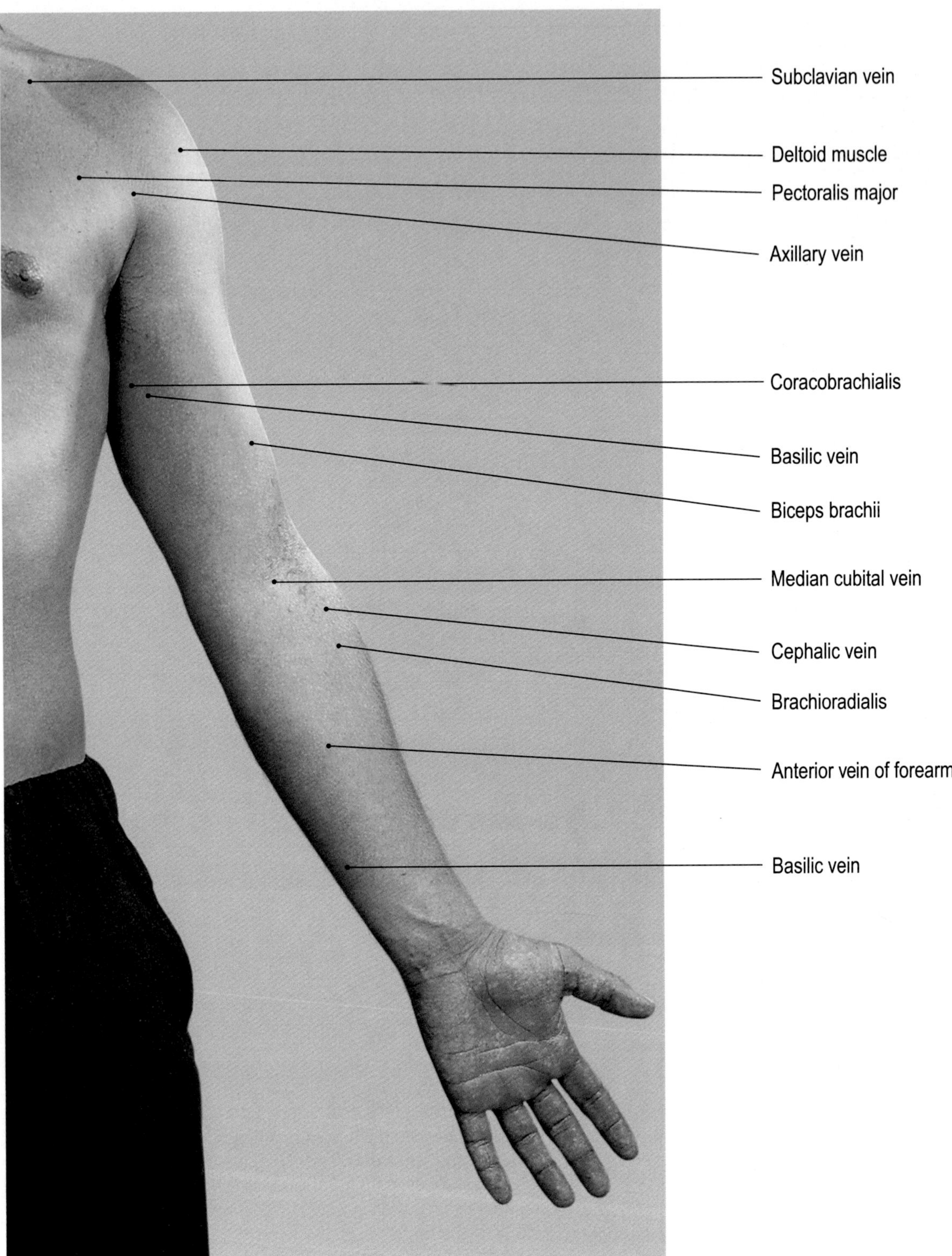

Fig. 2.25 (a) Veins of the left upper limb (anterior view)

VEINS (FIG. 2.25)

For convenience, the veins of the upper limb are divided into two groups: deep and superficial. The deep veins tend to follow the arteries deep within the limb, whereas the superficial veins lie within the superficial fascia forming a variable network. All veins in the upper limb possess valves, more numerous in the deep than in the superficial veins. The function of the valves is to facilitate venous return to the heart.

Palpation

The superficial veins are extremely difficult to palpate as they are normally thin-walled, variable in position, concealed within the superficial fascia and possess low internal pressure. Thus, only a few of the superficial veins are palpable in the normal limb. The deep veins are impossible to palpate.

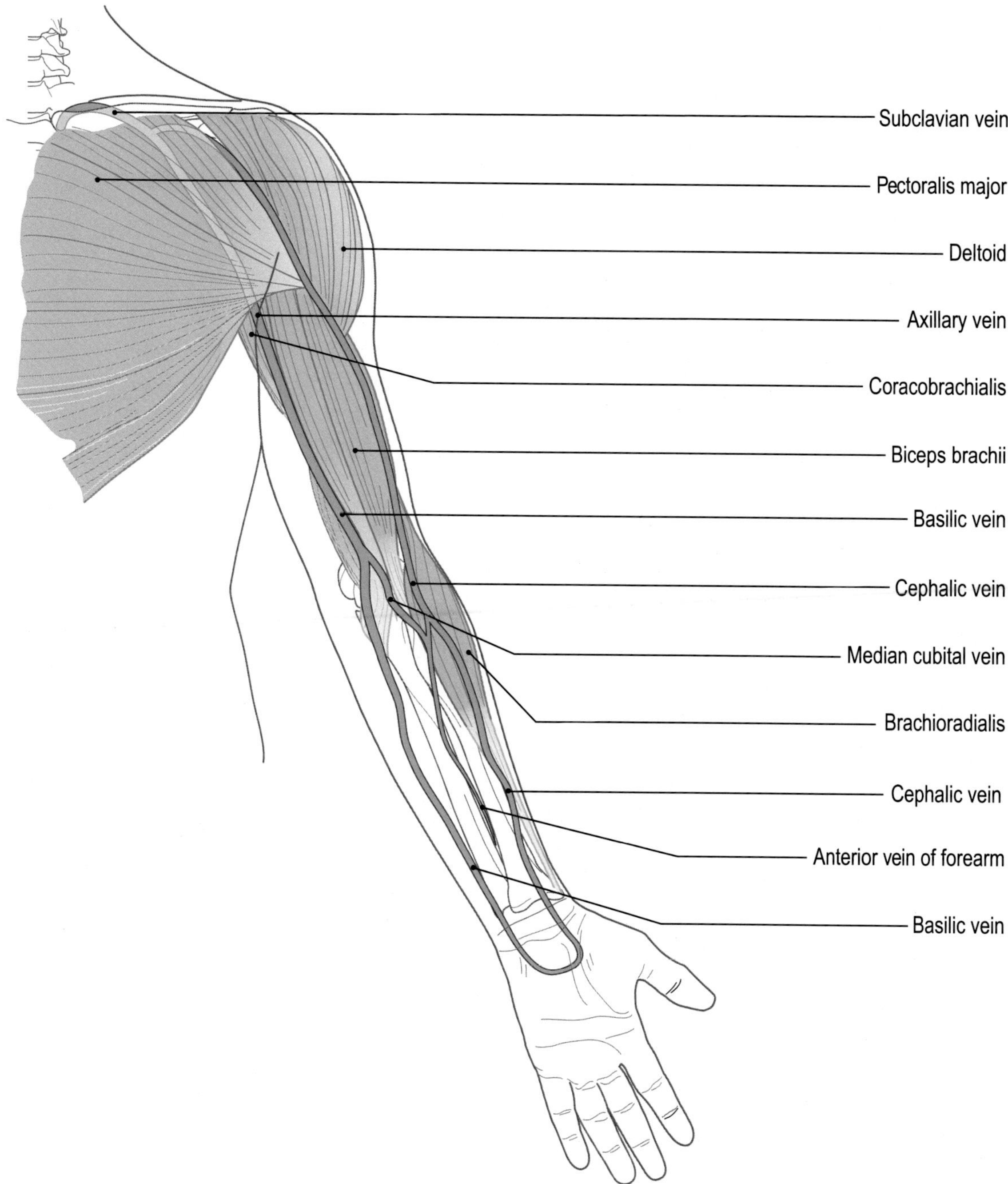

Fig. 2.25 (b) Veins of the left upper limb in relation to muscles (anterior view)

Gentle brushing of the skin surface may be all that is required to indicate the course of superficial veins. Some veins merely show as a bluish line just below the skin, while others are accompanied by raised areas. The appearance of the veins varies considerably in individuals. These variations are dependent on such factors as sex, body weight and age. In males the veins are usually more prominent. In individuals classified as obese, they are more difficult to find. Veins tend to show more clearly in elderly subjects, as the fascia becomes thinner and the veins themselves become tortuous and distended.

- The venous network on the dorsum of the hand. Palpation is facilitated if you ask the model to hang the arm by the side. Now apply firm pressure to the inner aspect of the arm anterior to the brachial artery.

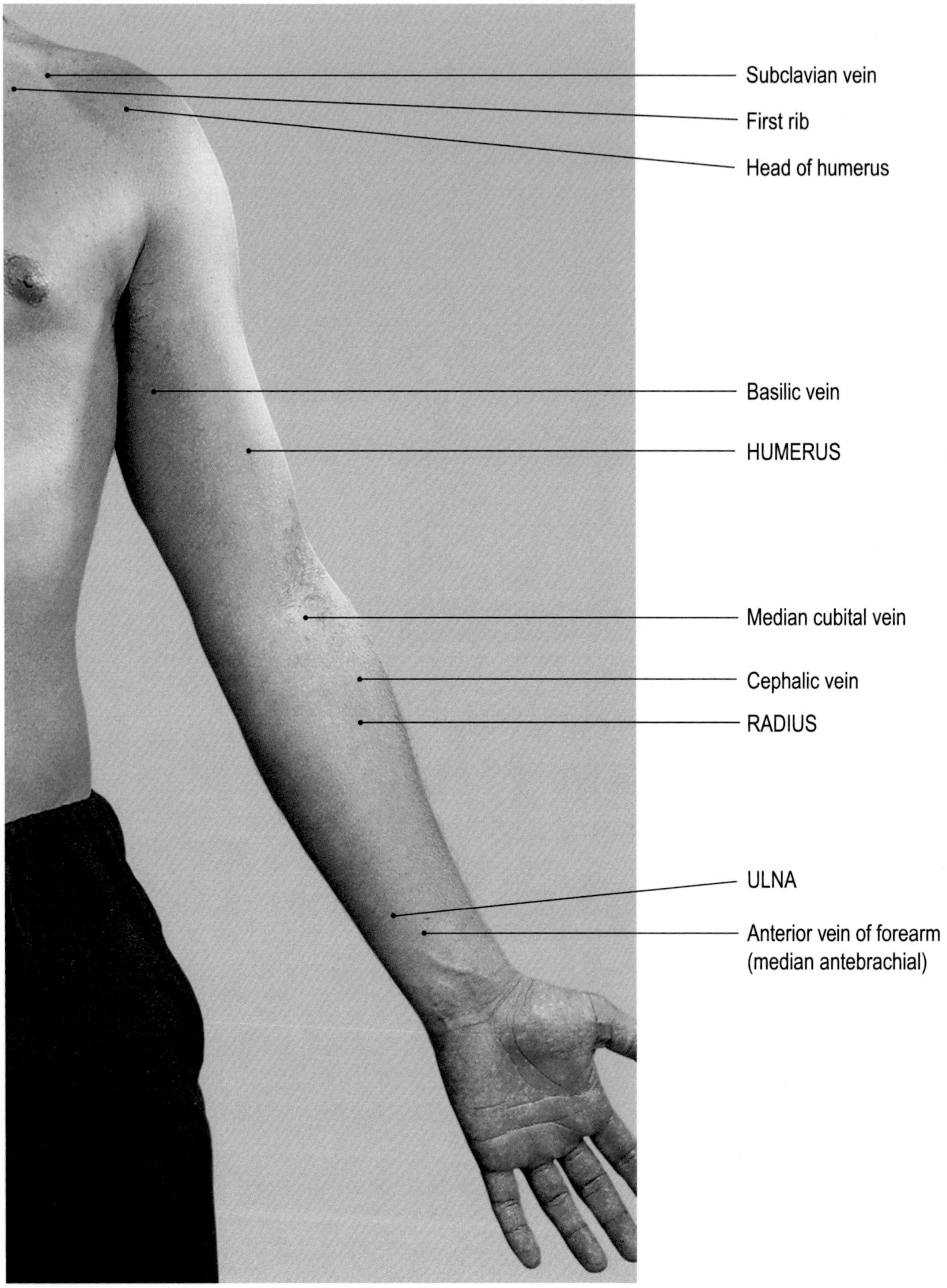

Fig. 2.25 (c) Veins of the left upper limb (anterior view)

Superficial drainage

- The cephalic vein (Fig. 2.25). Trace the vein from the posterolateral aspect of the dorsal venous network. From there it passes upwards around the lateral border of the forearm anterior to the head of the radius. It then ascends on the lateral side of biceps brachii to the groove between deltoid and pectoralis major (Fig. 2.25a, b). It ends in the infraclavicular fossa where it pierces the clavipectoral fascia to join the axillary vein.
- Note. Proximal to the head of the radius the vein is more difficult to identify.
- The basilic vein (Fig. 2.25). Trace the course of the vein from its beginning on the medial side of the dorsal venous network. It then passes up the medial aspect of the forearm, coming to lie anterior to the medial condyle of the humerus. It continues up the medial side of the arm, piercing the deep fascia, near the insertion of coracobrachialis, to accompany the brachial vessels before becoming the axillary vein.

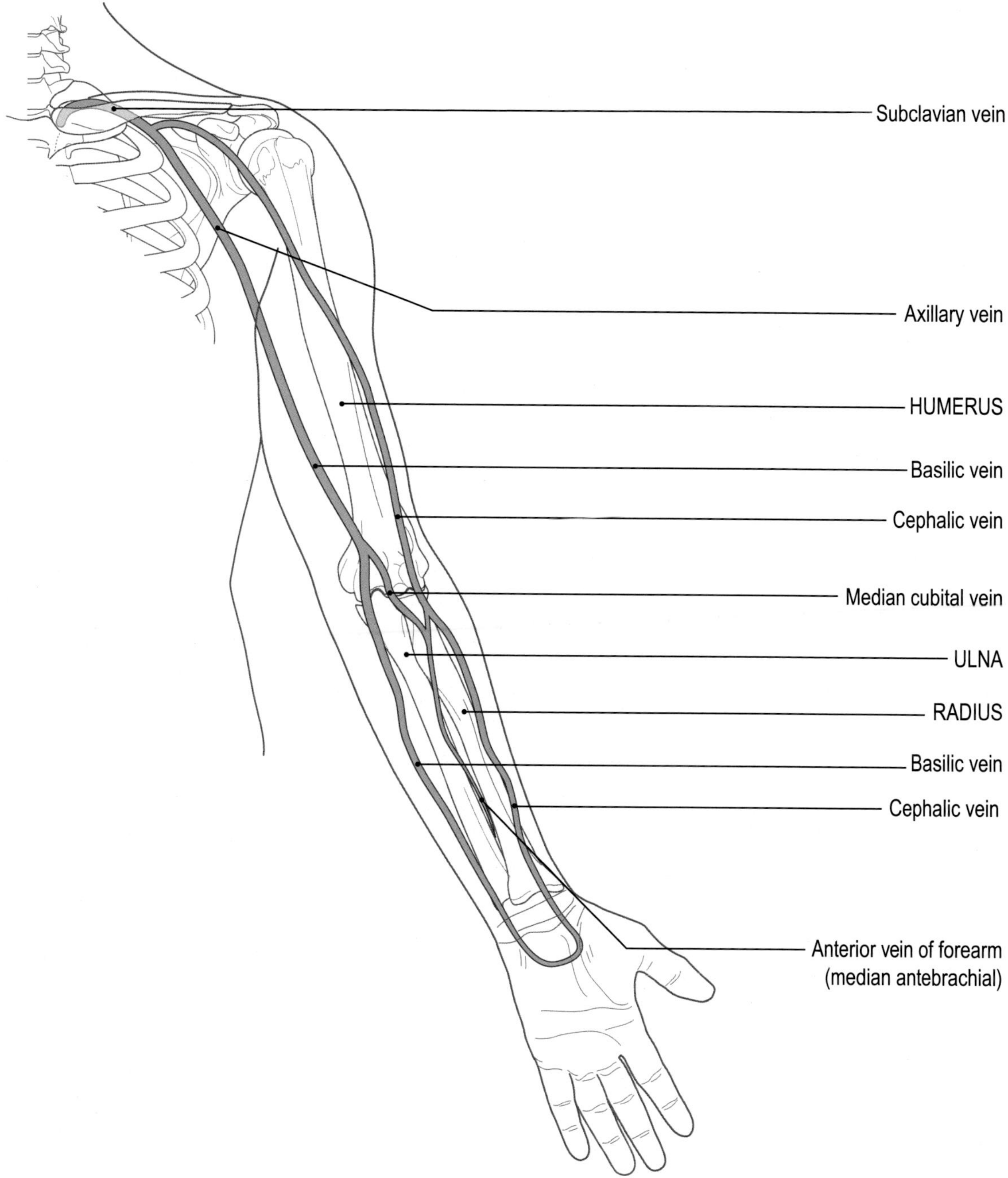

Fig. 2.25 (d) Veins of the left upper limb in relation to bones (anterior view)

- **Note.** The distal half of the vein can usually be palpated, whereas proximally it may only appear as a bluish line.
- The veins of the forearm. On the front of the forearm there is normally a midline vein, the **median antebrachial**, which commonly joins with the **median cubital vein**. The median cubital vein itself passes across the cubital fossa, uniting the cephalic and basilic veins. You should be able to palpate all of these veins. Palpation is facilitated if you apply pressure to the inner aspect of the arm.
- **Note 1.** The position and size of these veins varies considerably in individuals.
- **Note 2.** Compression of these superficial veins is easily achieved if you apply light pressure with your finger or thumb. This will emphasize the vein distal to the point of compression and may, on larger veins, indicate the position of the valves.

The lower limb 3

Contents

At the end of this chapter you should be able to:

1. Find, recognize the shape and position of the hip bone, femur, tibia, fibula, patella, tarsal, metatarsal bones and phalanges.
2. Recognize and palpate many of the bony features.
3. Name all the joints of the lower limb, recognizing the bones which form them.
4. Palpate and trace the lines of the joints, where possible, indicating their bony landmarks and surface markings.
5. Describe or carry out any accessory movements possible noting the ranges in which they are most obvious.
6. Note the ranges of each of the joints and indicate the factors limiting the movement.
7. Give the class and type of each joint, noting the axes of movement where possible.
8. Name and demonstrate the action of all the muscles palpable in the lower limb.
9. Indicate the shape of the muscle on the surface and palpate its contraction.
10. Palpate tendons and attachments where possible.
11. Name all the main nerves supplying the lower limb.
12. Demonstrate the course and distribution of each of the main nerves of the lower limb.
13. Name the main arteries of the lower limb, showing their course and giving their distribution.
14. Name the main veins of the lower limb, noting their drainage areas and course.

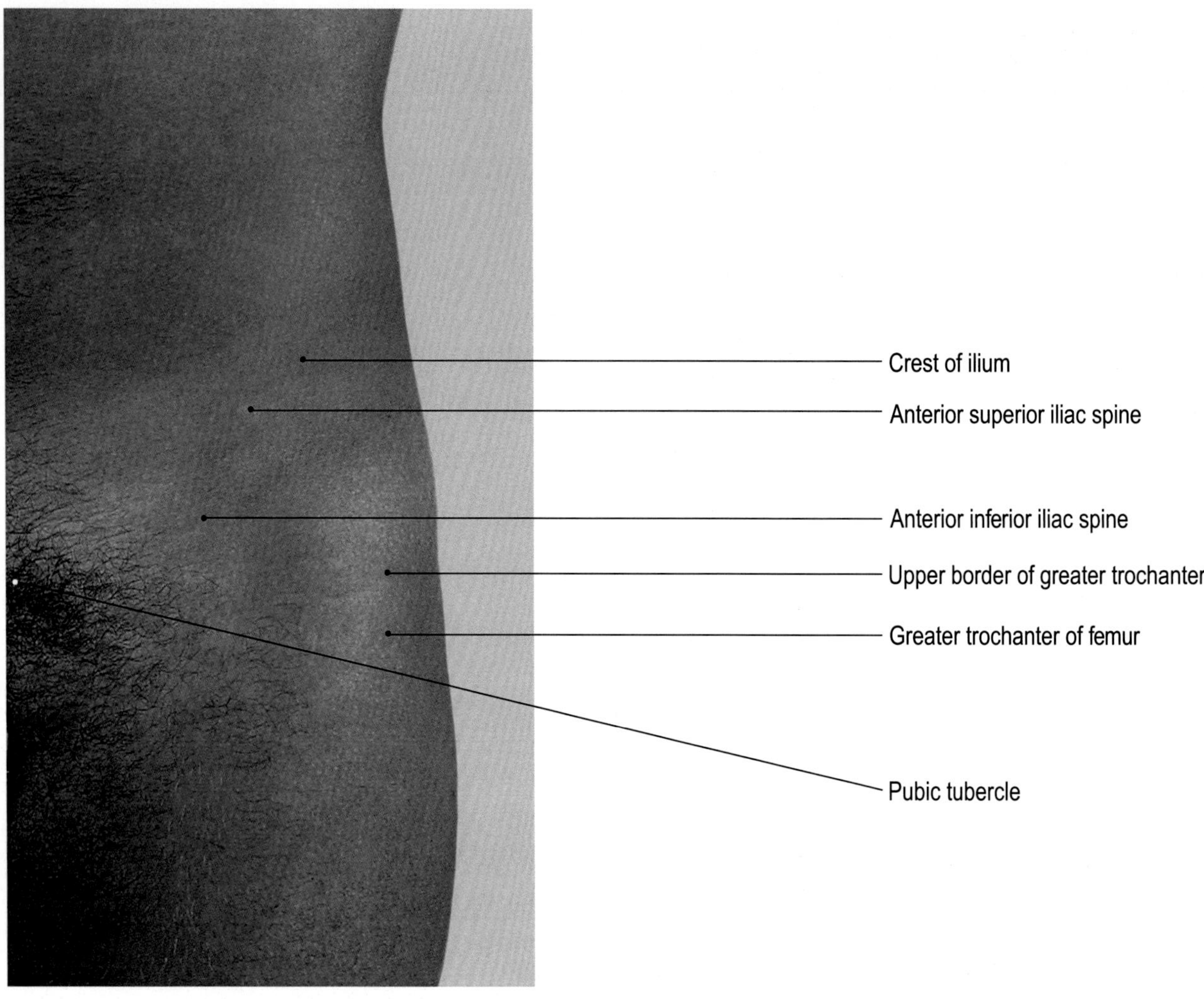

Fig. 3.1 (a) The left hip region (anterior aspect)

BONES

The hip region

The two hip bones on either side and the sacrum, posteriorly, form the pelvic girdle. In its lower section it forms a complete ring (the true pelvis) with the two pubic bones joined at the pubic symphysis, whereas in its upper part (the false pelvis) the two blades of the **ilium** leave a large space anteriorly.

The hip or innominate bone [*os innominatum* (L) = bone without a name] comprises the ilium, the **ischium** and the **pubis**. They are united at the acetabulum, a deep rounded hollow situated on the lateral side of the bone on the constricted area between two blades. The bone above and posterior is the ilium; the bones below and anterior are the pubis and ischium. The ilium has an inner and outer surface. It has a broad crest above a narrow border at the front and back. The upper part of the sciatic notch lies inferiorly just posterior to the ilioischial junction. The lower blade presents a large **foramen**. Medial to this is the flattened bone of the body of the pubis. The pubis has a superior ramus above and an inferior ramus passing downwards and laterally. The ischium is situated below the acetabulum. It forms the lateral part of the **obturator foramen** with its ramus passing from below upwards to join the inferior ramus of the pubis.

The upper end of the femur comprises the head, neck, greater and lesser trochanters. The head lies medially and articulates in the acetabulum. The greater trochanter lies at the lateral end of the neck. The lesser trochanter projects medially and backwards from just below the junction of the neck with the shaft.

Palpation

- **Preliminary note.** Owing to the size and thickness of muscle and fascia, you will find this region much more difficult to palpate than the shoulder. It is often covered by a layer of fat which makes palpation even more difficult.
- For palpation in this region, the model should be in the standing position.
- The **iliac** [*ilium* (L) = the flank] **crest**. Place both hands around the model's waist. Slide your hands downwards and identify a bony ridge on either side of the waist.
- **Note 1.** The iliac crest is convex laterally in its anterior two-thirds. It is broad and rounded, with inner and outer lips.
- **Note 2.** The posterior third of the iliac crest is concave laterally, less well defined and a little sharper on its superior border.
- The **anterior superior iliac spine** (ASIS) (Fig. 3.1). Trace each crest forwards until you identify a well-defined projection, the ASIS. Palpate the anterior superior iliac spines

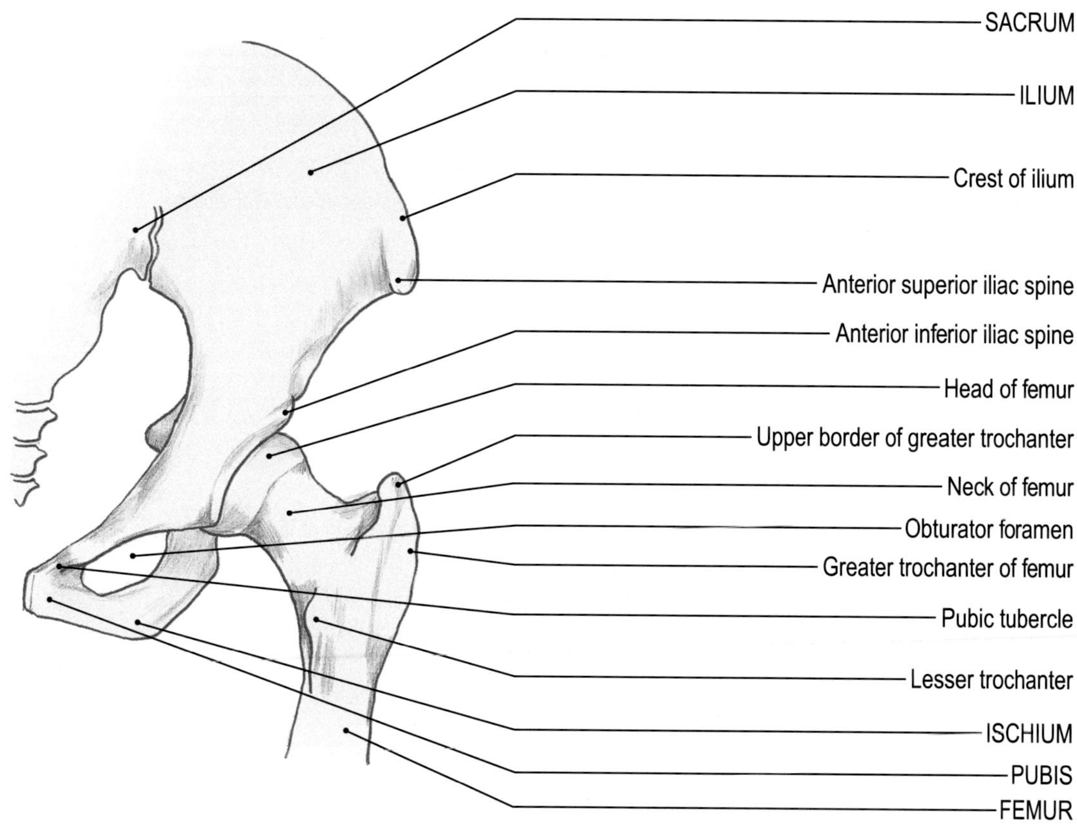

Fig. 3.1 (b) Bones of the left hip region (anterior aspect)

which are set approximately 30 cm apart (a little more in women), the abdomen usually protruding forwards between them.

- The posterior superior iliac spine (PSIS). Trace the iliac crest posteriorly to a small spine just prior to the bone angling downwards. This is the posterior superior iliac spine. In lean subjects the iliac crest is easily palpated from the ASIS to the PSIS.
- The tubercle of the iliac crest. Identify the tubercle of the iliac crest which lies approximately 5–7 cm posterior to the lateral lip of the ASIS.
- **Note.** The tubercle of the iliac crest gives attachment to the upper end of the iliotibial tract.
- The **anterior inferior iliac spine** (AIIS) (Fig. 3.1). From the ASIS, trace the sharp concave anterior border of the ilium downwards to another, less well-defined anterior projection, the AIIS. This lies approximately 2 cm above the rim of the acetablum.
- The anterior rim of the true pelvis (Fig. 3.1). Place the palm of your hand on the lower abdomen. Move it gently downwards where you will feel another ridge of bone approximately 4 cm above the genitalia. This is the anterior rim of the true pelvis.
- **Note.** This ridge is depressed centrally where the two pubic bones join: the pubic [*pubes* (L) = the growth of hair in the region in adulthood] symphysis. It is marked superiorly on either side by the **pubic tubercles**.
- The pubic tubercles. Palpate the pubic tubercles which lie approximately 1 cm on either side of the midline on the upper border of the pubis.
- **Note 1.** This area is quite tender on palpation.
- **Note 2.** It is frequently covered with a fatty pad of tissue which may make palpation of these tubercles difficult.
- The superior pubic ramus. Palpate the superior ramus of the pubis which is lateral to the pubic tubercles.
- **Note.** The superior pubic ramus gradually becomes hidden by muscle.
- The **greater trochanter of the femur** (Fig. 3.1). Trace a line along the pubic crest laterally beyond the region of the hip joint to the lateral aspect of the upper thigh. Palpate a hard, bony prominence. This is the greater trochanter of the femur. It lies approximately 10 cm below the most lateral aspect of the iliac crest.
- **Note.** The femoral trochanters are quadrilateral shape. Whilst they are surrounded by muscle, you should be able to identify them easily. They are the most lateral bony part of the hip region.
- From the back, the ease of palpation depends to a large extent on the build of the subject. The region is often covered with a thick layer of fat which may make it difficult to locate the bony points precisely.

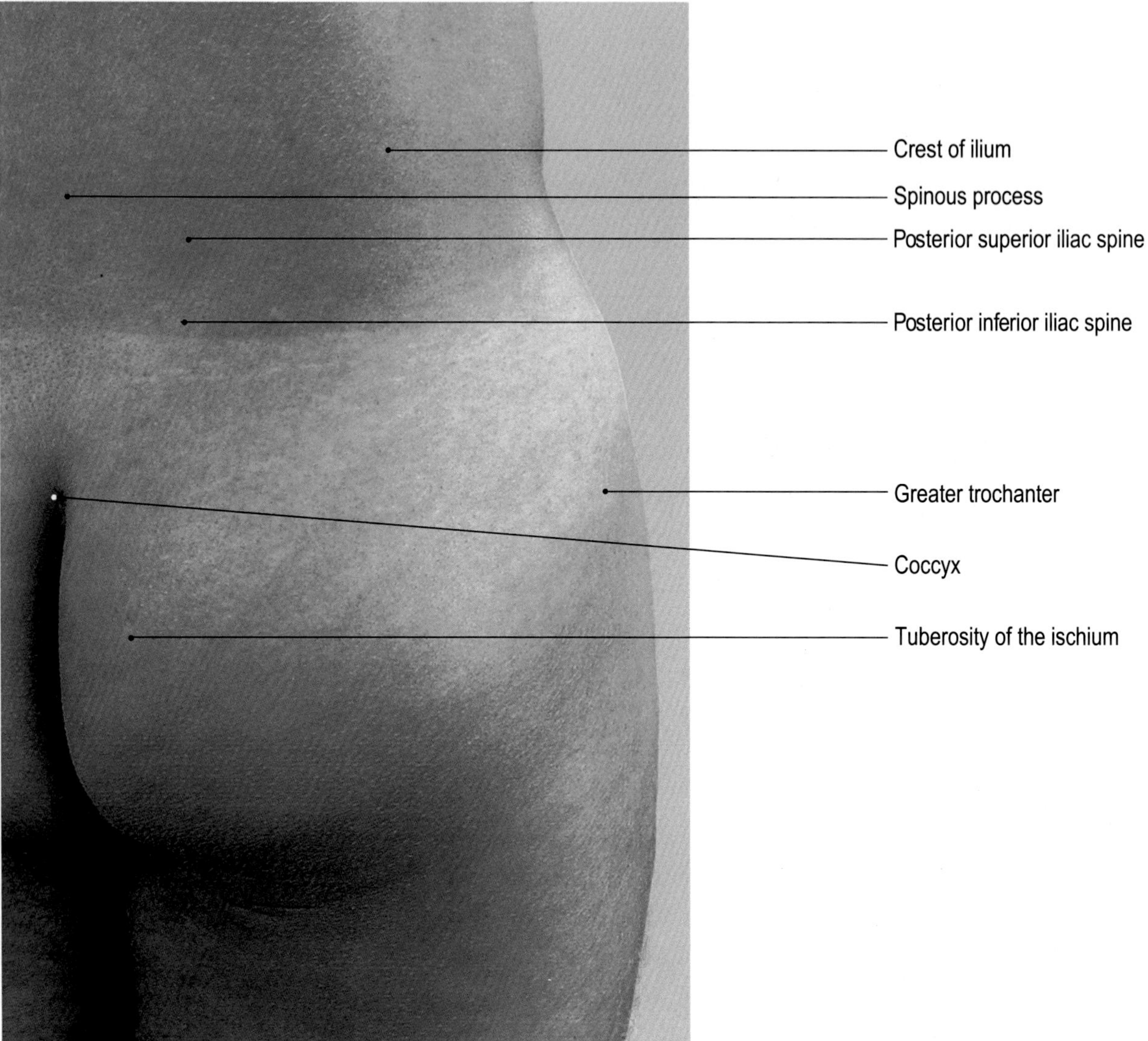

Fig. 3.2 (a) The right hip region (posterior aspect)

- The posterior superior iliac spine (PSIS) (Fig. 3.2). Return to the iliac crest. Trace the iliac crest backwards and medially until you reach the posterior superior iliac spine. You may find that this is more difficult to palpate than the ASIS.
- Note. In women, the PSIS is often located in a small dimple characteristic of this region.
- The posterior inferior iliac spine (PIIS). From the PSIS follow the posterior border downwards and slightly medially. It is concave posteriorly and terminates approximately 2.5 cm below at the PIIS.
- Note. From here the posterior border passes forwards. It forms the upper boundary of the greater sciatic notch. The notch itself is difficult to identify, except in lean subjects.

The sacrum [from *sacer* (L) = sacred], so-called because it is believed that this was the only bone to survive a sacrifice. Its lower lateral border (S4 and S5) forms the medial component of the sciatic notch. It can easily be identified running downwards and medially to the cleft between the buttocks and terminating at the coccyx, which is often tucked forwards towards the anal canal. The upper part of the sacrum is held between the two ilia posteriorly. Its upper border is on a line 2 cm above the level of the PSIS.

Palpation

- The sacral spinous processes (Fig. 3.2). Run your hand down the centre of the posterior surface of the sacrum. Palpate a series of up to five tubercles, gradually diminishing in size. The spinous processes lie in line with the spines of the lumbar vertebrae.
- The articular tubercles. Palpate the smaller tubercles which lie on either side of these spines. They are in line with the articular processes of the vertebrae above.
- Note. This area is often covered with a fatty pad of tissue which may make it difficult to identify these tubercles.
- The ischial tuberosity [*ischion* (Gk) = the socket in which the thigh bone turns] (Fig. 3.2). You will be able to palpate the ischial tuberosity when the model is in the standing or prone lying position. It is anterolateral to the lateral border of the sacrum and posteromedial to the greater trochanter of the femur. You will find it much easier to palpate the tuberosities if you ask the model to sit on your hands. Alternatively, ask the model to adopt the prone kneeling position. With the model in the sitting position, you will be able to feel large rounded processes carrying most of the weight of the trunk to the supporting surface. If you ask the model to move gently from side

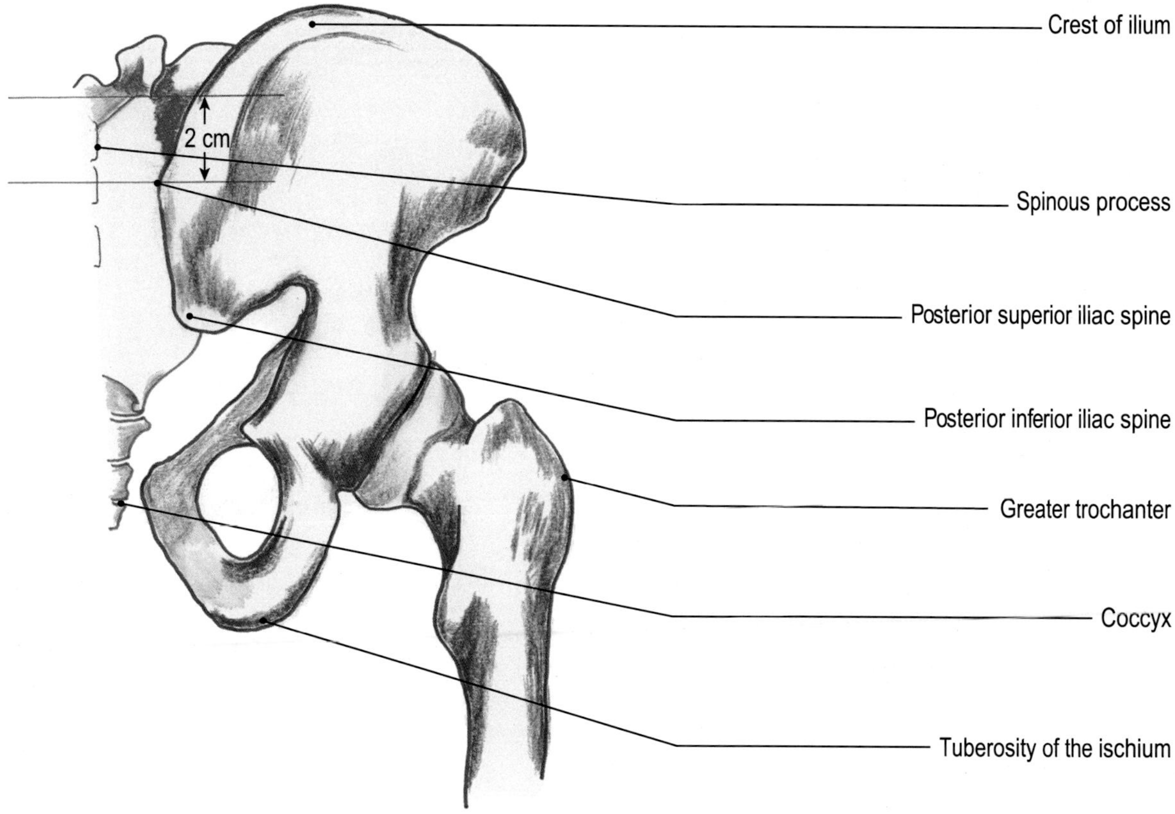

Fig. 3.2 (b) Bones of the right hip region (posterior aspect)

to side, you will be able to feel the transference of weight from one tuberosity to the other.

- Note 1. In sustained sitting on a hard surface, such as a wooden pew, these tuberosities become very tender and uncomfortable. The pressure is increased if the model sits upright, preventing the sacrum from sliding forward to take some of the weight.
- Note 2. The lower area of the tuberosities are covered partially by a bursa medially and the tendinous attachment of adductor magnus laterally. The bursa may become inflamed after long periods of sitting upright, causing acute pain over the area (bursitis).

Palpation on movement

Once the position and shape of the pelvis has been established by palpation it is useful to know how its position may change during movements. It is usual to consider the bony pelvis, i.e. the two hip bones and the sacrum, as one unit which moves as a whole.

- Forward tilting of the pelvis. Stand on the right side of the model. Place your right hand on the upper anterior part of the ilium and place your left hand on the sacrum. Now ask the model to drop the lower abdomen forwards by arching the lumbar spine. You will feel the pelvis tilting forwards.
- Backward tilting of the pelvis. Ask the model to pull in the lower abdomen and flatten the lumbar spine. You will feel the pelvis tilting backwards.
- Note. Both movements occur around a frontal axis running through the heads of both femora.
- Lateral tilting of the pelvis. Stand facing the model. Ask the model to stand on the right leg. Place one hand on the crest of both ilia. Ask the model to draw up the left side of the pelvis by using the left trunk side flexors of the same side and the hip abductors of the standing leg. If these muscles are then relaxed you will feel the pelvis drop on the left side.
- Note. This lateral tilting of the pelvis occurs around a sagittal axis through the right hip joint.
- Repeat the same procedure using the left leg as the standing leg.
- Rotation of the femoral trochanters. Stand behind the model. Place your fingers over the two greater trochanters. Ask the model to flex and extend the right hip rhythmically. Palpate the trochanter, rotating anticlockwise on flexion and clockwise on extension.

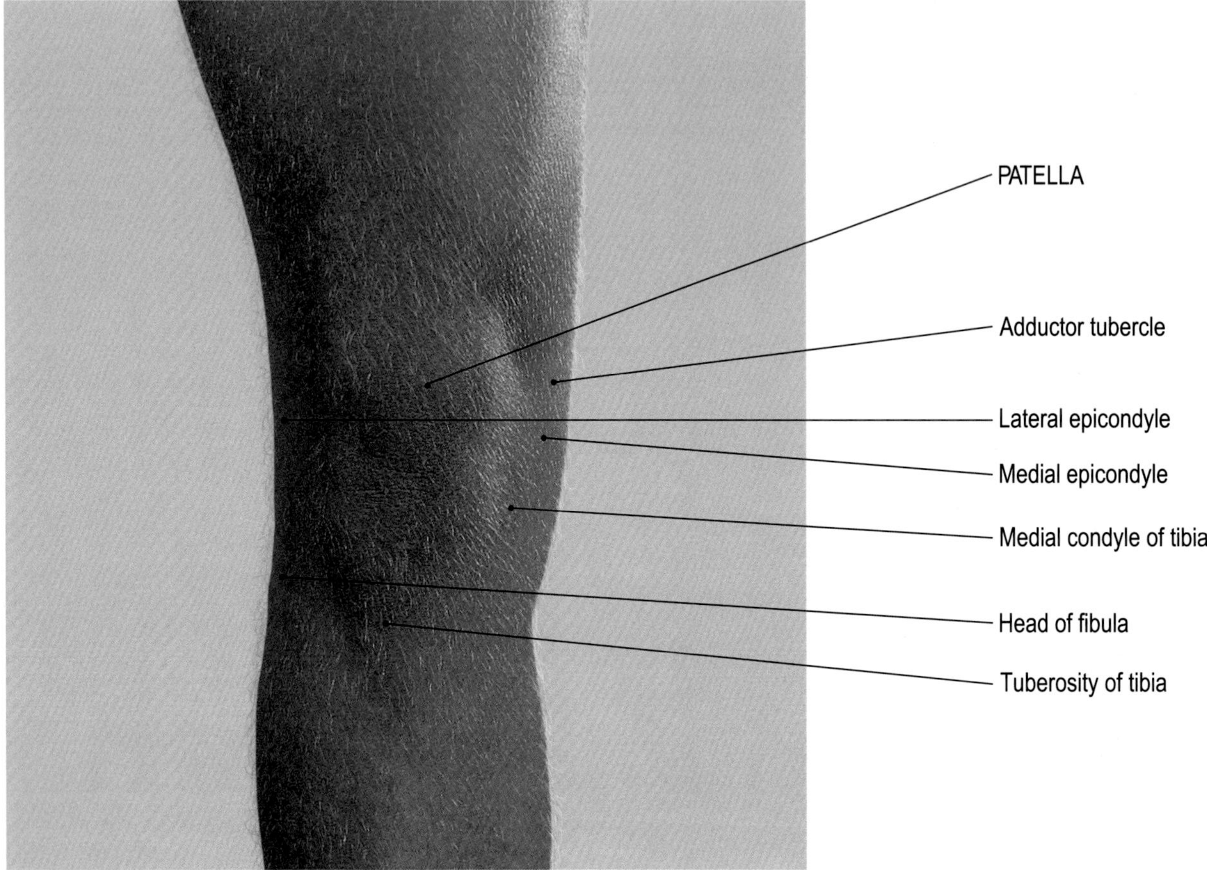

Fig. 3.3 (a) The right knee region (anterior aspect)

The knee region

There are four bones that can be palpated in this region: the **femur**, the **tibia**, the **fibula** and the **patella**.

The femur [*femur* (L) = a thigh] is the longest and strongest bone in the human body. It takes the weight from the hip and transfers it through the knee joint to the tibia. It narrows in its middle half and becomes more or less cylindrical with a very broad posterior border: the linea aspera. The bone broadens in its lower half, forming two large condyles at its lower end. These project backwards and are separated from each other by the intercondylar notch. The lateral condyle is stouter than the medial, which is slightly longer from front to back. Both condyles are smooth on their posterior, inferior and anterior surfaces. They are covered by articular cartilage in the living body. The smooth surfaces meet anteriorly at a triangular, patella, surface. The lateral surface of the lateral condyle is roughened and is marked just below its centre by a tubercle: the **lateral epicondyle**. The medial condyle is also roughened on its medial side and marked just below its centre by a slightly larger tubercle: the **medial epicondyle**. Each condyle has a sharp border above: the medial and lateral supracondylar ridges. The medial supracondylar ridge presents a tubercle at its lower end: the **adductor tubercle**.

The tibia [*tibia* (L) = a flute] is also a very strong stout bone. It carries the body weight to the ankle joint and foot. It is broader above and has two large condyles. Both condyles are flattened superiorly and slightly depressed centrally. They are separated by the intercondylar eminence and a roughened area anteriorly and posteriorly. The shaft narrows as it descends. It presents a large tubercle anteriorly: the tibial tuberosity. This is situated just below the level of the knee joint. The sharp anterior border (shin) passes vertically down from this tubercle.

The patella [*patella* (L) = a small plate], as its name implies, is a small flat bone situated on the front of the knee. It is triangular in shape with the apex downwards. It has a roughened anterior surface and a smooth posterior surface. This is divided into two articular facets with the roughened apex below.

The fibula [*fibula* (L) = a pin] is a long, thin bone situated lateral to the tibia. It has complex surfaces and a border mainly produced by the muscles attaching to it. It is expanded above and below. The upper expansion, the head, articulates with the undersurface of the lateral condyle of the tibia. It takes no part in the knee joint. The lower expansion forms the lateral malleolus and takes part in the formation of the ankle joint.

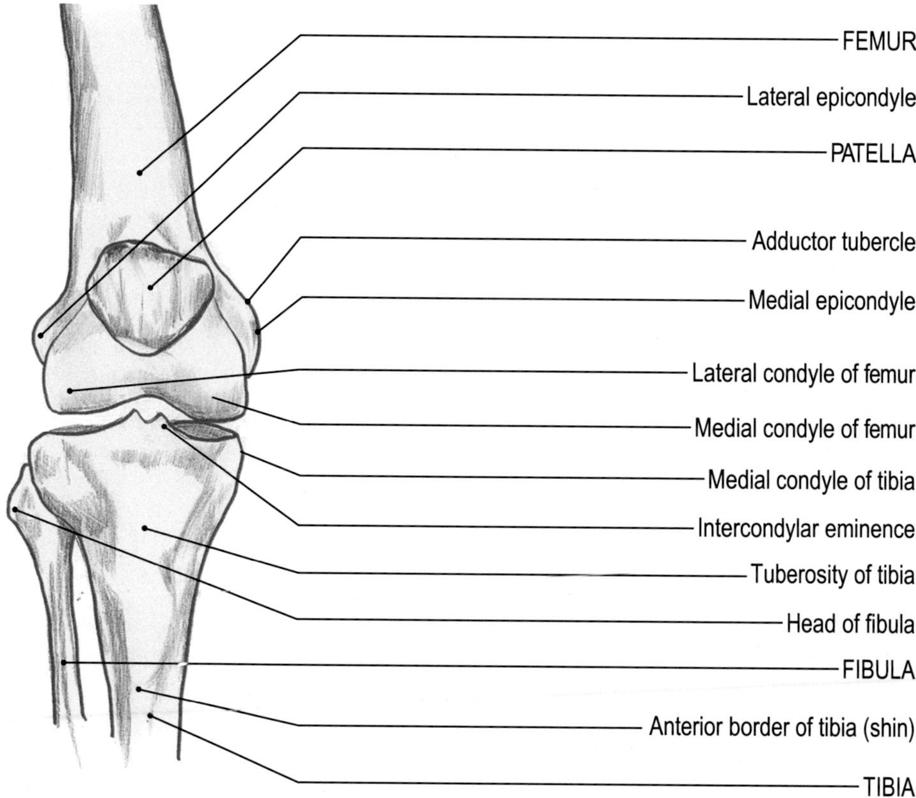

Fig. 3.3 (b) Bones of the right knee region (anterior aspect)

Anterior aspect

Palpation

For palpation in this region the model is in the sitting position.

- The patella (1). Place your fingers on the anterior surface of the patella. Palpate its surfaces and borders.
- Note 1. The patella is broader superiorly. It narrows to a rounded point below where it is continuous with the ligamentum patellae.
- Note 2. The borders of the patella are rounded. The anterior surface, although appearing slippery due to the presence of the prepatellar bursa, has rough vertical ridges in line with the fibres of the tendon of quadriceps femoris.
- The patella (2). Ask the model to flex the knee 90°. This will make the patella much more prominent and therefore easier to palpate.
- The femoral condyles. Palpate the medial and lateral femoral condyles on either side of the patella and on which the patella sits.
- Note 1. Each femoral condyle is convex forwards and is palpable on either side of the patella. It is narrower superiorly and broader inferiorly due to the shape of the patella.
- Note 2. These condylar surfaces pass posteriorly into the knee joint itself.
- The tibial condyles. Palpate the medial and lateral tibial condyles below the femoral condyles. Palpate their flattened upper surfaces which are marked by a sharp circumference separating them from the more vertical surfaces of the shaft.
- The tibial tuberosity (Fig. 3.3). Palpate the large tibial tuberosity below and centrally from the patella.
- Note 1. The lower part is smooth and slippery, due to the presence of the superficial infrapatellar bursa.
- Note 2. The upper part gives attachment to the ligamentum patellae.
- Note 3. The tibial tuberosity is particularly noticeable when the knee is extended.
- The tibial condyles. Ask the model to flex the knees to 90°. Place your fingers in the small triangular fossae on either side of the ligamentum patellae. Palpate the upper surfaces of the tibial condyles below and the undersurface of the femoral condyles above. Between your fingers lies the ligamentum patellae.
- Note. Directly posteriorly is the cleft of the knee joint, with the medial and lateral menisci between.
- The menisci. These are not always palpable. Ask the model to flex the knee to 90° and then medially rotate the joint. You may now be able to palpate the anterior edge of the medial meniscus bulging forwards on medial rotation of the tibia. Now ask the model to laterally rotate the knee joint. You may now be able to palpate the anterior edge of the lateral meniscus on lateral tibial rotation.

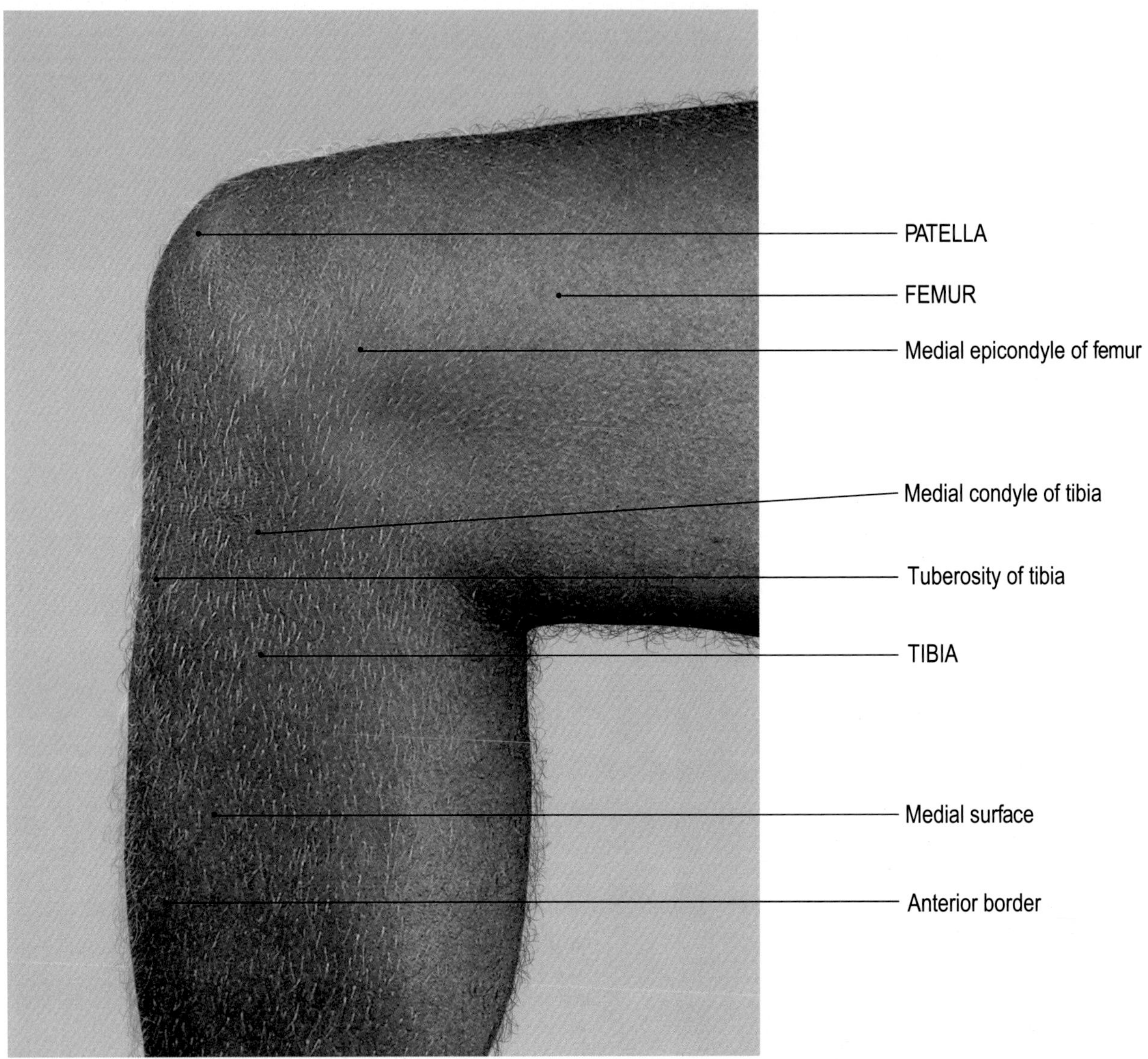

Fig. 3.3 (c) The right knee (medial aspect)

Medial aspect

On the medial side of this region the large, elongated medial condyle of the femur sits on top of the flattened plateau of the medial tibial condyle. The centre of the medial surface of the femoral condyle is marked by a tubercle: the medial epicondyle. Vertically above this is the medial supracondylar line marked at its lower end by the adductor tubercle.

Below the femoral condyle the flattened **medial tibial condyle** continues downwards as the **medial surface** of the tibial shaft, bounded in front by its **anterior border** and marked at its upper end by the **tibial tuberosity**.

Palpation

- The medial surface of the femoral condyle (Fig. 3.3). Palpate the medial surface of the femoral condyle and the epicondyle projecting from its mid point.
- The adductor tubercle. Palpate the adductor tubercle, which is approximately 2 cm proximal to the medial epicondyle. You may find this difficult because it is hidden to a certain extent by the attachment of the tendinous part of adductor magnus.
- **Note.** This tubercle represents the most distal part of the medial supracondylar ridge, little of which can be palpated.

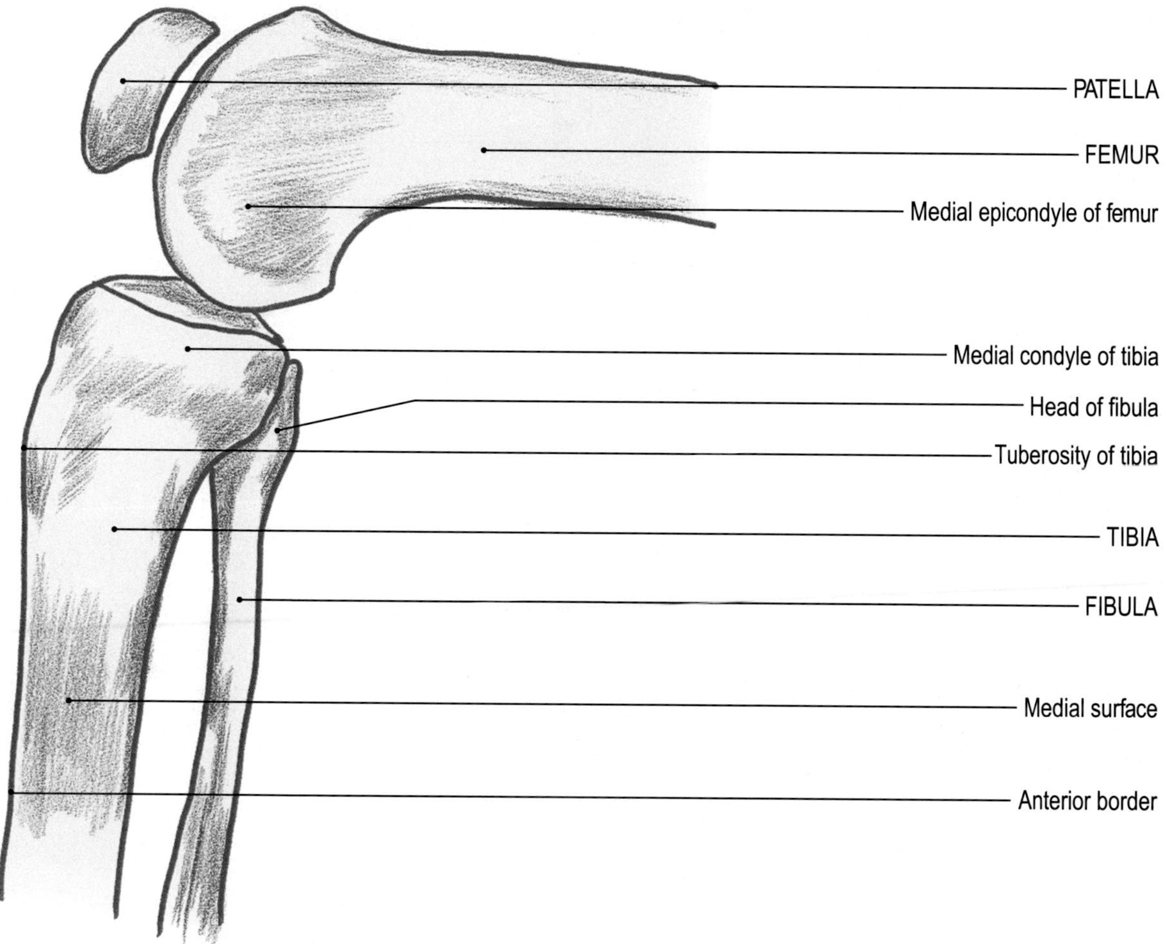

Fig. 3.3 (d) Bones of the right knee (medial aspect)

- The medial tibial condyle (Fig. 3.3c, d). Palpate the medial tibial condyle below the femoral condyle.
- Note. It appears to be larger than the lateral tibial condyle.
- The medial surface of the tibial shaft. From the medial tibial condyle, trace around the medial side and then downwards where the condyle becomes continuous with the medial surface of the shaft of the tibia.
- The anterior tibial border. Palpate the subcutaneous anterior tibial border (the shin) and follow it down as far as the medial malleolus.

Palpation on movement

- The patella. Ask the model to extend the knee. Place the fingers of one hand on the medial condyle of the femur. Place the fingers of the other hand on the medial border of the patella. Now ask the model to flex the knee. Palpate the patella, sliding downwards and backwards on the femoral condyle until it lies inferiorly. Ask the model to return to the extended position.
- The medial tibial condyle. Now move your fingers from the patella and place them on the upper part of the medial surface of the medial condyle of the tibia, close to the joint line. Ask the model to flex the knee. Palpate the tibial condyle, moving backwards and upwards on to the posterior aspect of the femoral condyle.
- Note. As in the case of the lateral condyles, in this position the anterior part of the tibial condyle appears to part from the femoral condyle. This is due to the smaller articular surface at the posterior part of the femoral condyle.

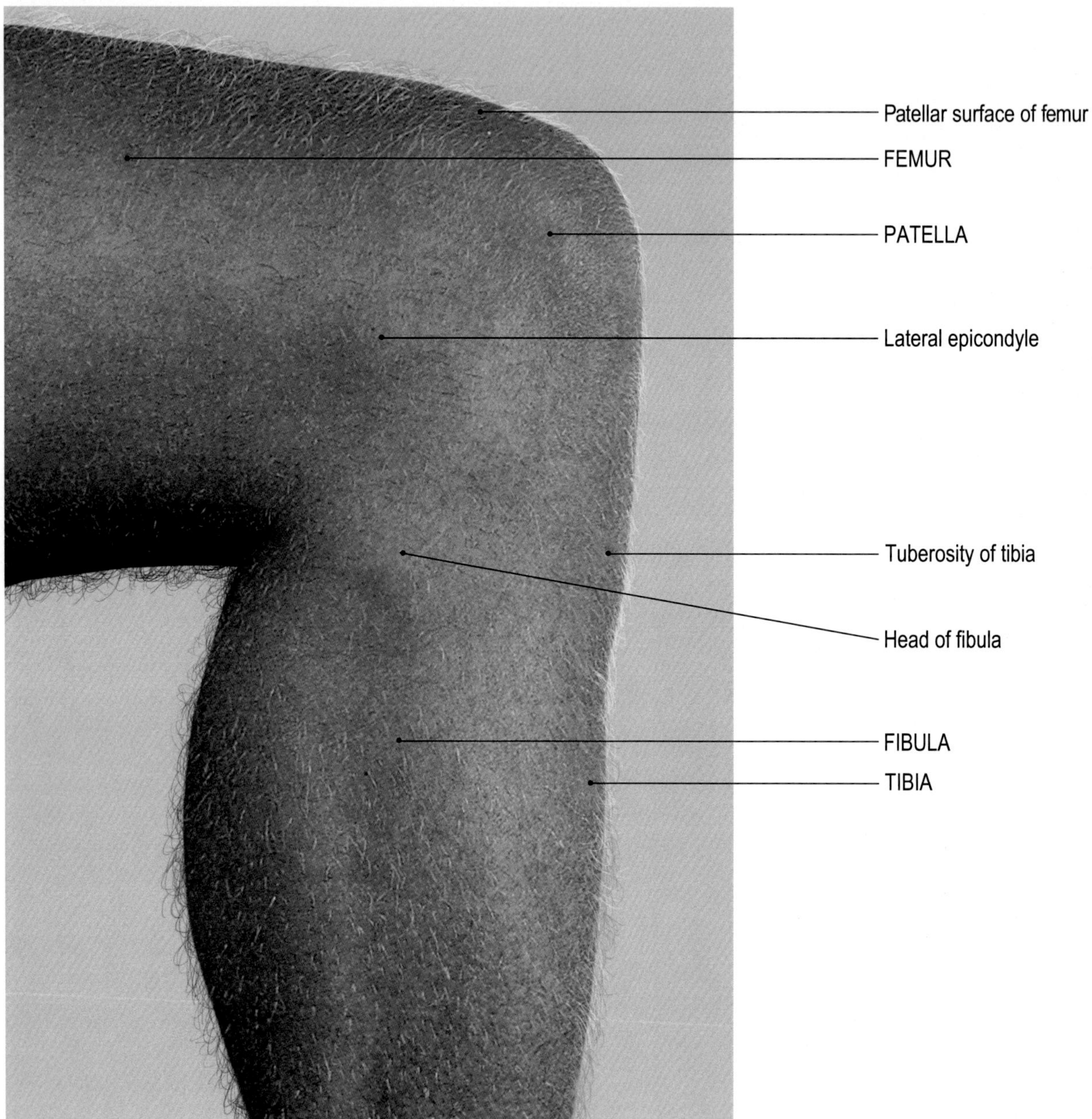

Fig. 3.4 (a) The right knee (lateral aspect)

Lateral aspect

On the lateral side of this region the stout lateral condyle of the femur sits on top of the plateau of the lateral condyle of the tibia. Posteriorly, the two condyles are close together. Anteriorly, however, they diverge into a small hollow which is bounded at the front by the lower section of the **patella** and the ligamentum patellae. The **head of the fibula** lies below and posterior to the knee joint.

Palpation

- The lateral femoral condyle. Palpate the flat lateral surface of the lateral femoral condyle, lying posterior to the lateral border of the patella. It is marked by a tubercle at its centre (the lateral epicondyle).
- The lateral supracondylar ridge of the femur. Run your fingers upwards from the **lateral epicondyle**. You may be able to palpate the lateral supracondylar ridge running vertically upwards.
- **Note.** This is difficult to palpate as the iliotibial tract tends to follow the same line.
- The lateral tibial condyle. Palpate the upper border of the lateral tibial condyle which lies approximately 2 cm below the lateral epicondyle and the lower border of the lateral femoral condyle running horizontally and diverging anteriorly.

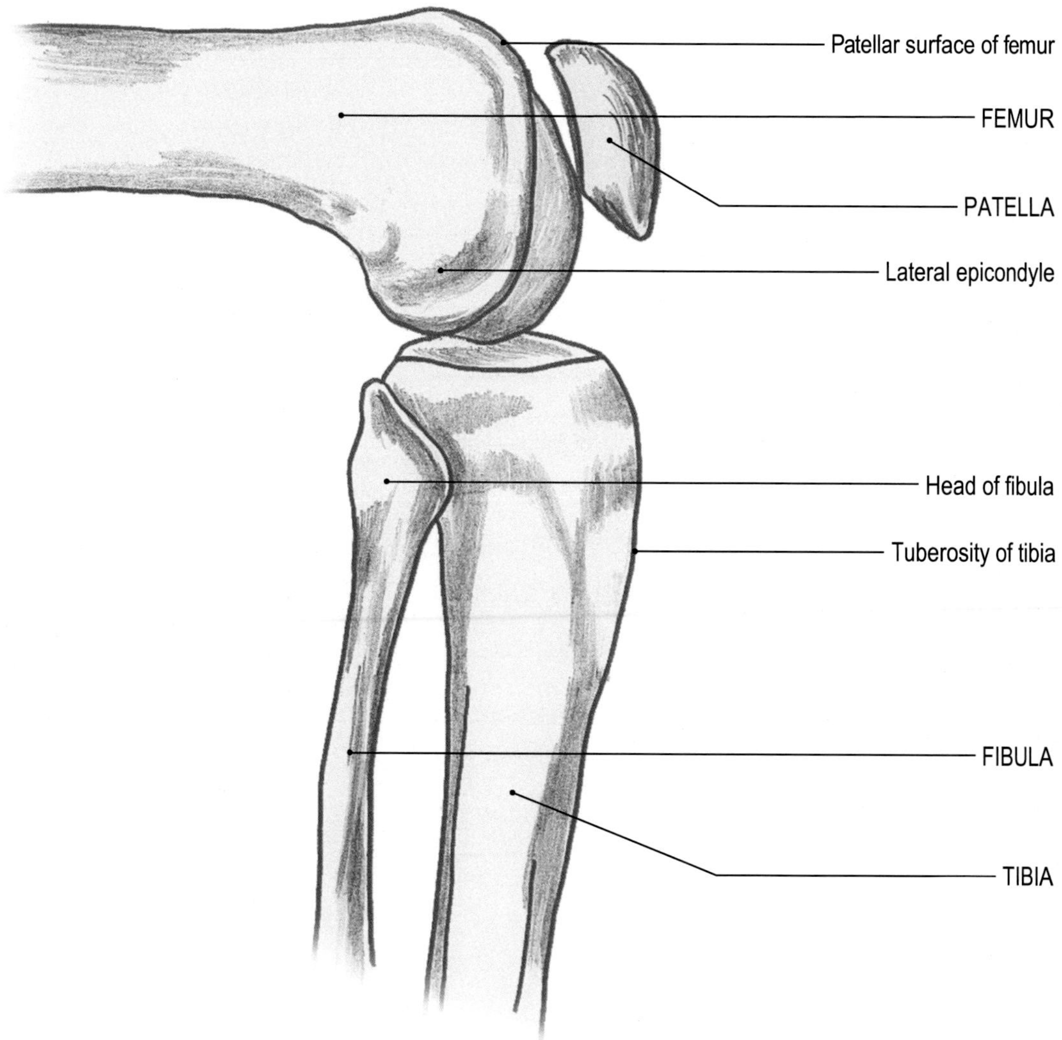

Fig. 3.4 (b) Bones of the right knee (lateral aspect)

- The head of the fibula (Fig. 3.4). Palpate the head of the fibula situated approximately 1 cm below the rim of the tibia. Run the palm of your hand up the lateral aspect of the model's leg.
- The styloid process of the fibula. Palpate the styloid process of the fibula projecting upwards from the head; the narrower neck lies just below the head.
- Note. The remainder of the upper end of the shaft of the fibula is surrounded by muscles and is therefore not palpable.

Palpation on movement

- Movements of the patella. Ask the model to extend the knee fully. Place the fingers of one hand on the lateral side of the patella and the fingers of the other hand on the lateral surface of the femoral condyle. Ask the model to flex the knee. Palpate the patella, sliding downwards and backwards under the condyle, finally ending up inferiorly. Ask the model to return to the extended position.
- Movements of the tibia. Place your fingers on the lateral condyle of the tibia close to the knee joint. Now ask the model to flex the knee. Palpate the tibia, gliding backwards and upwards on to the posterior surface of the femoral condyles.
- Note. At this position the anterior part of the tibial condyle appears to part from the femoral condyle. This is due to the posterior surface of the femoral condyle being smaller than that of the tibia.

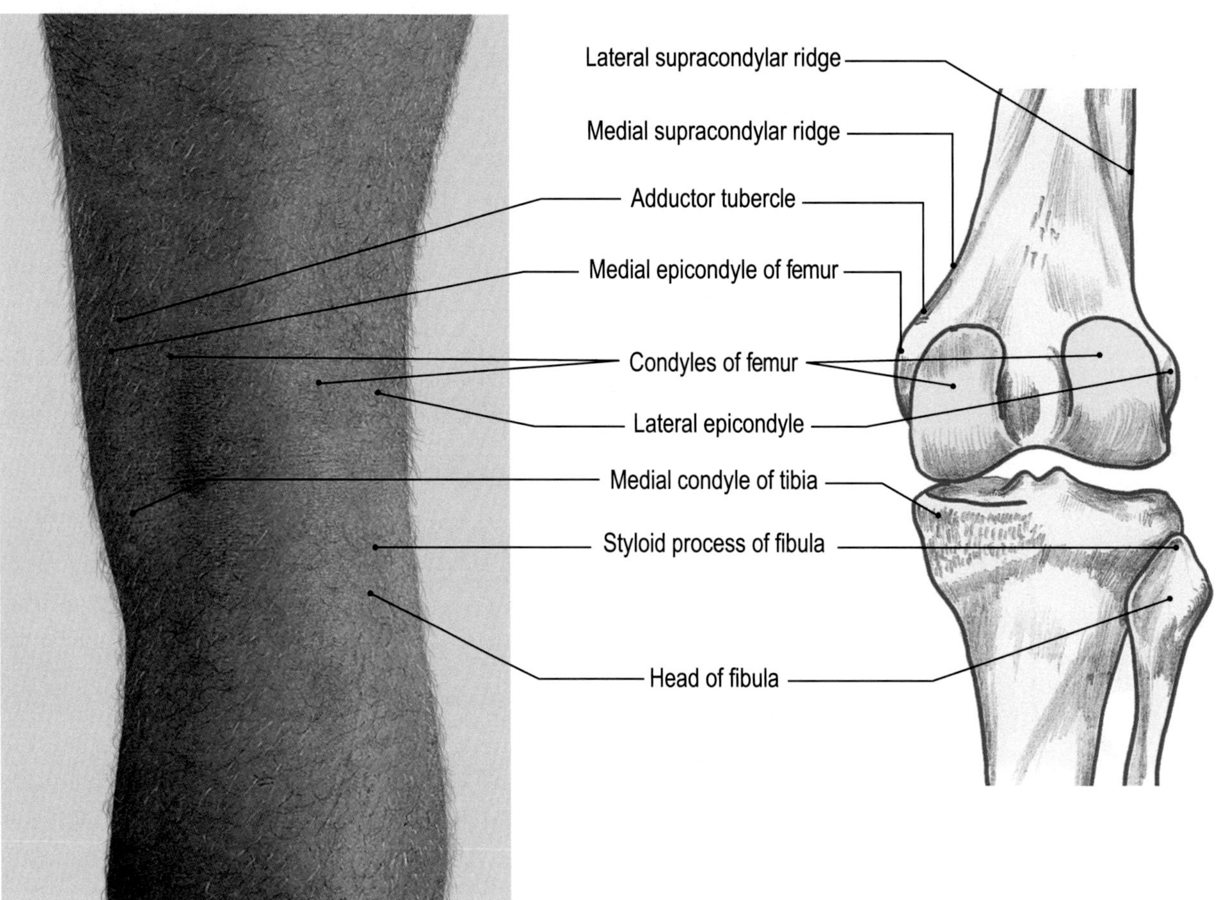

Fig. 3.4 (c, d) The right knee (posterior aspect)

Posterior aspect

Virtually no bony features can be palpated on the posterior aspect of the knee, either when it is flexed or extended. The posterior aspect of the sides of each femoral condyle and the medial surfaces of the tibia soon become hidden by the fascia and muscles at the back of the knee.

- The head of the fibula (Fig. 3.4). Palpate the head of the fibula on the lateral side of the popliteal fossa, with the tendon of biceps femoris attaching to its upper section.
- **Note.** Care must be taken when palpating in this area because the common peroneal nerve passes down the back of the head of the fibula en route to its passage around the lateral side of the neck.

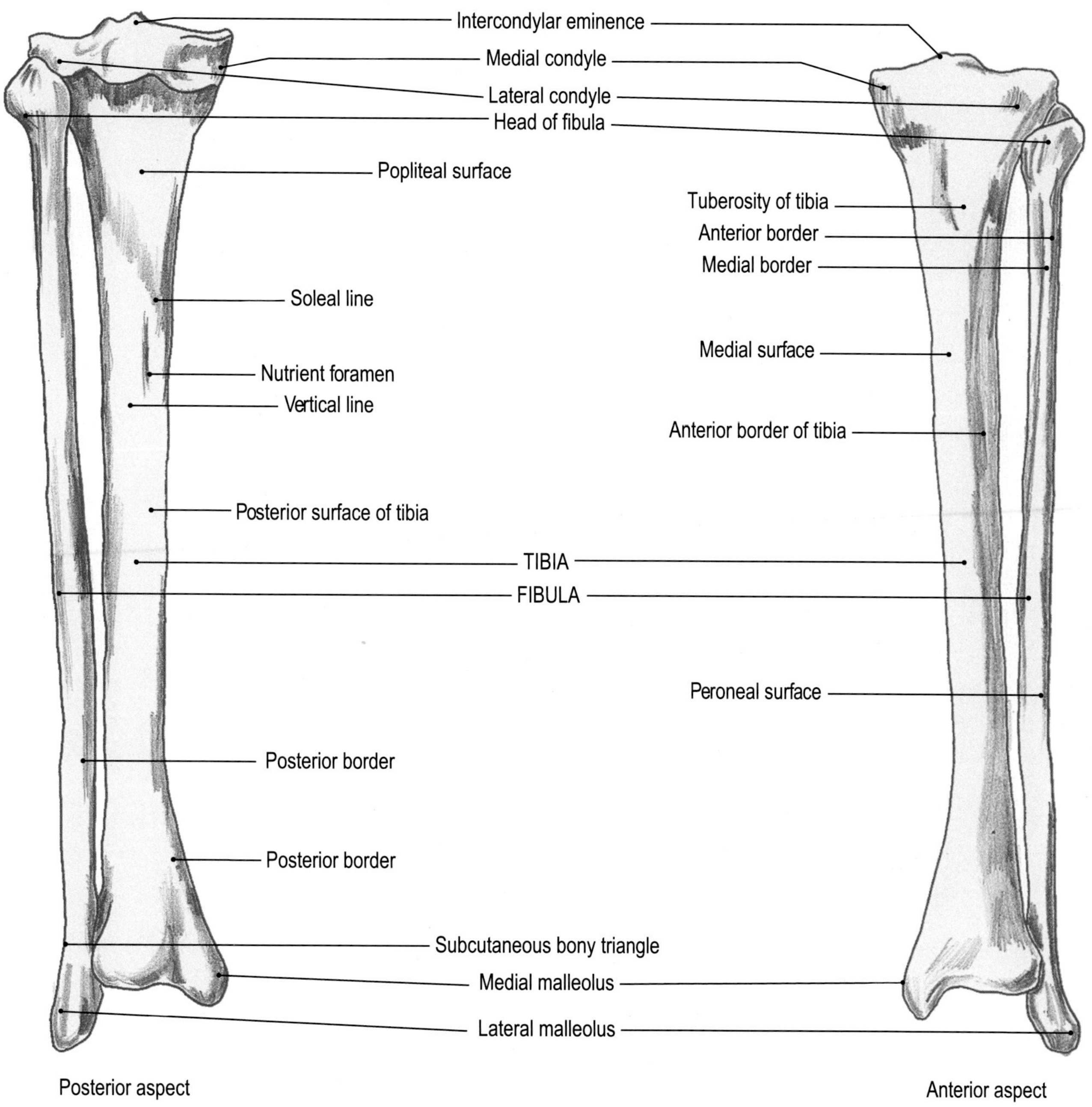

Fig. 3.4 (e, f) The tibia and fibula

- The patella. The model is in the supine lying position. Ask the model to extend the knee and relax the quadriceps femoris. Now move the patella from side to side.
- Note 1. This produces a knocking effect as the patella crosses either side of the grooved patellar surface of the femur.
- Note 2. This manoeuvre is classified as an accessory movement. It exposes a strip of the patellar surface of the femur on the side away from the direction of the movement. Hold the patella to one side. Now palpate the articular surface of the bone on that side for approximately 1 cm on its posterior surface.

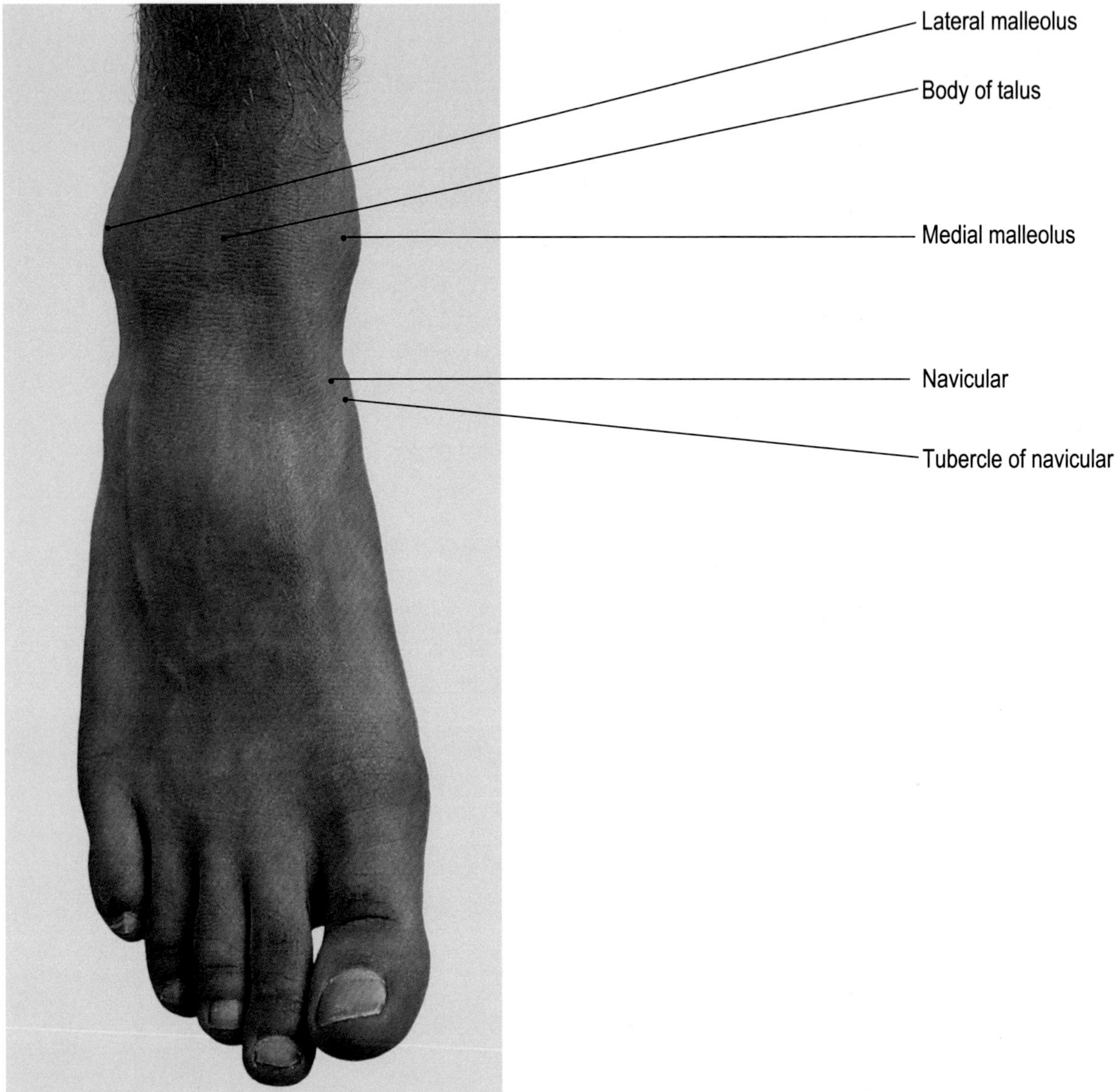

Fig. 3.5 (a) The right ankle region (anterior aspect)

The ankle region

Four bones participate in the formation of this area: the lower ends of the tibia and fibula, the talus and the calcaneus.

The lower end of the tibia

From its narrowest cross-section, two-thirds of the way down the shaft, the tibia expands to form part of the mortice for the formation of the ankle joint. Its medial side presents a large projection downwards: the medial malleolus. On its lateral side there is an elongated triangular area for the attachment of an extremely strong interosseous ligament which binds the two bones together. Its undersurface and the lateral side of the malleolus are smooth for articulation with the talus in the ankle joint.

The lower end of the fibula

The slender shaft of the fibula expands below to form the pointed lateral malleolus. This forms the lateral section of the mortice of the ankle joint. It is flattened from side to side. It has a smooth articular surface on its medial side and a roughened surface on its lateral, subcutaneous side.

The talus

The talus comprises a body, a neck and a head. The body is narrower at the back and wider anteriorly. It is pulley-shaped superiorly and slightly concave inferiorly. It has smooth, articular surfaces on its superior, inferior, lateral and the upper part of its medial surface.

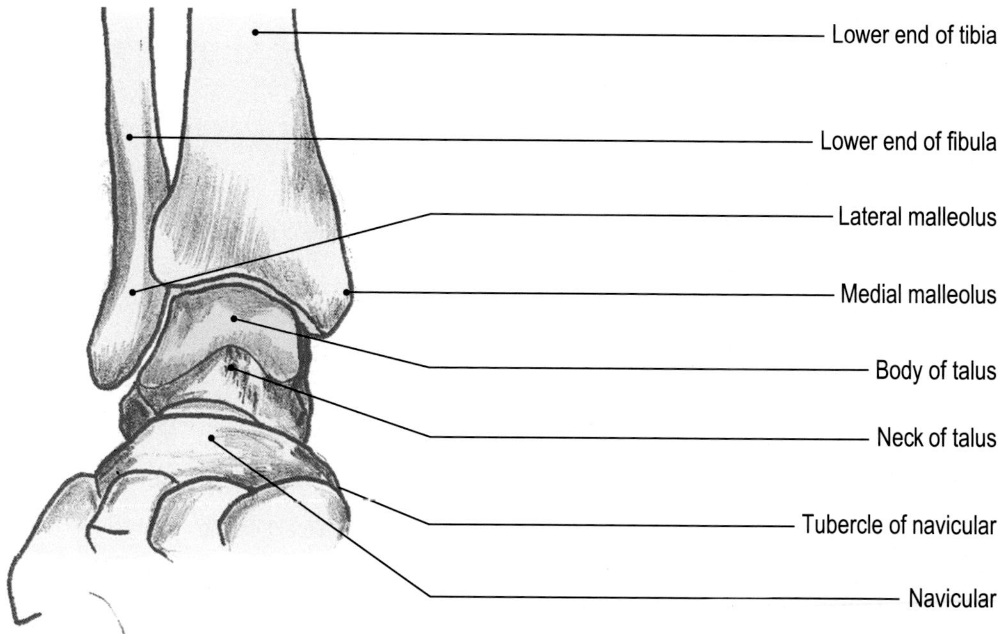

Fig. 3.5 (b) Bones of the right ankle region (anterior aspect)

The neck passes forwards and medially to expand into the head, which articulates with the posterior surface of the navicular bone.

Palpation

At the ankle the muscles of the leg have become tendinous and thus the bones are easier to palpate and identify between and deep to the tendons and retinacula.

Anterior aspect

- The medial malleolus [*malleolus* (L) = a small hammer] (Fig. 3.5a, b). Place your hands on the subcutaneous medial surface of the tibia. Trace down the anterior border of the tibia (shin) which appears to form the anterior part of the malleolus. Palpate its anterior border and tip. The posterior border may be more difficult to palpate because it is partially hidden by tendons and the flexor retinaculum.
- **Note.** The anterior border of the malleolus continues upwards and laterally under the extensor tendons and extensor retinacula, marking the line of the ankle joint.
- The lateral malleolus (Figs 3.4e, f and 3.5). The lateral malleolus of the fibula is the most outstanding feature on the lateral side of the ankle.
- From the tip of the lateral malleolus, trace both the anterior and posterior borders upwards, encompassing the large prominence of the malleolus.
- **Note.** The tip of the lateral malleolus lies at a lower level than that of the medial malleolus.
- The shaft of the fibula. From just above the level of the ankle joint, at approximately 2.5 cm, palpate the fibula where it narrows to a triangular subcutaneous lateral surface. From here, trace the shaft upwards for approximately 15 cm.
- **Note.** At this point it becomes hidden by peroneus tertius anteriorly and peroneus brevis and the tendon of peroneus longus posteriorly.
- The head and neck of the talus [*talus* (L) = the ankle bone]. With your right hand over the front of the ankle region, place your index finger on the lateral malleolus and your thumb on the medial malleolus of the model's left ankle. Draw your finger and thumb forward into a small hollow on either side. Between your thumb and finger you will feel the head of the talus. Now ask the model to plantarflex the foot. Palpate the neck of the talus.
- The navicular. Immediately anterior to this point, palpate the narrow gap of the talonavicular joint and posterior part of the navicular with its prominent **tubercle**, medially.
- The upper surface of the calcaneus [*calx* (L) = a heel]. Ask the model to plantarflex the foot. Deep beneath the tip of your index finger, just lateral to the head of the talus, you will feel the anterior section of the upper surface of the calcaneus.
- **Note.** Extensor digitorum brevis arises from this point.

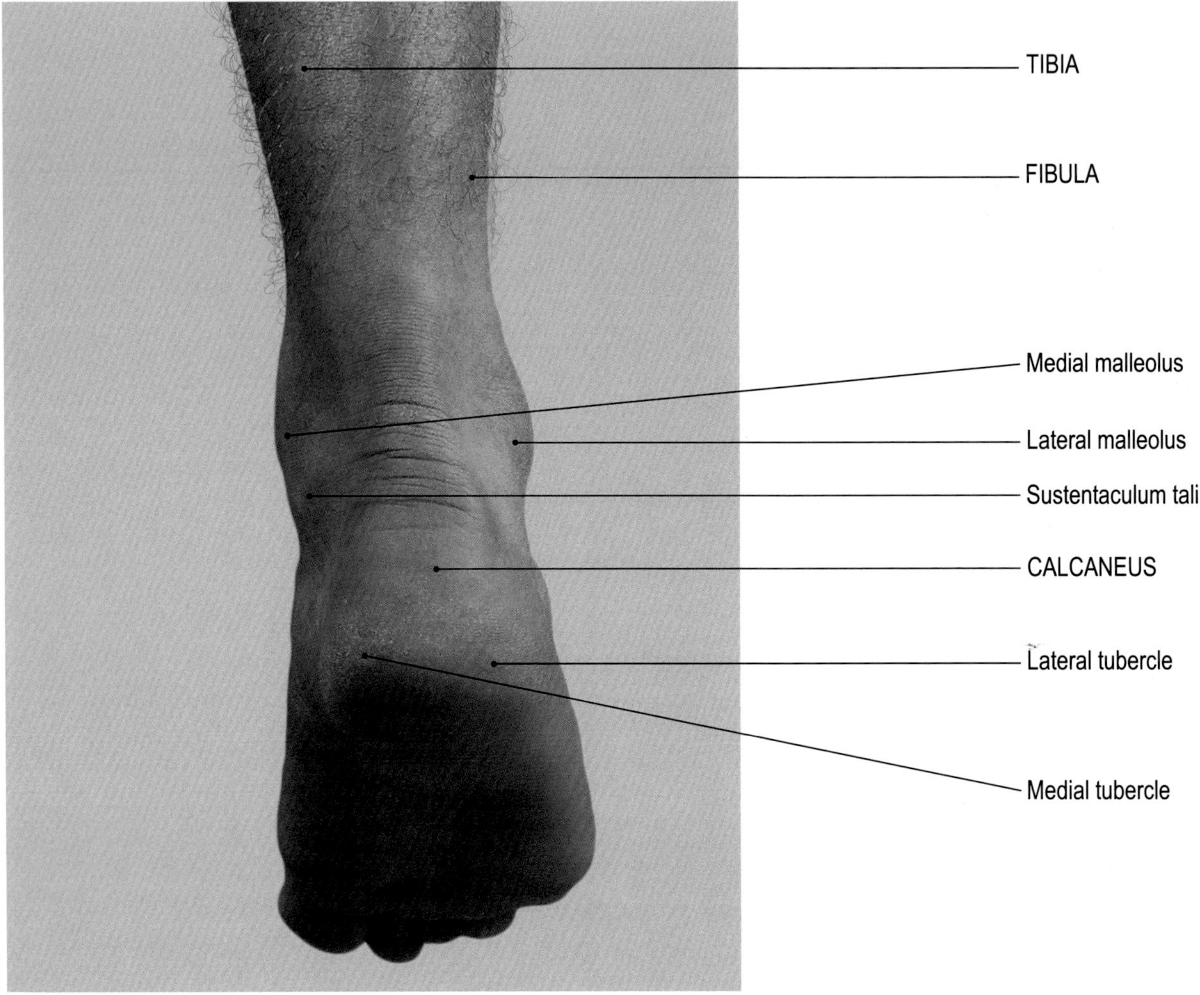

Fig. 3.5 (c) The right ankle region (posterior aspect)

Posterior aspect

From the posterior aspect very little of the talus can be seen as the body has narrowed down to just two tubercles and a groove running downwards and medially. The mortice of the ankle joint is formed by the two malleoli and the inferior border of the tibia. Both the malleoli are marked posteriorly by a fossa for the attachment of ligaments.

The calcaneus

This is the largest of the tarsal bones and is situated below the talus and behind the navicular and cuboid. It is oblong in shape, projecting forwards and backwards beyond the talus. The backward projection forms the heel. It has six surfaces:

- anterior, which is smooth
- superior, marked by a smooth articular surface centrally
- medial, which is fairly smooth and converted into a hollow by the projection medially from its upper section of the sustentaculum tali
- lateral, which is roughened, presenting two tubercles
- posterior, which is rounded and roughened across its centre for the attachment of the tendo calcaneus
- inferior, which is slightly concave downwards and is roughened for the attachment of muscles and fascia. It is marked by three broad, rounded tubercles; two posteriorly and one anteriorly.

Palpation

- The sustentaculum tali of the calcaneus. Ask the model to evert the foot. Place your hands at the tip of the medial malleolus. Move your fingers 1 cm down from this tip. You will feel the horizontal ridge of the sustentaculum tali. Trace the ridge as it runs for approximately 2–3 cm and is clearer anteriorly and posteriorly.
- The tubercle of the navicular. At the anterior end of this ridge identify a small gap. You will now be able to palpate the tubercle of the navicular.
- **Note.** This gap is spanned by the 'spring ligament'.
- The malleolar fossae. You will find it difficult to identify many bony features posteriorly because the tendo calcaneus lies almost 2 cm clear of the ankle joint. If you pay particular attention to the posterior borders of the lateral and medial malleoli, you will be able to palpate small depressions. These are the malleolar fossae.
- **Note.** The posterior surface of the medial malleolus is continuous with the posterior border of the medial surface of the tibia (Fig. 3.5c, d).

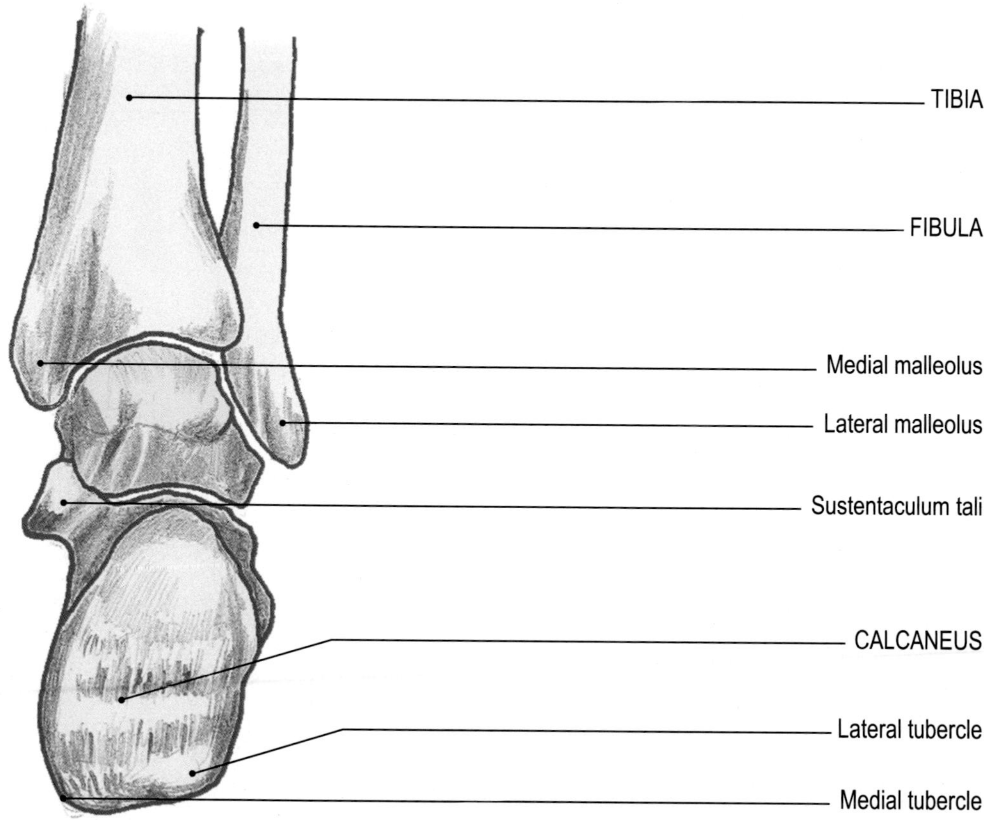

Fig. 3.5 (d) Bones of the right ankle region (posterior aspect)

Palpation on movement

- Movements of the talus 1. Stand facing the lateral side of the model's ankle region. With your left hand, grip the two malleoli with your fingers on the medial and your thumb on the lateral. With your right hand, grip the anterior part of the body and neck of the talus with your fingers in the hollow just anterior to the medial malleolus and your thumb in the hollow just anterior to the lateral malleolus. Both sets of fingers and both thumbs should be close to each other. Starting from the fully plantarflexed position, ask the model to dorsiflex the foot. You will feel the anterior part of the body of the talus disappearing into the gap between the two malleoli. In fact, the fingers of your right hand will now be gripping the neck and head of the talus. At this point the ankle is in its close-packed position and no side-to-side movement is possible.
- Movements of the talus 2 – rocking. When the model fully plantarflexes from the dorsiflexed position the head and neck of the talus will move forwards and downwards and the anterior section of the body will reappear from within the mortice. At this point you can rock the head and neck of the talus from side to side. This is an accessory movement.
- Movements of the calcaneus 1. Ask the model to return the ankle to the mid position. Adopt the same procedure as described above. This time, move the fingers of your right hand to just below the tip of the medial malleolus. Identify the horizontal rim of the sustentaculum tali. Ask the model to plantar- and dorsiflex the ankle rhythmically. You will feel the sustentaculum tali moving forwards and backwards, describing a shallow arc around the medial malleolus.
- Movements of the calcaneus 2. Adopt the same position with your left hand. Place your right thumb on the two tubercles below the lateral malleolus. You will feel movement forwards and backwards around the malleolus when plantar- and dorsiflexion is performed.
- Movements of the calcaneus 3. Adopt the same position as described above. Grip the two malleoli with your left hand. Place your right hand under the heel with your fingers resting on the posterior aspect of the calcaneus on either side of the tendo calcaneus. Ask the model to dorsi- and plantarflex the ankle. You will feel the calcaneus moving forwards and backwards away and towards the posterior part of the tibia.
- **Note.** When the calcaneus passes downwards it is nearly impossible to move from side to side. This is because the anterior part of the talus moves into the mortice of the ankle joint.

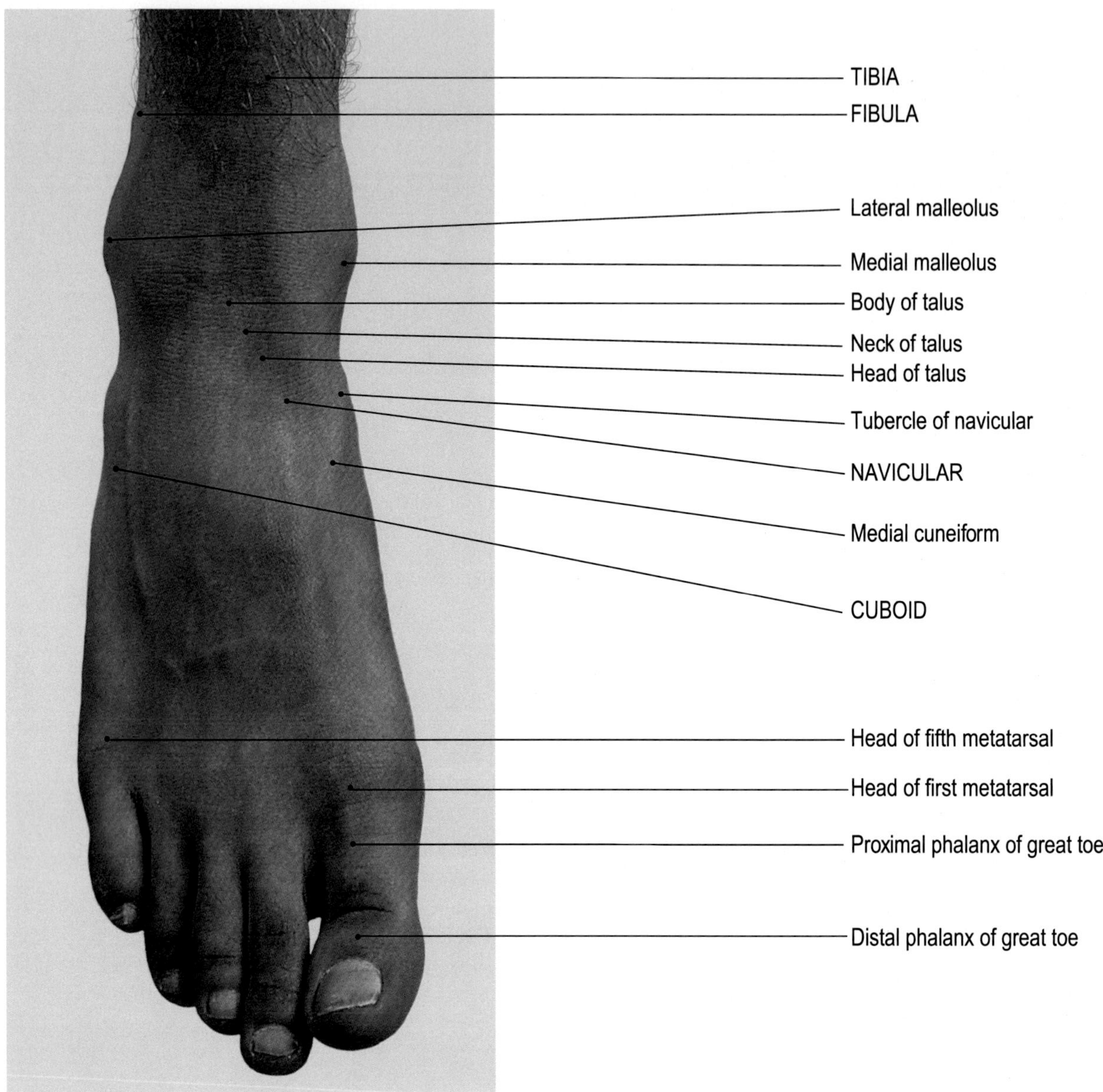

Fig. 3.6 (a) The right foot (dorsal aspect)

The foot

Three main groups of bones form the skeleton of the foot (Fig. 3.6).

- Posteriorly. The tarsus, comprises large irregular bones.
- Anteriorly. The phalanges: miniature long bones that form the toes.
- Linking the above groups are the metatarsals: also miniature long bones.

The calcaneus forms the heel. It is the largest and most posterior of the group of tarsal bones. In front and to the lateral side is the **cuboid** [*kubgides* (Gk) = cube shape]. Sitting on the middle section of the upper surface of the calcaneus is the **body of the talus**. Its **neck** and **head** passes forwards and medially, medial and slightly above the level of the cuboid. The **navicular** lies in front of the head of the talus. The three cuneiform bones [*cuneus* (L) = a wedge] are interposed between the anterior surfaces of the navicular and the three medial metatarsal bones. The two lateral metatarsals lie anterior to the cuboid.

Palpation

For palpation in this region, the model is in the sitting position.

Dorsal aspect

- The talocalcaneonavicular joint. Locate the medial and lateral malleoli. Run your index finger and thumb forwards until you can grip the head of the talus between them. Now palpate the upper part of the talocalcaneonavicular joint.
- The tuberosity of the navicular (Figs 3.5a, b, and 3.6). Trace the roughened dorsal surface of the navicular medially to its large tuberosity. This projects downwards and medially and is approximately 2.5 cm downwards and forwards from the tip of the medial malleolus.
- The medial cuneform bone. Immediately distal to the navicular, palpate the **medial cuneiform** bone which projects downwards.
- The middle and lateral cuneform bones. Identify the dorsal surfaces of the middle and lateral cuneiform bones on the

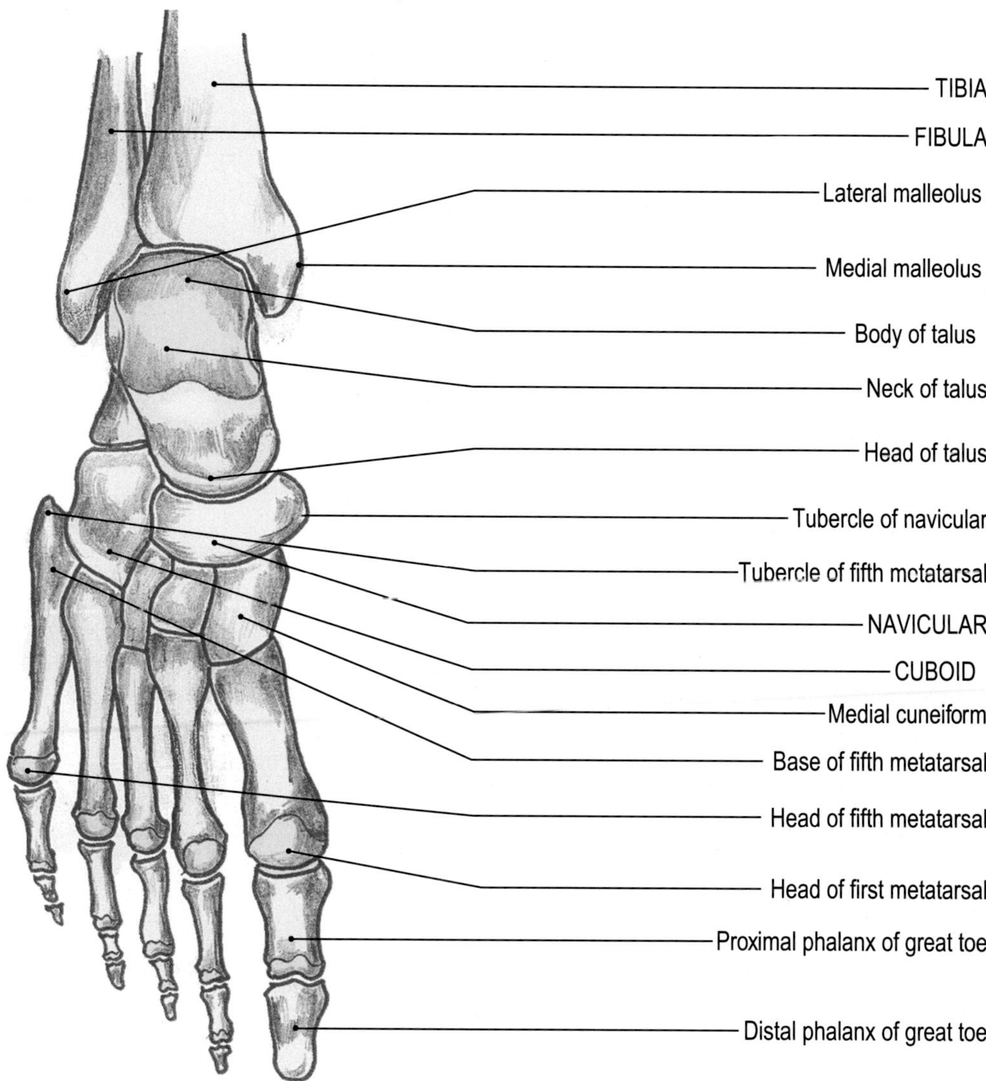

Fig. 3.6 (b) Bones of the right foot (dorsal aspect)

dorsum of the foot which lie lateral to the medial cuneiform bone.

- The first metatarsal bone. You will find it easy to identify the base, shaft and **head of the first metatarsal bone**.
- **Note.** The first metatarsal bone is much stouter than the other four. In some individuals the head projects medially, carrying the base of the toe with it. This causes inflammation of the bursa on its medial side which is often accompanied by pain and swelling. Such medial deviation of the metatarsal head commonly progresses to a condition termed 'hallux valgus'.
- The second, third, fourth and fifth metatarsal bones. Run the pads of your fingers carefully over the dorsum of the foot. Now palpate the base, shaft and head of each of the remaining metatarsal bones. You can trace the base of the second metatarsal further proximally than the others to the middle cuneiform, the third to the lateral cuneiform and the fourth and fifth to the cuboid (Fig. 3.6).
- **Note.** The **base of the fifth metatarsal** is more expanded than the rest. It has a **tubercle**, or **styloid process**, which projects proximally on its lateral side.
- The base of the fifth metatarsal bone. Trace backwards along the shaft of the fifth metatarsal. Palpate the large lateral projection which is elongated proximally and overlies the lateral side of the cuboid.
- The peroneal tubercle. Identify the peroneal tubercle on the lateral side of the calcaneus. It is 1 cm below and just anterior to the tip of the lateral malleolus. This tubercle is elongated downwards and forwards. Ask the model to evert the foot. Two tendons appear to pull clear.
- **Note 1.** The tendon above the tubercle is peroneus brevis; the one below is peroneus longus.
- **Note 2.** This tubercle must not be confused with that of the calcaneofibular ligament. This can be found if you carefully palpate just below and posterior to the tip of the lateral malleolus.

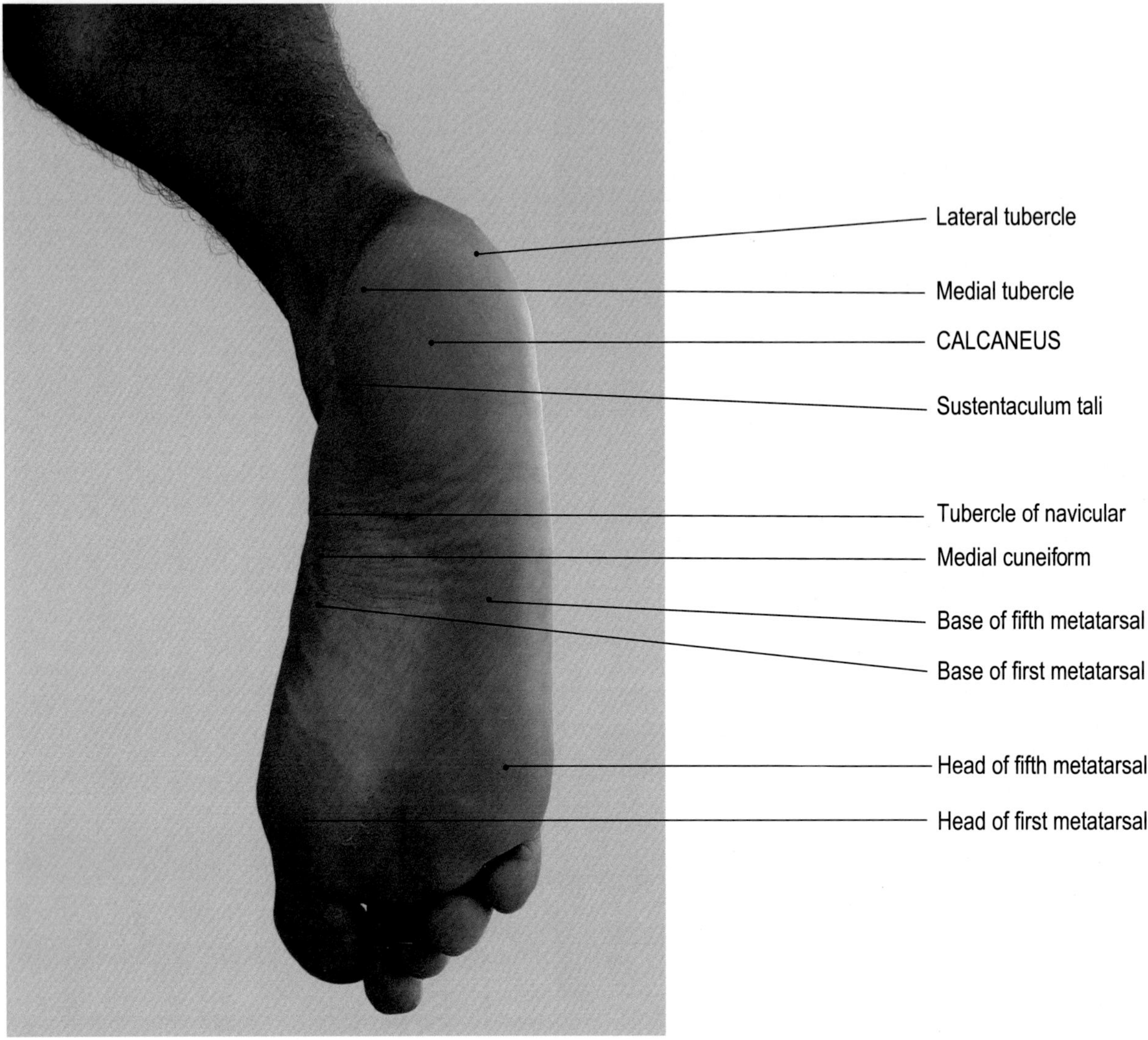

Fig. 3.7 (a) The right foot (plantar aspect)

Plantar aspect

As in the palm of the hand, very few bony points are palpable in this region. This is due in part to the presence of overlying muscles and in part to the existence of a dense and thick layer of plantar fascia: the 'plantar aponeurosis'.

Palpation

For palpation in this region, the model is in the supine lying position.

- The **calcaneus**. Identify the heel, which is the most posterior and inferior aspect of the calcaneus. Palpate the large, broad **tubercles** (**medial** and **lateral**) on either side of the bone.
- **Note 1.** The tubercles give attachment to the more superficial of the plantar muscles.
- **Note 2.** There is often a horizontal raised area on the posterior aspect of the heel to which the tendo calcaneus attaches (see Fig. 3.22b).
- **Note 3.** Below this the posterior surface of the calcaneus is covered with a pad of tough fibrous tissue and fat.
- The peroneal tubercle. Locate the area below and in front of the tip of the lateral malleolus. Palpate the elongated tubercle (the peroneal tubercle) on the calcaneus.
- **Note.** The tendon of peroneus brevis is above; the tendon of peroneus longus is below.
- The sustentaculum tali of the calcaneus. Palpate the horizontal ridge immediately below the tip of the medial malleolus: the sustentaculum tali.
- **Note.** This is slightly hidden by the tendon of flexor digitorum longus.
- The tuberosity of the navicular. Palpate the inferior surface of the navicular tuberosity on the medial side of the foot 3 cm anteroinferior to the tip of the medial malleolus.
- **Note.** The base of the fifth metatarsal and its tubercle are covered by the plantar fascia and muscles.
- The **heads** of the metatarsals (Fig. 3.7). You will find these relatively easy to identify.
- **Note.** The heads of the **first** and **fifth metatarsals** lie deep to a pad of harder skin at the broadest part of the foot on the medial and lateral side, respectively.
- The heads of the second, third and fourth metatarsals. You will find these are less easy to palpate. They lie on a well-formed anterior metatarsal arch. Palpation is facilitated if the arch is flattened. Grasp the model's toe between your finger and thumb of one hand. Passively extend the joint. Now palpate the metatarsal head on the plantar surface proximal to the base

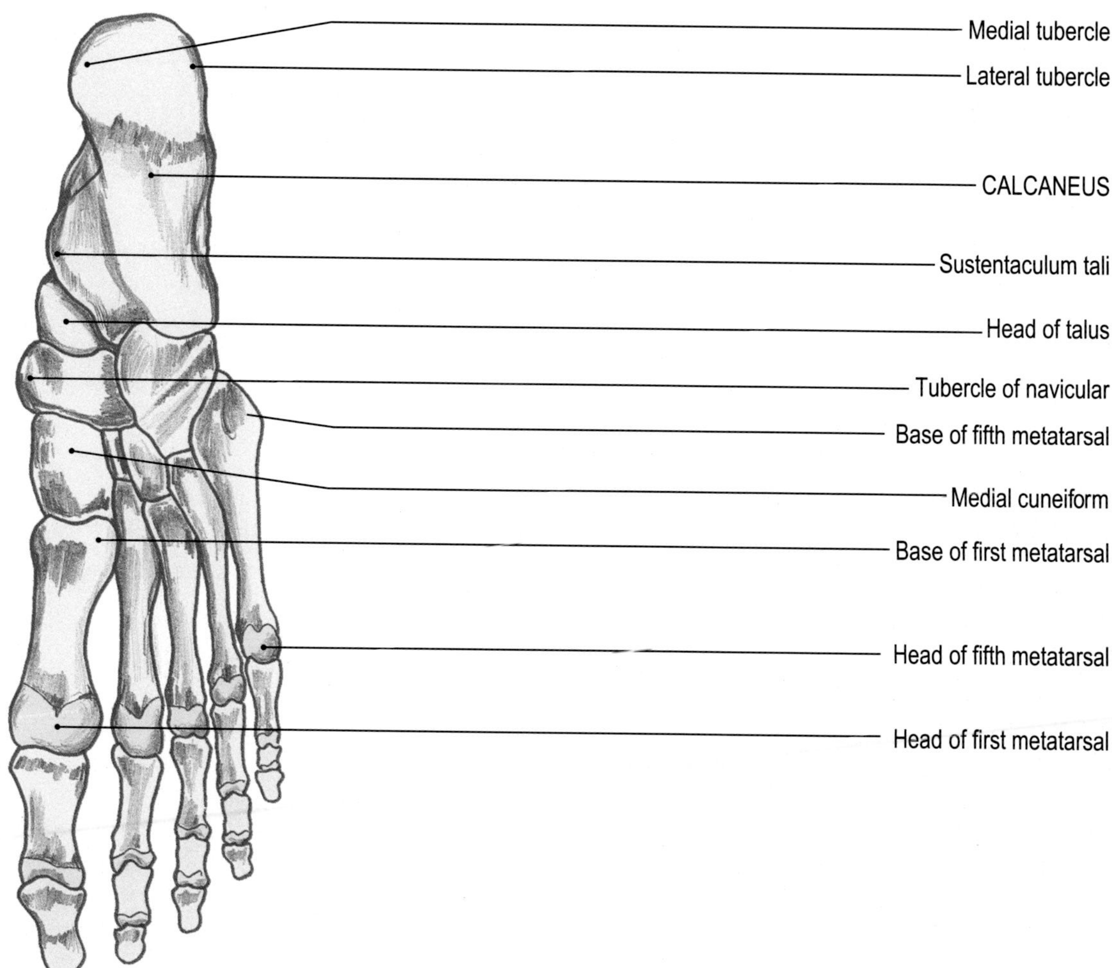

Fig. 3.7 (b) Bones of the right foot (plantar aspect)

of the toe. If you ask the model to flex the toe at the metatarsophalangeal joint, you will feel the metatarsal head on the dorsum of the foot, as the knuckles would in the hand.

- The phalanges. Identify the base of the proximal phalanx just beyond the corresponding metatarsal head.
- **Note.** The heads of the proximal phalanges, particularly those of the second, third and fourth, are often flexed and project dorsally. They are covered by hard skin and a bursa which often swells and becomes inflamed. If not treated, the inflamed bursa may lead to a condition known as 'hammer toes'.
- The proximal interphalangeal joints (Fig. 3.7). Ask the model to extend the toes at the proximal interphalangeal joint. Now identify the small bicondylar head of the bone.

Palpation on movement

- The head of the talus. Adopt the same position and the same hand holds as for palpation on movement, anterior aspect (see p. 95). Ask the model to plantarflex the ankle and then move the foot into adduction and abduction. Palpate the **head of the talus** moving from side to side.
- **Note.** This will not occur in dorsiflexion due to the close-packed nature of the ankle joint.
- The tubercle of the navicular. Now move your hands down and grip the head of the talus in your left hand. With your right hand, grip the foot, with your fingers over the tubercle of the navicular and your thumb over the base of the fifth metatarsal bone. Ask the model to evert the foot. Feel the tubercle descending and the metatarsal rising. Now ask the model to invert the foot. Feel the tubercle rising and the metatarsal bone descending.
- **Note.** The navicular is rotating around an axis running through the neck and head of the talus.
- The metatarsophalangeal joints. Move your hands down to the base of the great toe. Grip the first metatarsal just proximal to the head with fingers and thumb of your left hand. Grip the proximal phalanx with fingers and thumb of your right hand. Ask the model to extend the toe. Palpate the head with the phalanx moving towards the dorsum of the head. Now ask the model to flex the toe. Palpate the phalanx, moving downwards around the head.
- **Note.** This movement can be observed in all the metatarsophalangeal joints, but to a lesser extent.
- The interphalangeal joints. You will be able to feel a similar movement in the interphalangeal joints. Ask the model to flex the toes. You will now be able to feel the head of the phalanx.

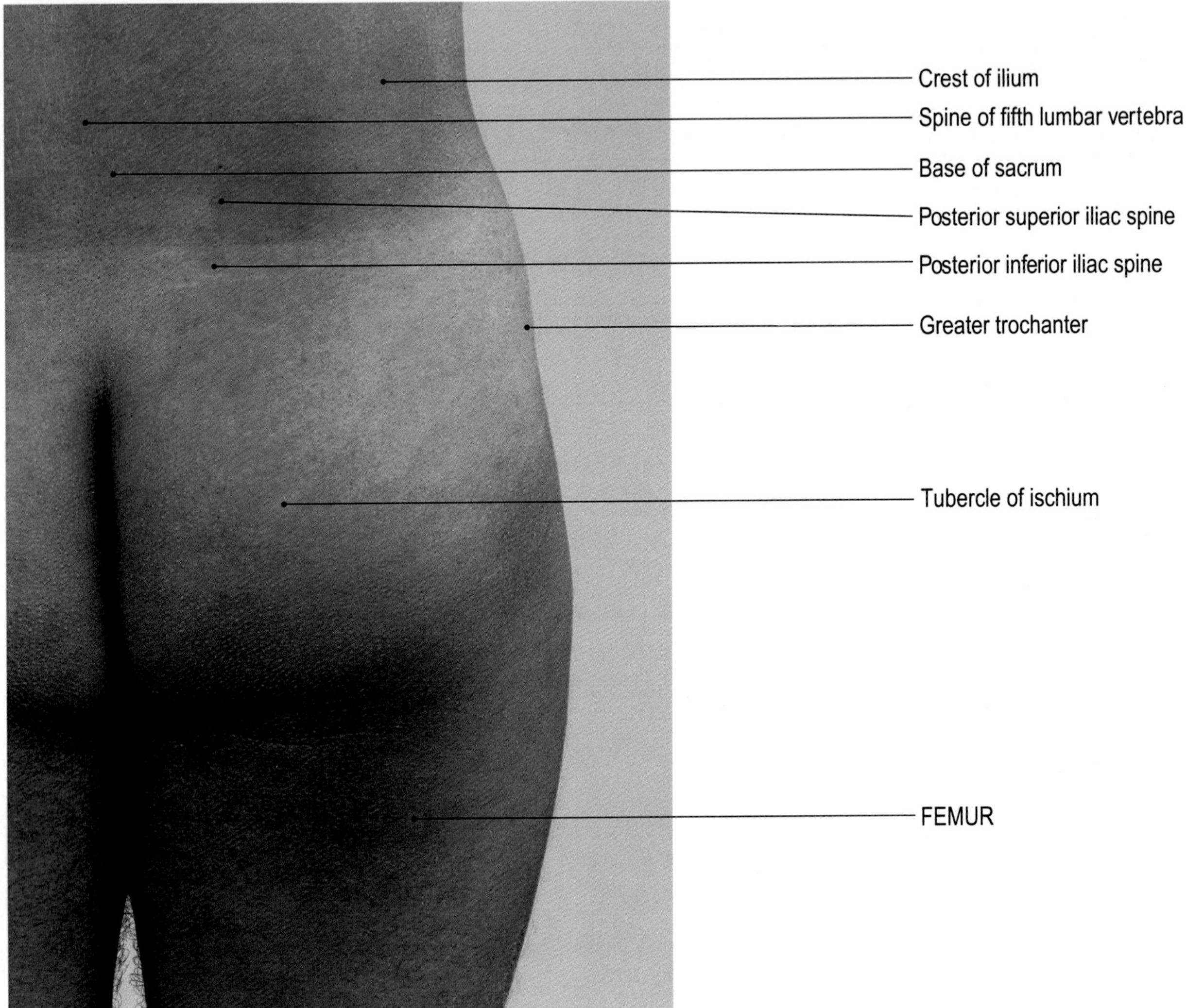

Fig. 3.8 (a) The right sacroiliac joint (posterior aspect)

JOINTS

Although the joints of the lower limb are structurally similar to their counterparts in the upper limb, they tend to be more stable. Movement at the lower limb joints is more limited, with the weight transmitted across them being considerably more than in the upper limb. The sacroiliac joint and the pubic symphysis are really associated with the pelvis, but as this is the region from which the lower limb functions, they are included in this section.

The sacroiliac joint

Structure

This joint is situated deep within the posterior aspect of the pelvis. It is formed by the auricular surface on the lateral side of the sacrum and the sacropelvic surface of the hip bone. It is a synovial joint surrounded by a capsule and lined with synovial membrane. The capsule is supported by anterior, posterior and interosseous ligaments. The joint is further supported by two accessory ligaments: the sacrotuberous and the sacrospinous ligaments.

Palpation: surface marking

For palpation in this region, the model is in the prone lying position.

The sacroiliac joint (Fig. 3.8) is set deeply at the back of the pelvis and is thus difficult to palpate. Nevertheless, certain landmarks can be identified, giving an accurate indication of its position.

- The joint line. Find the **posterior superior** and **inferior iliac spines**, as outlined above (see p. 88). Draw an oblique line passing downwards and medially from a point 5 cm lateral to the **spine of the fifth lumbar vertebra** to a point just lateral to the posterior inferior iliac spine.
- **Note.** The joint is, however, in a plane running forwards and laterally under the posterior part of the ilium. It reaches as far forward as the apex of the greater sciatic notch (Fig. 3.9b).

Accessory movements

There is much controversy concerning the movements that may occur at this joint. The fact that it is a synovial joint with plane,

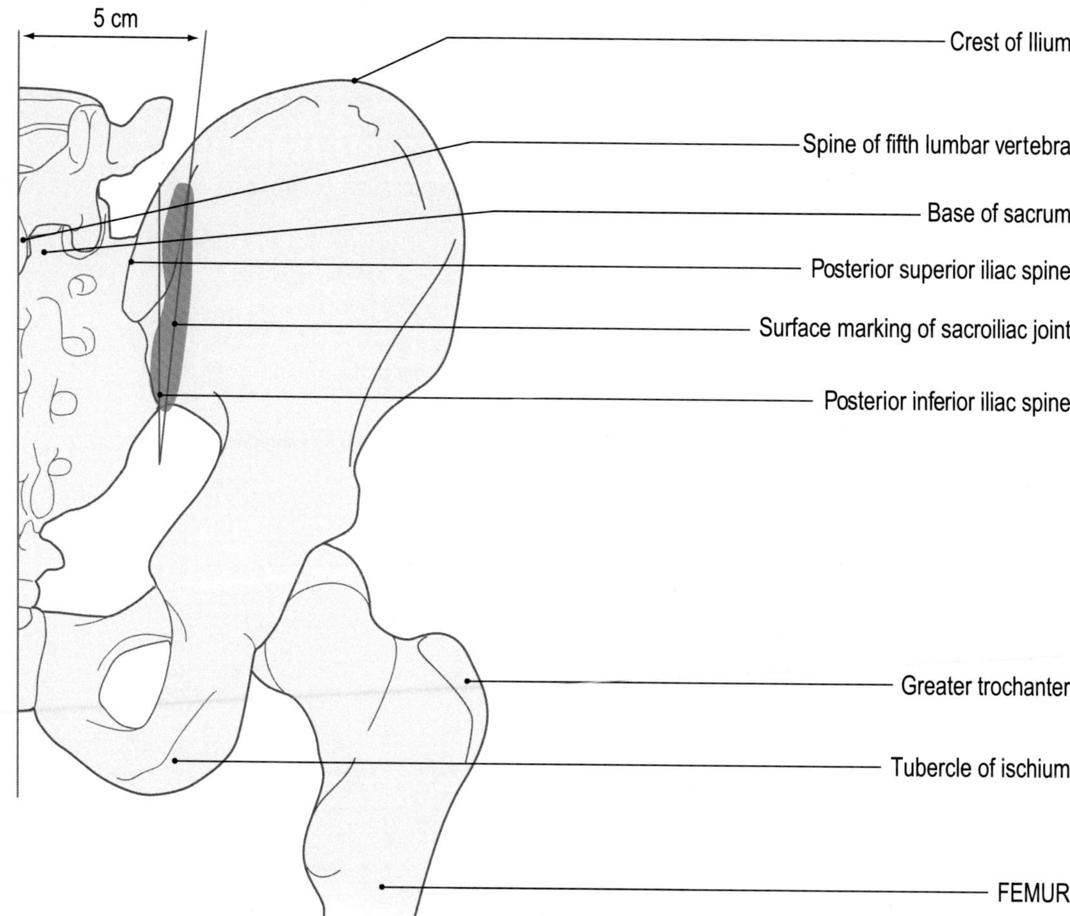

Fig. 3.8 (b) The right sacroiliac joint (posterior aspect)

although irregular, articular surfaces suggests that it is designed for movement. The irregularity of the articular surface, together with the presence of extremely strong, short interosseous ligaments, means that in reality little movement is possible.

- **Note 1.** In young females, due to the laxity of the surrounding ligaments, some movement is possible; in elderly males, there is little or no movement.
- **Note 2.** The two joints on either side of the **sacrum** and the symphysis pubis anteriorly allow slight rotation and gapping movements to occur. This reduces the stresses imparted on the pelvis from the trunk and lower limbs.

Palpation

- Rotation of the sacrum. Slight rotation of the sacrum forwards and backwards around a frontal axis running through its interosseous ligament may be regarded as normal physiological movement. This movement is facilitated if you apply pressure alternately on the upper and lower aspects of its posterior surface, so rocking the sacrum between the ilia.
- Rotation of the ilium. The model is in the side lying position. Enhance the movement by using the **femur** as a lever and localize the movement of the joint with your other hand. Stand behind the model's hip region. Take the upper femur into extension. Place your other hand on the posterior aspect of the **iliac crest**. Ask the model to hold the underneath knee up to the chest. This fixes the pelvis. Flex the femur on the pelvis. Feel the backward rotation of the ilium on the sacrum. To enhance the movement, ask the model to extend the alternate leg. Now apply pressure from the front on the anterior superior iliac spine.
- Gapping of the sacroiliac joint. The model is in the supine lying position. Ask the model to flex the hip and knee of the lower limb on the opposite side to which you are standing. Rotate the pelvis and the flexed lower limb towards you. Apply a downward and inward pressure on the femur, towards the hip. This produces a slight gapping of the posterior part of the sacroiliac joint.
- **Note.** Movements of the pubic symphysis. During the above movements, associated gapping and twisting occur at the pubic symphysis. For additional information consult the manipulation literature.

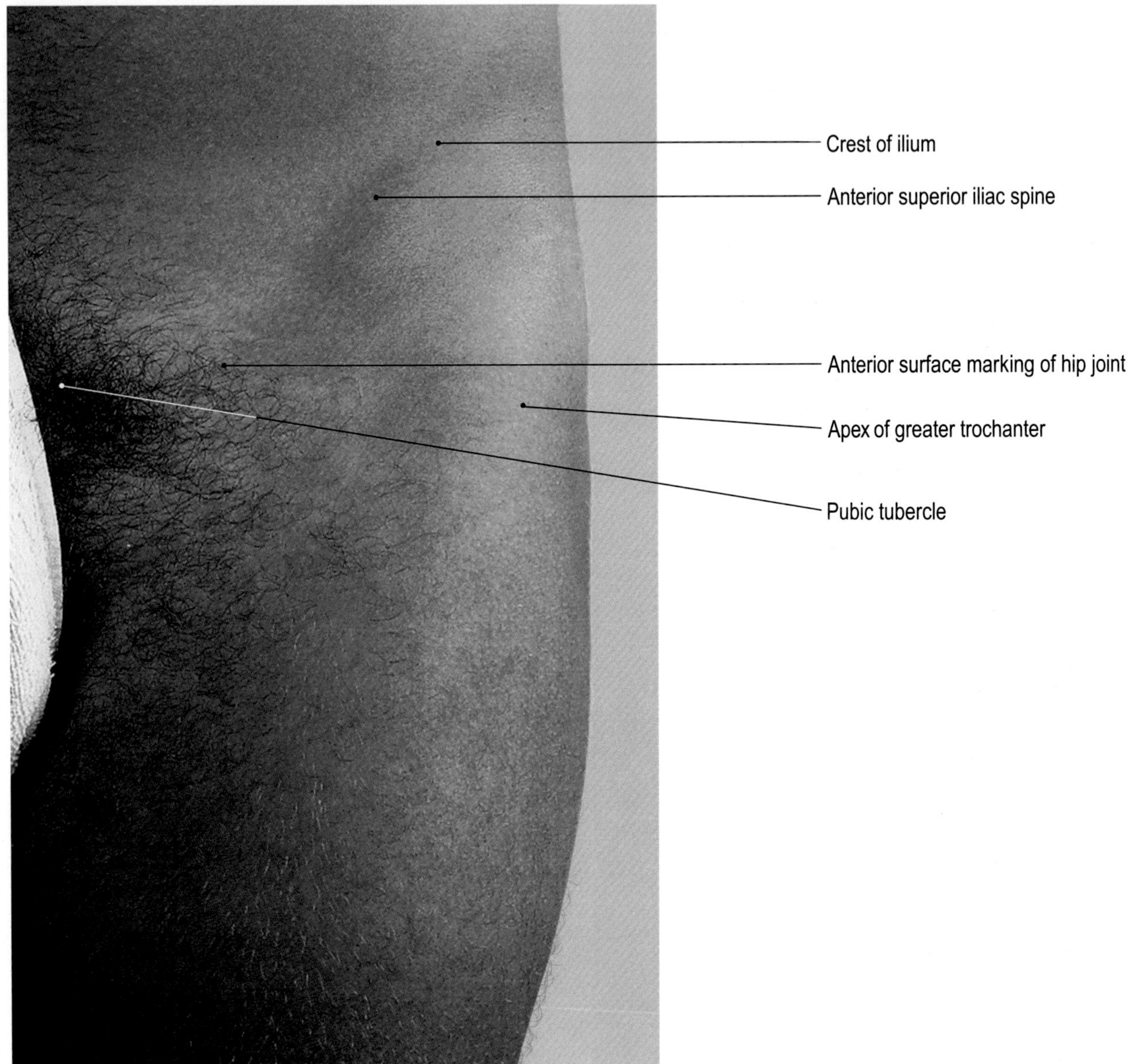

Fig. 3.9 (a) The left hip joint (anterior aspect)

The hip joint (Fig. 3.9)

This is a large synovial ball-and-socket joint between the head of the femur and the acetabulum of the hip bone. It lies on the anterolateral aspect of the pelvis and affords a considerable amount of mobility to the lower limb. It is surrounded by a capsule which encloses a large part of the femoral neck, both lined with synovial membrane. The capsule is supported, externally, by the very powerful iliofemoral, ischiofemoral and pubofemoral ligaments. Further support is afforded internally by the ligament of the head of the femur deep inside the joint and the acetabular labrum. The labrum attaches to the rim of the acetabulum and transverse ligament, thus surrounding the head.

Palpation: surface marking

For palpation in this region, the model is in the supine lying position.

- The hip joint. Draw the joint line which lies in the groin some 1.5 cm below the mid point of the inguinal ligament, i.e. halfway between the **anterior superior iliac spine** and the **pubic tubercle** (see p. 81).
- **Note.** The acetabulum extends 4 cm vertically below this point deep to the head of the femur. Midway between the upper and lower limits, i.e. at the mid point of the joint, the acetabulum extends 2 cm either side of this vertical line (Fig. 3.9).
- Alternative method. Trace a line horizontally and medially from the upper border of the **greater trochanter** to a point

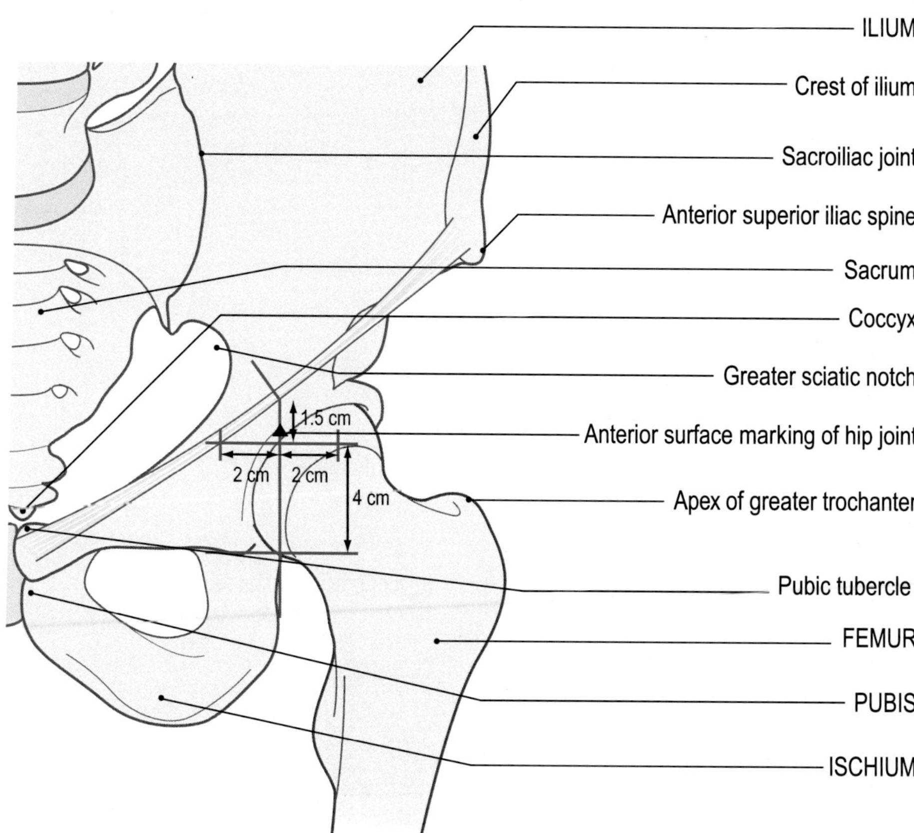

Fig. 3.9 (b) Bones of the left hip joint (anterior aspect)

below the mid point of the inguinal ligament. This identifies the centre of the joint. When viewed posteriorly, the centre of the hip joint lies 5 cm above and 3 cm lateral to the ischial tuberosity.

Palpation

Palpation of the joint from any aspect is virtually impossible because it is covered by thick muscle which crosses it, in particular, posteriorly and laterally. Only if the hip is fully extended can movement be detected and then only anteriorly.

The model is in the side lying position.

- The head of the femur. Ask the model to extend the limb to approximately 15°. Place your fingers on the anterior surface marking of the joint. You will now palpate the head of the femur projecting forwards under the anterior covering of iliopsoas and pectineus.

Accessory movements

Palpation

The model is in the supine lying position.

- Note. Very little accessory movement is possible at this joint.
- Parting of the articular surface. Ask the model to flex the hip to approximately 30°. Kneel with your legs on either side of the model's leg. Cup your hands around the upper calf and lean backwards. This will allow you to apply strong traction to the hip joint. This produces slight parting of the articular surfaces.
- Combinations of movement. By combining the three components of movement, i.e. flexion/extension, abduction/adduction and medial/lateral rotation, you can test the joint movement and function to extremes.
- Note. Testing these combined movements is often referred to as the 'quadrants'. For further information consult the manipulation and mobilization literature (Maitland 1991).

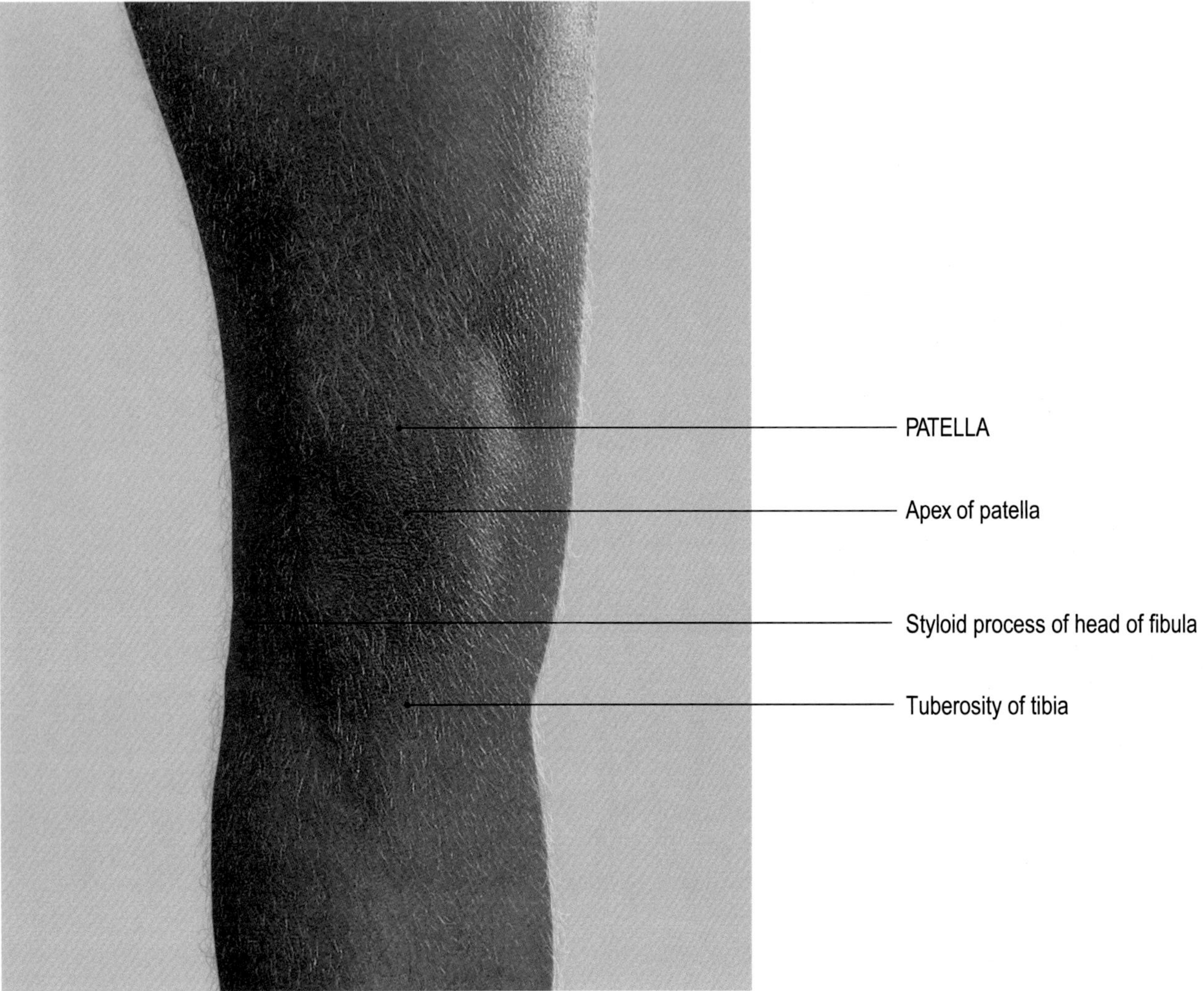

Fig. 3.10 (a) The right knee joint (anterior aspect)

The knee joint (Fig. 3.10)

The knee joint is a synovial composite joint. It comprises the bicondylar section between the condyles of femur and tibia and the plane joint between the patella and the patellar surface of the femur. The joint functions as a modified hinge. Its main movements are flexion and extension. Rotation can be produced in the semiflexed position and in the final few degrees of full extension.

The knee joint is the largest joint in the human body and perhaps the most complex (see Palastanga et al 2002).

The articular surfaces are covered with articular cartilage, but are not congruent. Those on the femur cover the superior, posterior, inferior and anterior surfaces of the large condyles. They come together anteriorly to form a triangular surface which is narrow at the top and is called the patellar surface. The articular surfaces of the tibia only cover the central section of the upper surface. Its outer sections are covered by two crescentic-shaped menisci.

The joint is supported on its posterior, lateral and medial side by a fibrous capsule. Anteriorly the capsule is formed by the lower section of the quadriceps femoris, the patella and the ligamentum patellae. The joint is lined by an extensive and complex synovial membrane. It is supported by numerous ligaments. Externally:

- the oblique popliteal
- the tibial collateral
- the fibula collateral.

Internally:

- the anterior cruciate
- the posterior cruciate
- the coronary.

The joint also relies heavily on the powerful surrounding muscles for its stability.

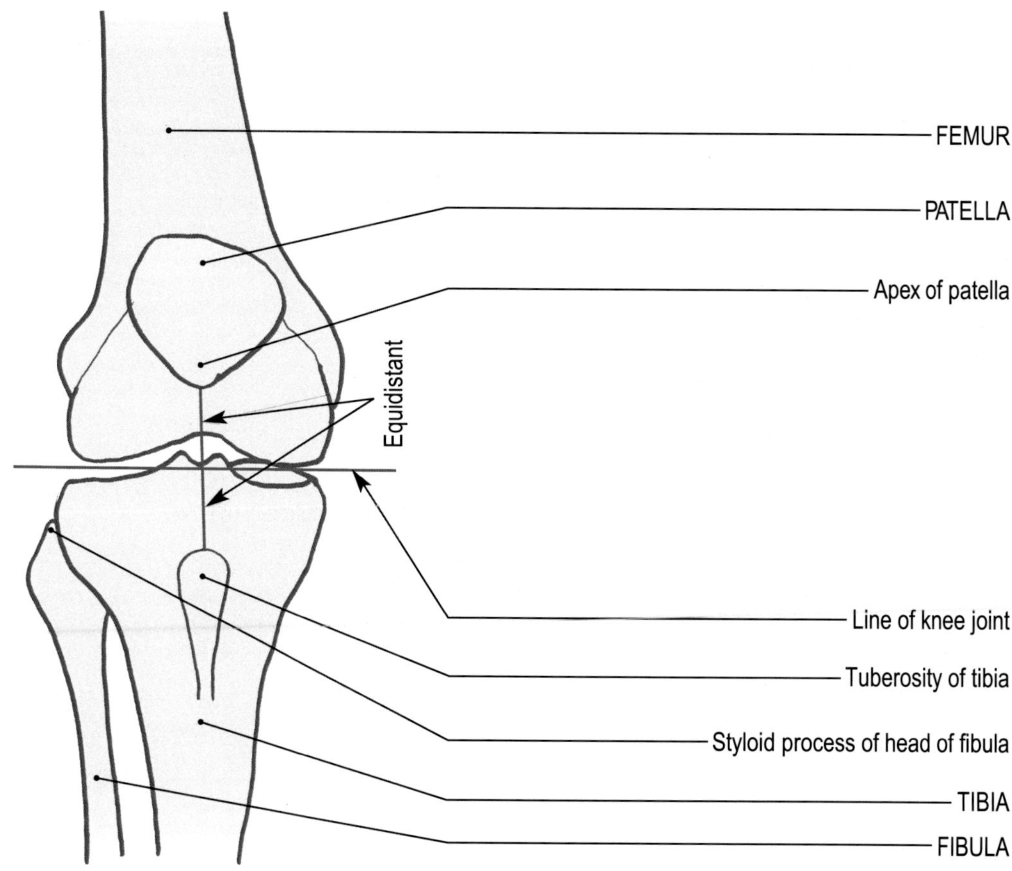

Fig. 3.10 (b) The right knee joint (anterior aspect)

The patellofemoral joint is anterior to the condylar section. This is between the posterior surface of the patella and the patellar surface of the femur. It is a synovial plane joint. Whilst it is separate from the knee joint, it shares the same joint space and synovial membrane.

The knee joint appears at first sight to be a very unstable joint with the two rounded condyles of the femur sitting on top of the two flattened surfaces of the tibia. This, however, is not so. This joint rarely dislocates and even then only under extreme force, such as a car or aeroplane crash. It is, however, subject to many stresses and strains, particularly in sport.

Palpation: surface marking

For palpation in this region, the model is in the sitting position with the leg dependent.

- The knee joint (Fig. 3.10b, d). Draw a line which bisects the ligamentum patellae horizontally **halfway between the lower tip of the patella and the tibial tuberosity**.
- Alternative method. Draw a line horizontally 1 cm above the tip of the styloid process of the fibula.

Palpation

- The menisci. Place your fingers on either side of the ligamentum patellae. Identify two triangular depressions. These are bounded by the tibia below, the femur above and the ligamentum patellae centrally. Locate the apex of the depression with the knee joint space running horizontally. Your fingers are now resting against the anterior aspect of the medial and lateral menisci. Ask the model to rotate the knee medially and laterally. Palpate the menisci moving forwards during rotation at the joint. The lateral meniscus moves on lateral rotation; the medial meniscus moves on medial rotation.
- Lateral aspect. Trace the joint posteriorly. Notice that the space becomes narrower until just behind the mid point, where it becomes hidden by the medial collateral ligament medially and the lateral part of the joint capsule laterally.
- **Note 1.** Posteriorly, the joint is impossible to palpate due to the presence of muscle, tendon and fascial coverings.
- **Note 2** (Fig. 3.10f). The joint can be represented by a horizontal line drawn across the back of the popliteal fossa 1 cm above the tip of the styloid process of the head of the fibula.

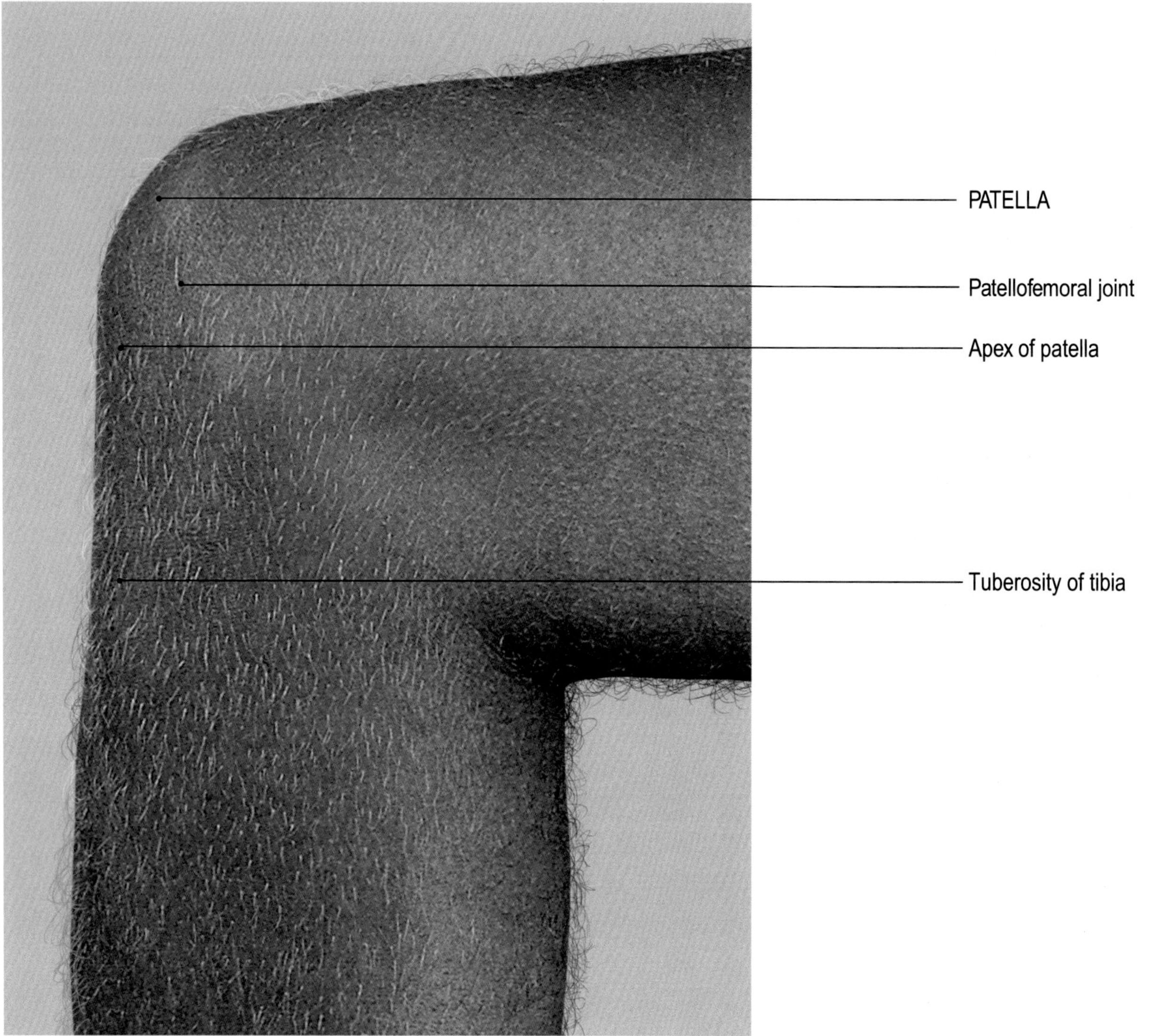

Fig. 3.10 (c) The right knee joint (medial aspect)

Accessory movements

- **Note.** The knee joint becomes 'close packed' on full extension; therefore, accessory movements should only be performed avoiding the extreme of extension.

Palpation

For palpation in this region, the model is in the supine lying position.

- Anterior and posterior movement of the tibial condyles. Ask the model to flex the knee to 90° with the foot firmly fixed on the supporting surface. For stability, you may need to sit on the model's foot. Place both hands around the knee with your thumbs resting on the tibial tuberosity. Draw the tibial condyles forwards (anterior draw test). Now push them backwards (posterior draw test). This produces a gliding movement of the tibial condyles on the femoral condyles.
- **Note.** There should be only a slight movement in either direction. Forward movement of the tibia is limited by the anterior cruciate ligament; posterior movement is limited by the posterior cruciate ligament.
- Side-to-side movement of the tibial condyles. Ask the model to flex the knee to 15°. Stabilize the undersurface of the model's thigh with one hand and grasp the lower end of the leg just above the ankle with the other. Now produce a side-to-side movement.
- Distraction of the joint surfaces. The model is sitting on a high plinth with the leg dependent. Ask the model to take the joint to the mid position. Now pull downwards on the leg.
- The **patellofemoral joint** (Fig. 3.10c, d). The joint lies deep to the **patella**, between it and the patellar surface of the femur, 1 cm deep to its anterior surface. It shares the same joint space as the bicondylar articulation. It is easily marked by tracing around the perimeter of bone.
- Movements of the patella. The model is in the supine lying position with the knee in an extended and relaxed position. Move the patella from side to side across the patellar surface of the femur which results in a rocking effect. Now move the

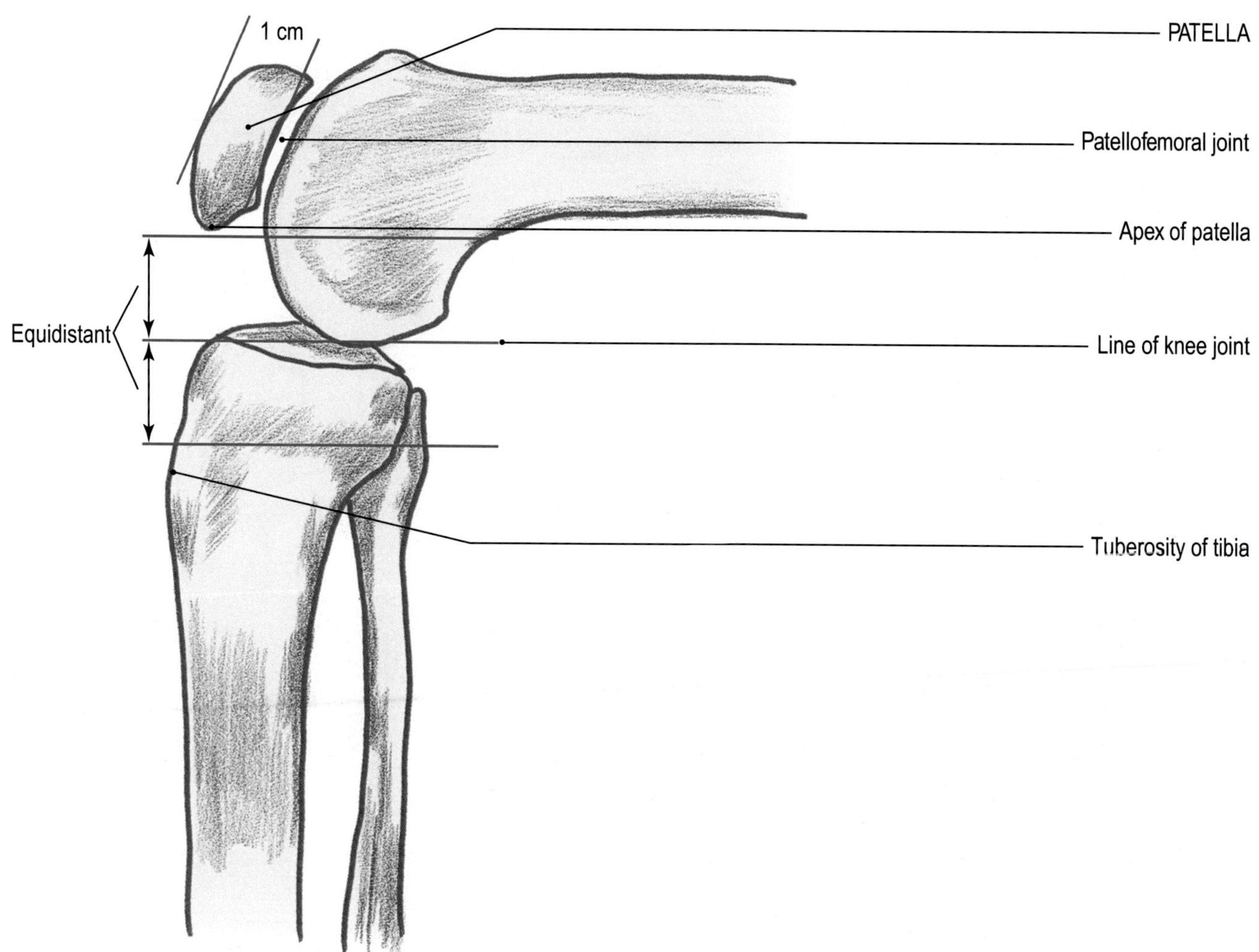

Fig. 3.10 (d) The right knee joint (medial aspect)

patella up and down as a gliding movement along the vertical groove of the femoral surface. If you move the patella laterally, you will be able to palpate the medial edge of the patellar surface of the femur. This is marked by a sharp ridge. In this position, you can also palpate the undersurface of the lateral edge of the patella. Conversely, if you move the patella medially, you will be able to palpate the lateral edge of the patellar surface of the femur and the medial undersurface of the patella.

Functional anatomy

Little stress is applied to the structural components of the knee joint, on which it relies for its stability during normal activities, such as walking, running, jumping, swimming, etc. Enormous tension is, however, applied to these components during sporting activities where the lower limbs are used for varied directional propulsion and kicking. Lateral or medial forces applied to the knee, particularly when the knee is in its extended 'close-packed' position, may cause strains, partial tears or even complete ruptures to medial or lateral ligaments. Violent over-extension of the knee may rupture the anterior cruciate ligament. The posterior cruciate ligament may rupture when enormous force is applied to the anterior aspect of the proximal end of the tibia. When the knee is over-rotated in a flexed position the menisci, especially the medial, sometimes get trapped between the rolling condyle of the femur on the tibia, producing a tear in the meniscus.

In addition to all the ligamentous problems, the very powerful muscle surrounding the joint, on which stability is also dependent, may be partially torn or even completely ruptured. On a violent extension force such as kicking a stationary object, or falling from a height on to the feet, the quadriceps femoris tendon may rupture, causing complete dysfunction of the joint.

Considering all the fractures that may occur through direct or indirect violence to the bones of the joint and the degeneration due to age and all the stresses applied by virtually the whole body weight being transferred through the joint during movement, it is hardly surprising that the knee joints are a source of much pain and suffering, for many, in their senior years.

(For detailed study of structure, stability, function, dysfunction, remedies, etc., see Palastanga et al 2002.)

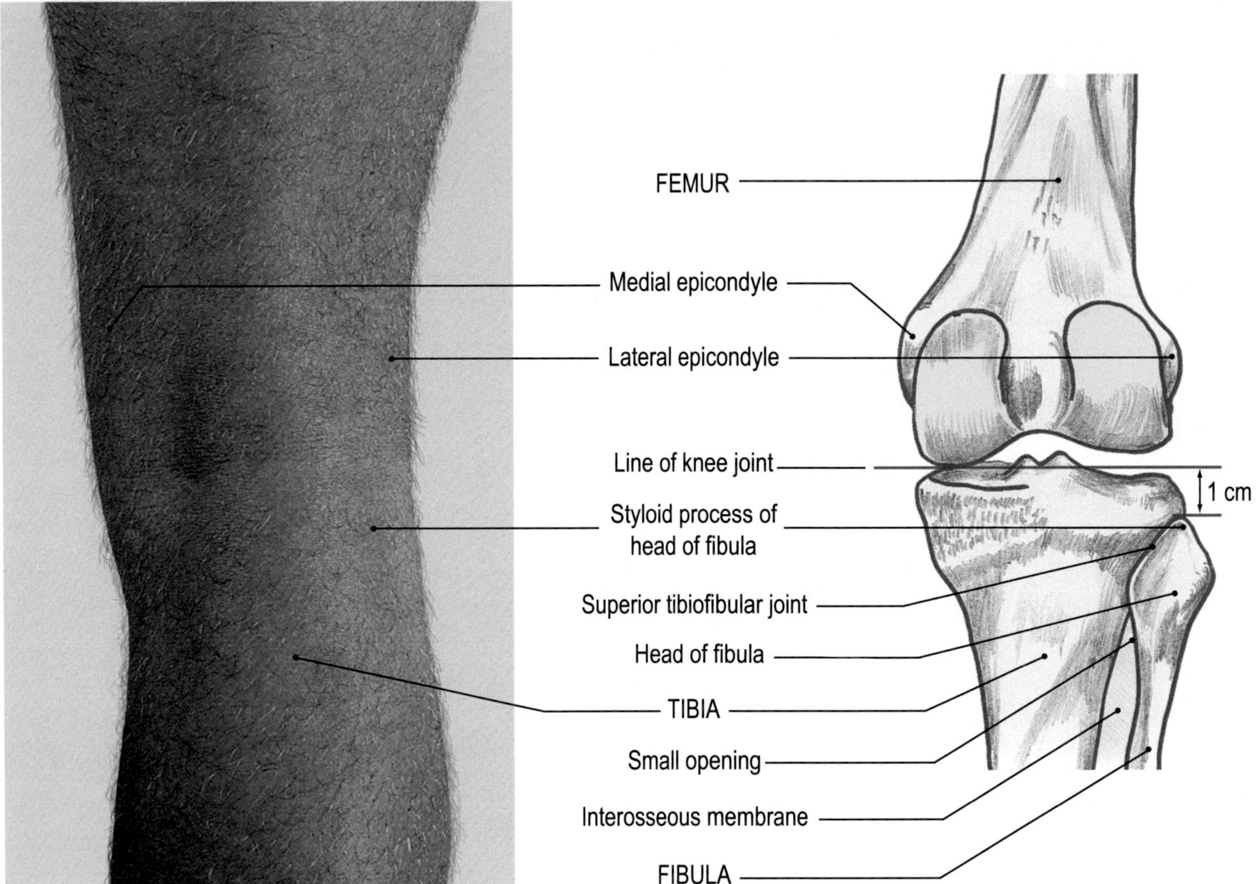

Fig. 3.10 (e, f) The right knee joint (posterior aspect)

The tibiofibular union

The tibia and fibula are united by two joints: the superior tibiofibular joint and the inferior tibiofibular joint, and an interosseous membrane. They unite the bones so tightly that very little movement occurs between the two.

The interosseous membrane is composed of strong fibrous tissue with its fibres passing downwards and laterally. There is a small opening above (see Fig. 3.10f), with an additional group of fibres passing in the opposite direction just below the superior tibiofibular joint.

The superior tibiofibular joint

This is a synovial joint, with its surfaces covered with articular cartilage. It is surrounded by a capsule lined with synovial membrane. The capsule is supported by the anterior and posterior tibiofibular ligaments.

Palpation: surface marking

For palpation in this region, the model is in the supine lying position.

- This joint can be represented, both anteriorly and posteriorly, by a line 1.5 cm in length running downwards and slightly medial to the head of the fibula (Fig. 3.11a, b).

Palpation

- Stand on the right side of the model just below the level of the knee. Place the index finger of your left hand on the styloid process of the head of the fibula. From that point your thumb can trace downwards and medially along the anterior aspect of the joint. Your middle finger is just behind the joint, and can also trace downwards and medially along the posterior joint line. This is a little more difficult to palpate as it is covered by the lateral head of gastrocnemius.

Accessory movements

Although the head of the fibula can be felt gliding up and down during dorsiflexion and plantarflexion of the ankle joint, accessory movement between the two bones is virtually impossible.

Palpation

- Movements of the head of the fibula. The model's ankle joint should be plantarflexed. Direct pressure, applied by your

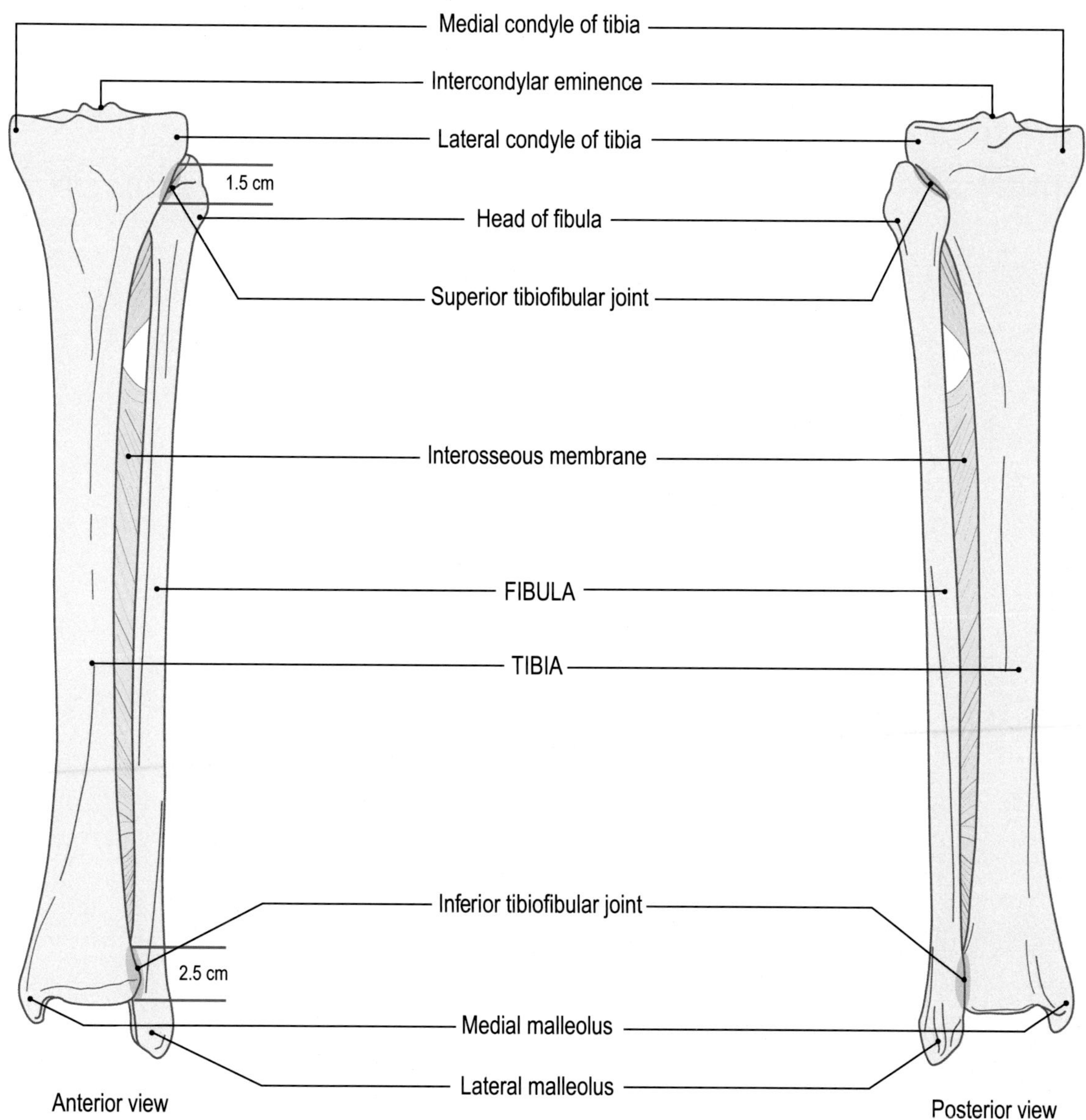

Fig. 3.11 (a, b) The superior and inferior tibiofibular joints and union of the left side

thumb, on the head of the fibula can produce a slight backward gliding.

- Forward gliding can be achieved using the same technique but with the model in the prone lying position. Extreme care must be taken, when performing this procedure, to avoid the common peroneal nerve as it winds around the neck of the fibula.

The inferior tibiofibular joint

This joint is a fibrous syndesmosis [*syndesmos* (Gk) = a band] between the lower lateral rough triangular surface on the tibia and a similar surface on the lower medial side of the fibula. The surfaces are bound together by a very strong interosseous ligament which is a continuation downwards of the interosseous membrane. The joint is further supported by an anterior, posterior and transverse tibiofibular ligament, the latter forming part of the socket of the ankle joint.

Palpation: surface marking

For palpation in this region, the model is in the supine lying position.

- Draw a vertical line 2.5 cm long running superiorly from the line of the ankle joint (see p. 110) on the medial side of the **lateral malleolus**.

Palpation

Again this joint is difficult to palpate, except for its upper edge, as it is mostly covered by the superior extensor retinaculum and extensor digitorum longus tendons. Posteriorly, little can be palpated owing to the presence of the tendo calcaneus.

Accessory movements

Accessory movement of the inferior tibiofibular joint is not possible, except when diastasis (a parting of the inferior tibiofibular joint) has occurred. It is unwise to increase the unwanted movement in this injury, as this leads to even further instability of the ankle joint.

The fibrous interosseous ligament between the two bones holds the two bones together and is referred to by some as a fibrous syndesmosis.

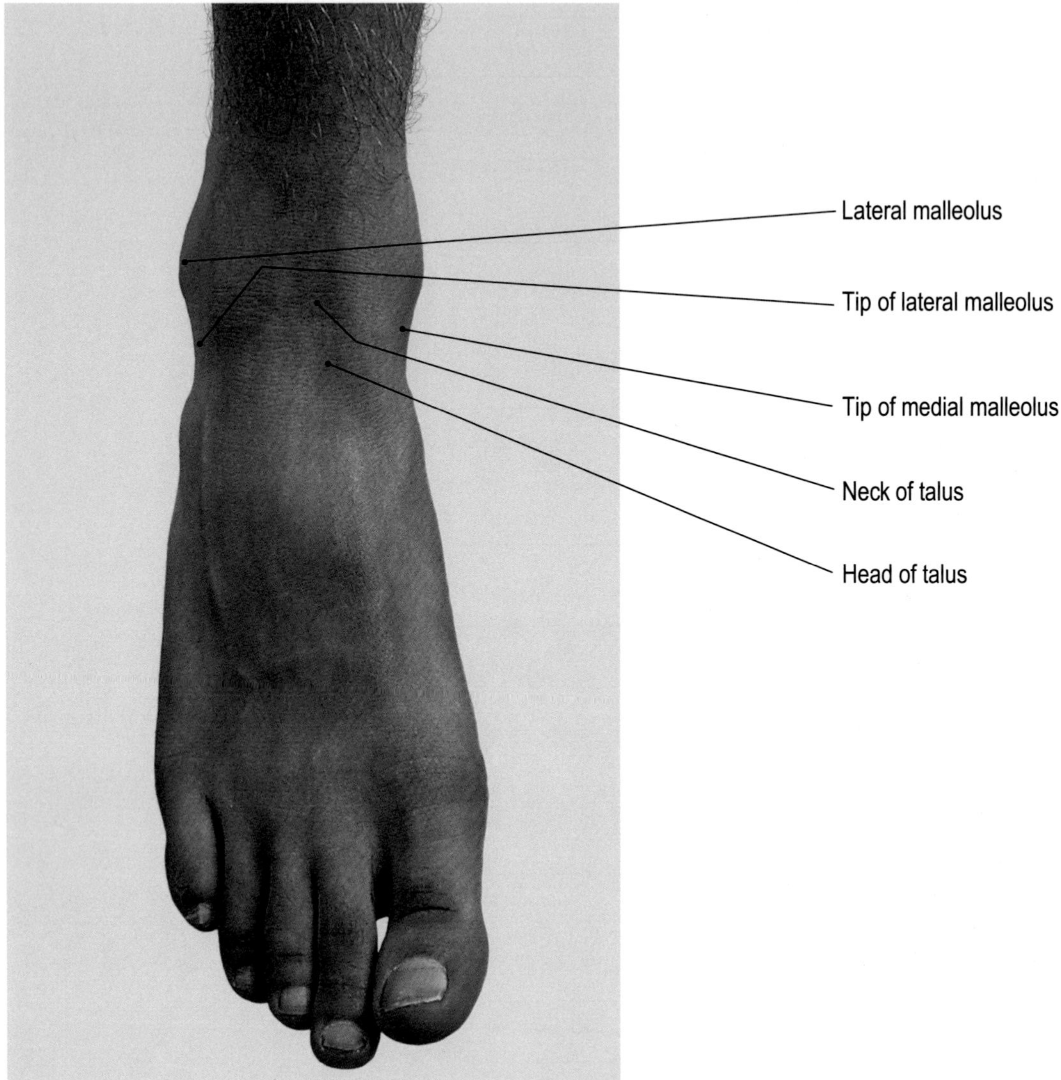

Fig. 3.12 (a) The right ankle joint (anterior aspect)

The ankle joint (Fig. 3.12)

The ankle joint is a synovial hinge joint involving the distal ends of the tibia and fibula proximally and the body of the talus distally. The weight-bearing surfaces are the trochlear surfaces of the tibia and talus. The stabilizing surfaces are those of the medial and lateral malleoli, which grip the body of the talus. The articular surfaces are composed of, above, the inferior surface of the tibia, the medial surface of the lateral malleolus and lateral surface of the medial malleolus, and, below, the superior, lateral and upper part of the medial surface of the talus. The surfaces are covered with articular cartilage. The joint is surrounded by a capsule lined with synovial membrane and is supported by very powerful lateral and medial (deltoid) ligaments. These two ligaments are delta-shaped, being narrower above and broader below. Above they are attached to the anterior and posterior borders, tip and fossae of each malleolus. Below, the medial attaches to the navicular, calcaneonavicular 'spring' ligament, sustentaculum tali and medial tubercle of talus, with a deep section attaching to the medial surface of the talus. The lateral has three portions, the anterior and posterior attaching to the talus and the middle portion to the calcaneus. The transverse tibiofibular ligament which passes across the posterior of the ankle joint, forming part of its socket, attaches to both malleoli and the lower border of the tibia.

Palpation: surface marking

For palpation in this region, the model is in the supine lying position.

- Draw a horizontal line across the anterior surface of the ankle 2 cm above the tip of the medial and 3 cm above that of the lateral malleolus. This marks the superior limit of the joint. It is continued down the medial side of the lateral malleolus and the lateral side of the medial malleolus to their tips which completes the joint line (Fig. 3.12b, d, f).

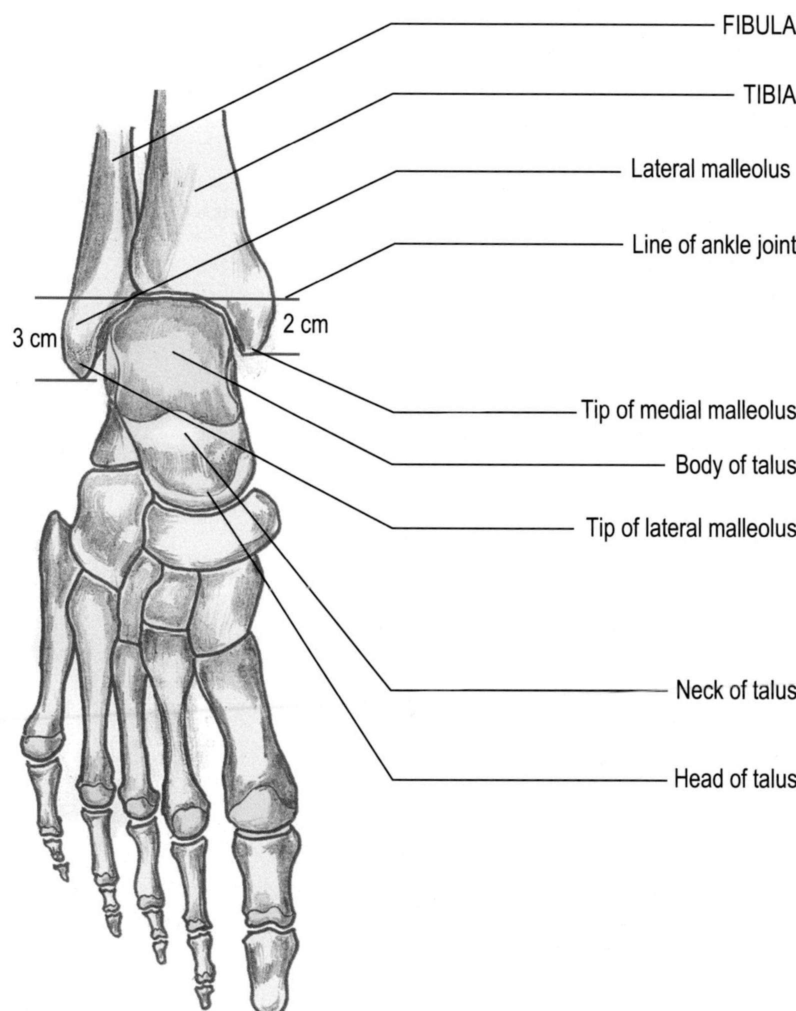

Fig. 3.12 (b) The right ankle joint (anterior aspect)

- Anteriorly. With care, palpate between the extensor tendons in the region of the horizontal part of the joint line; this reveals the lower border of the tibia.
- Medially. Trace the joint line from the anterior border of the medial malleolus down to the tip.
- Posteriorly. Trace the joint line up the posterior border of the medial malleolus, above the malleolar fossa where it is hidden by tissue which lies between the tendo calcaneus and the joint.
- Laterally. Palpate the joint line between the talus and lateral malleolus anteriorly from where it can be traced down to the tip of the malleolus. As on the medial side, its posterior border can be traced upwards above the malleolar fossa until it too is lost under similar fascia.
- Ask the model to plantarflex the ankle. You can feel the body of the talus, i.e. its upper, lateral and medial surfaces, gliding forwards (Fig. 3.12c, d). Posteriorly the joint is hidden by tendons and fascia.

Accessory movements

The ankle joint allows the movements of dorsiflexion and plantarflexion. Side-to-side movement is limited by the presence of the two malleoli, there being no movement possible when the joint is dorsiflexed and 'close packed' as the body of the talus is gripped between the two malleoli.

Palpation

- Movements of the talus. Ask the model to plantarflex the ankle. Grip the foot with one hand and stabilize the leg with the other. You can now move the narrower part of the body of the talus from side to side and forwards and backwards.
- **Note.** The lateral (and less frequently the medial) malleolus is commonly fractured by a lateromedial or mediolateral force. Unless the malleolus is replaced exactly, the talus is able to move sideways and the joint becomes less stablc. The same mechanical problem will occur if the two bones are parted at the inferior tibiofibular joint (diastasis – see p. 109).

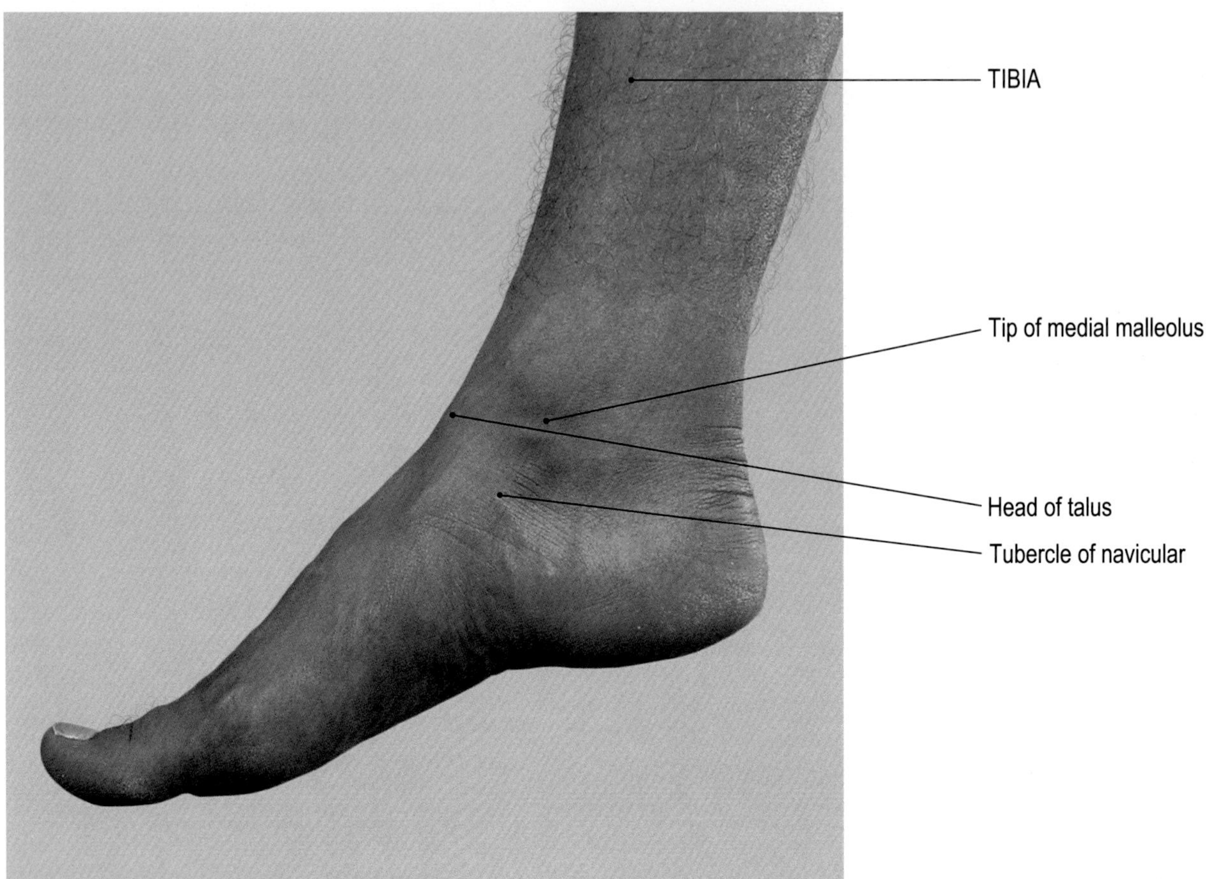

Fig. 3.12 (c) The right ankle joint (medial aspect)

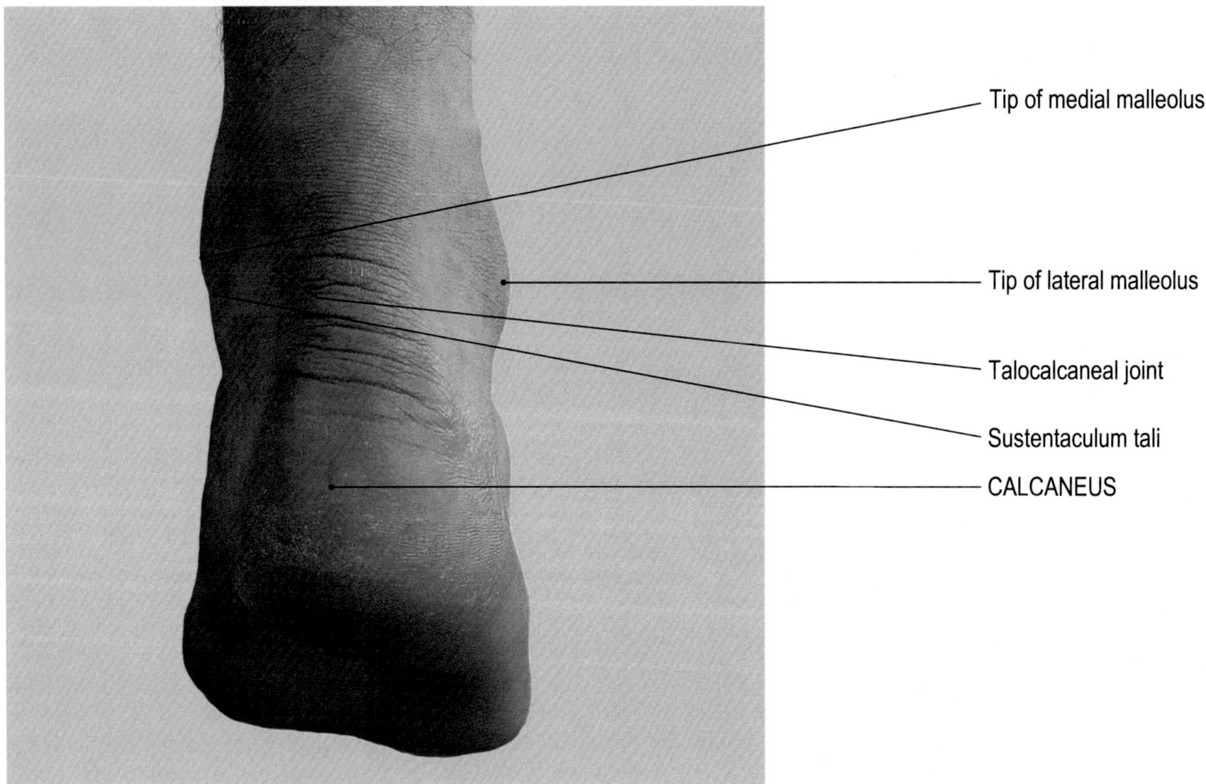

Fig. 3.12 (e) The right ankle joint (posterior aspect)

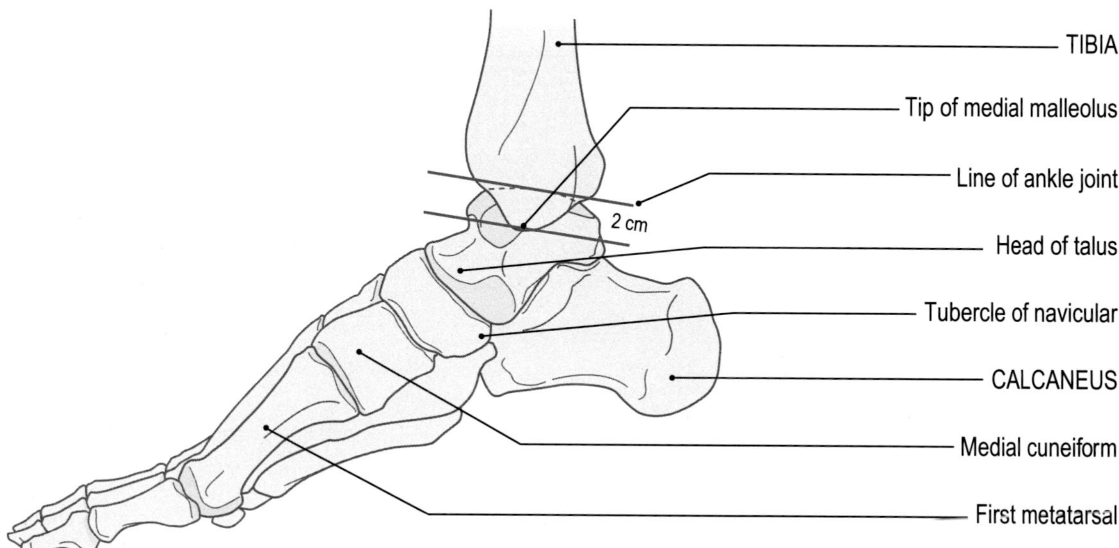

Fig. 3.12 (d) The right ankle joint (medial aspect)

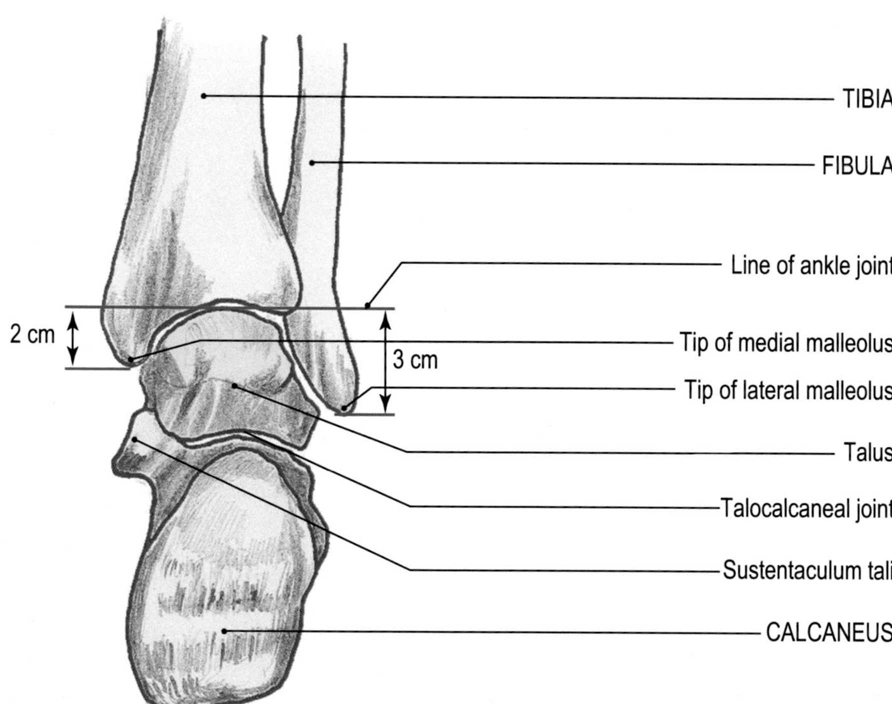

Fig. 3.12 (f) The right ankle joint (posterior aspect)

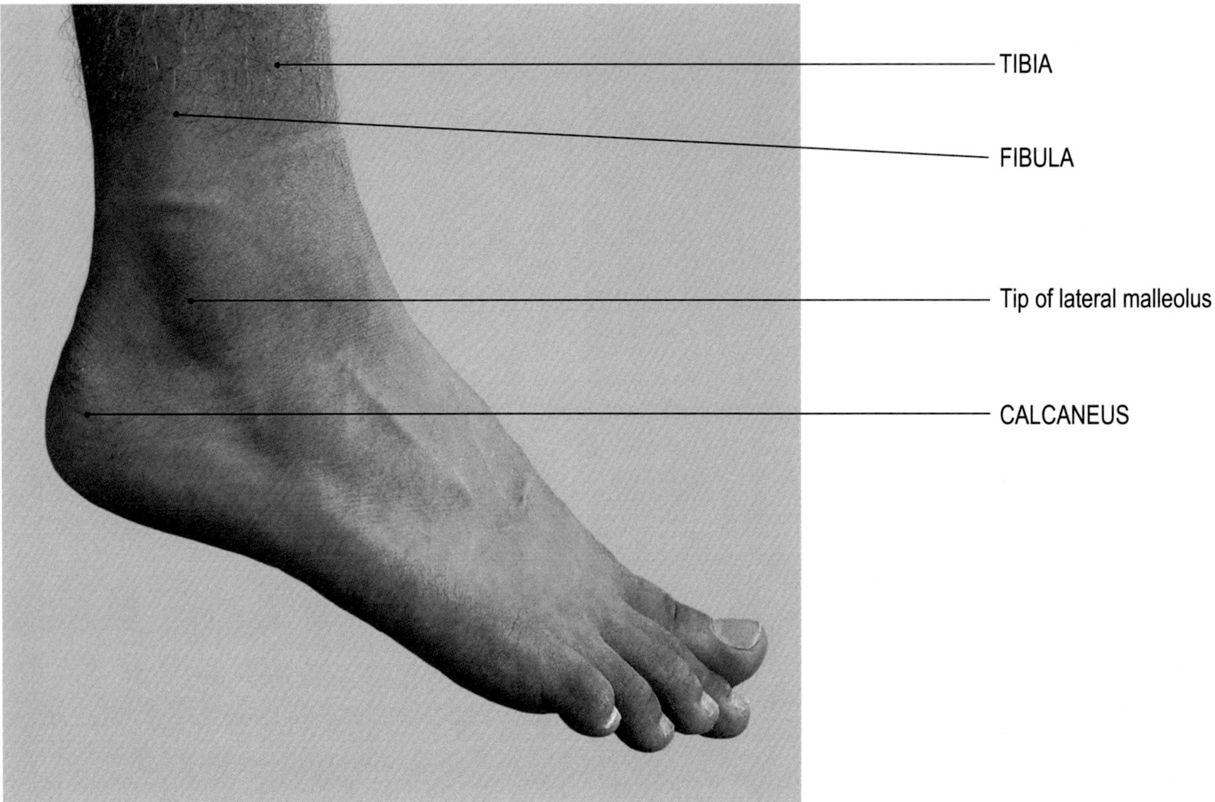

Fig. 3.13 (a) The talocalcaneal (subtalar) and ankle joint of the right foot (lateral aspect)

The foot

The joints of the foot are divided into those between the tarsal bones (the intertarsal joints) and the tarsal and metatarsal bones (the tarsometatarsal joints); between the metatarsal bases (the intermetatarsal joints); between the metatarsals and phalanges (the metatarsophalangeal joints) and those between the phalanges (the interphalangeal joints). Most of the joints are readily identifiable on the dorsum of the foot as they are only covered by thin fascia and the tendons of the long extensor muscles, whereas the plantar aspect of the foot is covered by numerous intrinsic muscles, in four layers, and very thick layers (up to 80) of plantar fascia.

The talocalcaneal (subtalar) joint (Fig. 3.13)

The **talocalcaneal joint** lies below the **talus** and is often referred to as the subtalar joint. The surfaces participating in this joint are the inferior surface of the talus and the middle section of the superior surface of the calcaneus. Both surfaces are covered with articular cartilage and the joint is surrounded by a fibrous capsule lined with synovial membrane. The capsule is supported by medial, posterior, lateral and interosseous ligaments. The interosseous ligament lies anterior to the joint and separates it from the talocalcaneonavicular joint. There is also a short ligament which joins the neck of the talus to the sustentaculum tali at the lateral end of the sinus tarsi.

Palpation: surface marking

- Draw a line across the front of the joint running horizontally 1 cm below the tip of the lateral malleolus on the lateral side to a point 1.5 cm below the tip of the medial malleolus on the medial side (Fig. 3.13b).

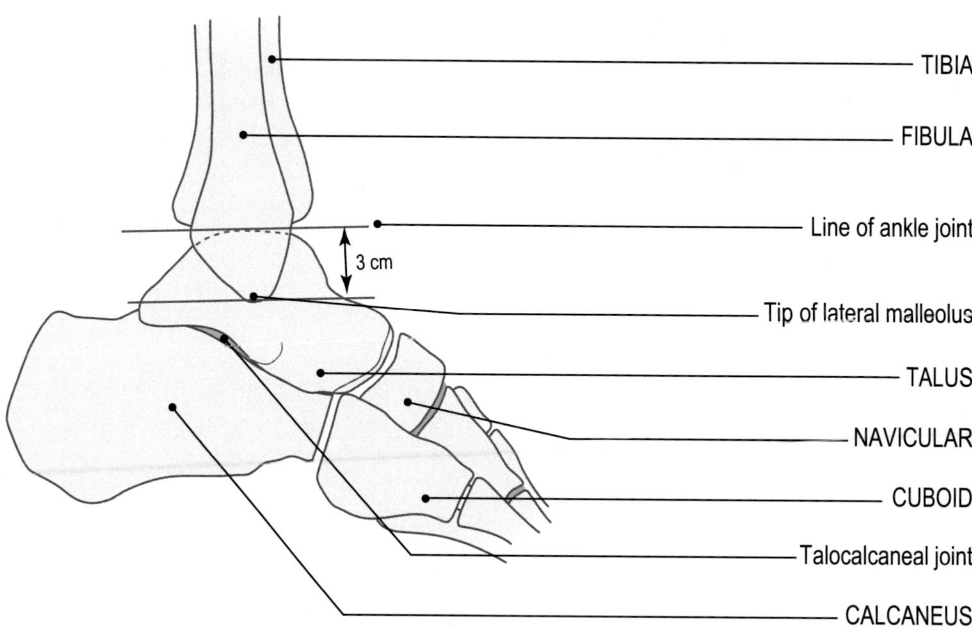

Fig. 3.13 (b) The talocalcaneal (subtalar) and ankle joint of the right foot (lateral aspect)

Palpation

This is a very difficult joint to palpate due to the fact that the medial and lateral malleoli and the powerful ligaments tend to hide the joint.

- The anterior part of the lateral side of the joint. Find the tip of the lateral malleolus and move forward into the hollow. Below your finger you will feel the sharp edge of the upper border of the **calcaneus**. This is the anterior part of the lateral side of the joint.
- The medial side of the joint. On the medial side find the tip of the **medial malleolus**. Move down 2 cm and you will be able to palpate a horizontal ridge. This is the medial edge of the **sustentaculum tali** and its upper border is the lower boundary of the subtalar joint.

Accessory movements

Palpation

- Movements of the calcaneus. Stand to the lateral side of the right foot (similar to the position adopted for accessory movements of the ankle joint). With your left hand grip the neck of the talus with your fingers on the medial side and thumb laterally. Fit the model's heel into the palm of your right hand. Wrap your fingers around the back of the calcaneus. You can now glide the calcaneus very slightly backwards and forwards. It can also be rocked from side to side, producing a slight gapping of the lateral and medial side of the joint alternately.

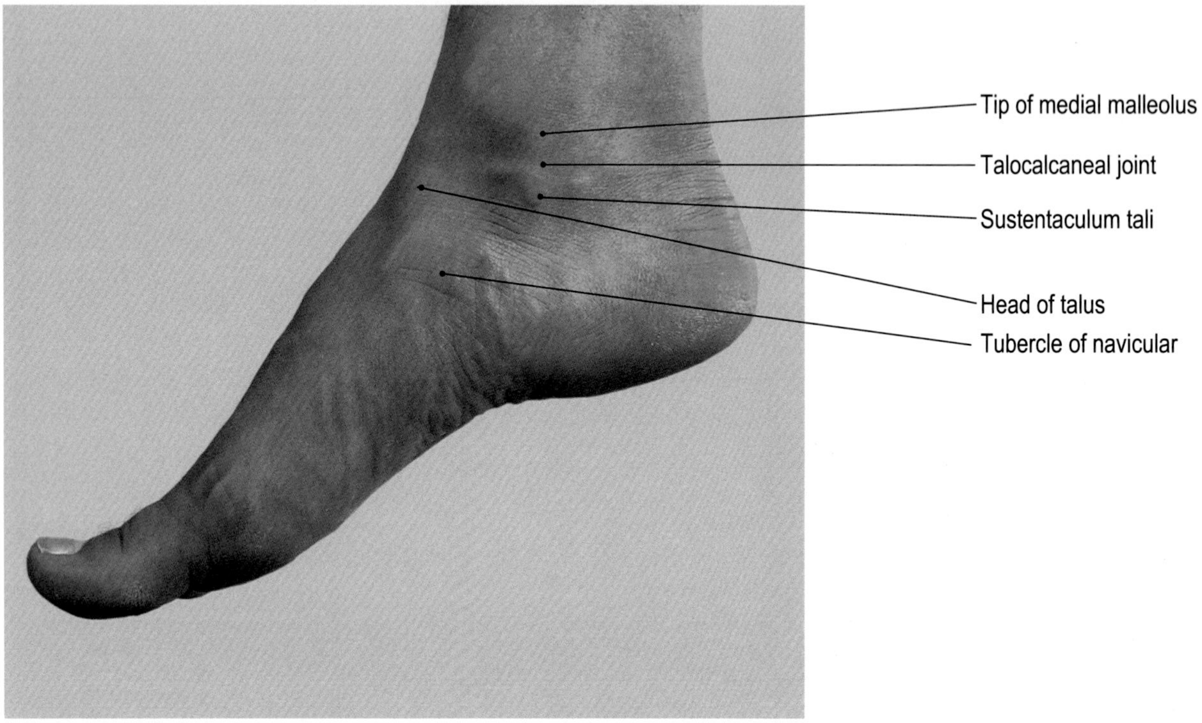

Tip of medial malleolus
Talocalcaneal joint
Sustentaculum tali
Head of talus
Tubercle of navicular

Fig. 3.13 (c) The right talocalcaneal (subtalar) joint (medial aspect)

TIBIA
FIBULA
TALUS
Medial malleolus
Lateral malleolus
3 cm
1 cm
Sustentaculum tali
CALCANEUS
Talocalcaneal joint

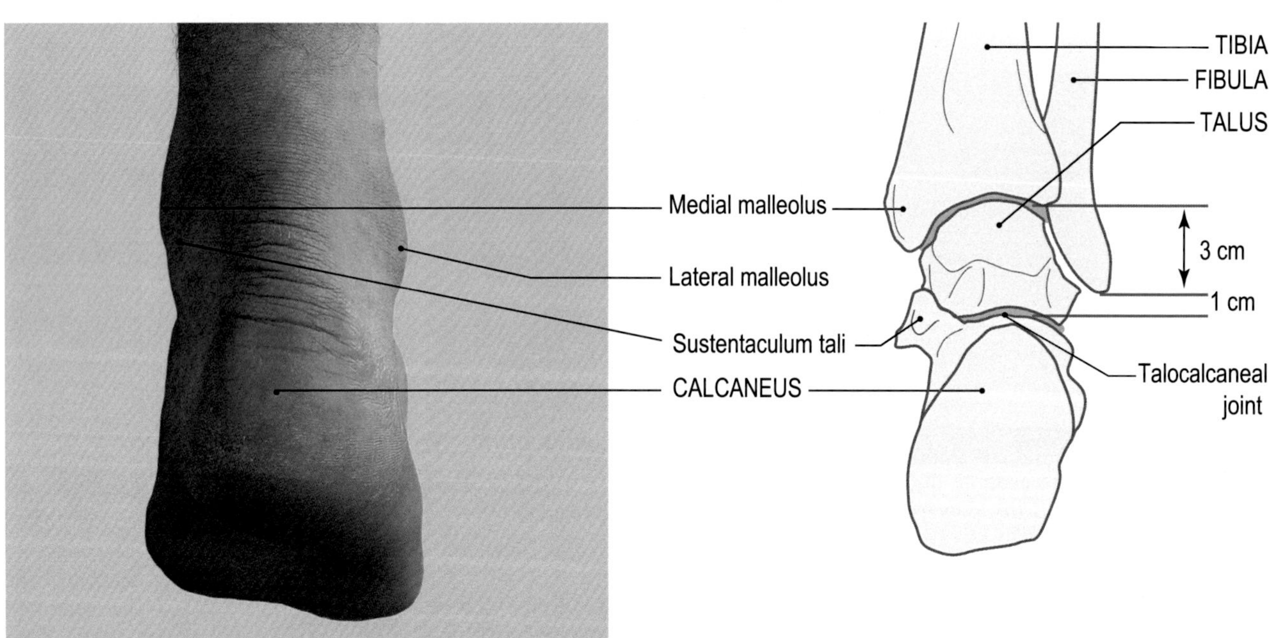

Fig. 3.13 (e, f) The talocalcaneal (subtalar) joint (posterior aspect)

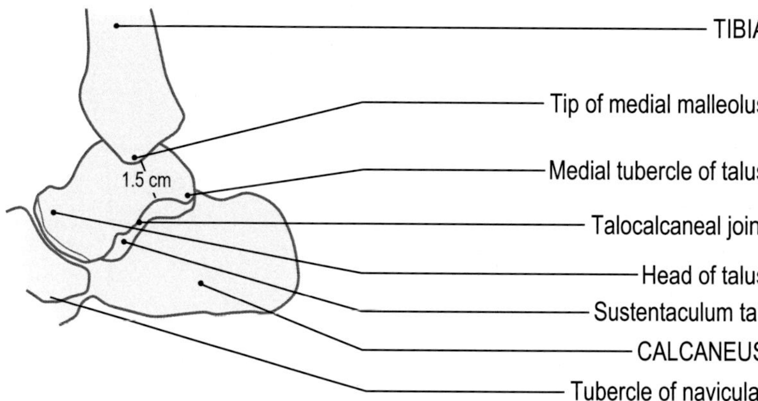

Fig. 3.13 (d) The right talocalcaneal (subtalar) joint (medial aspect)

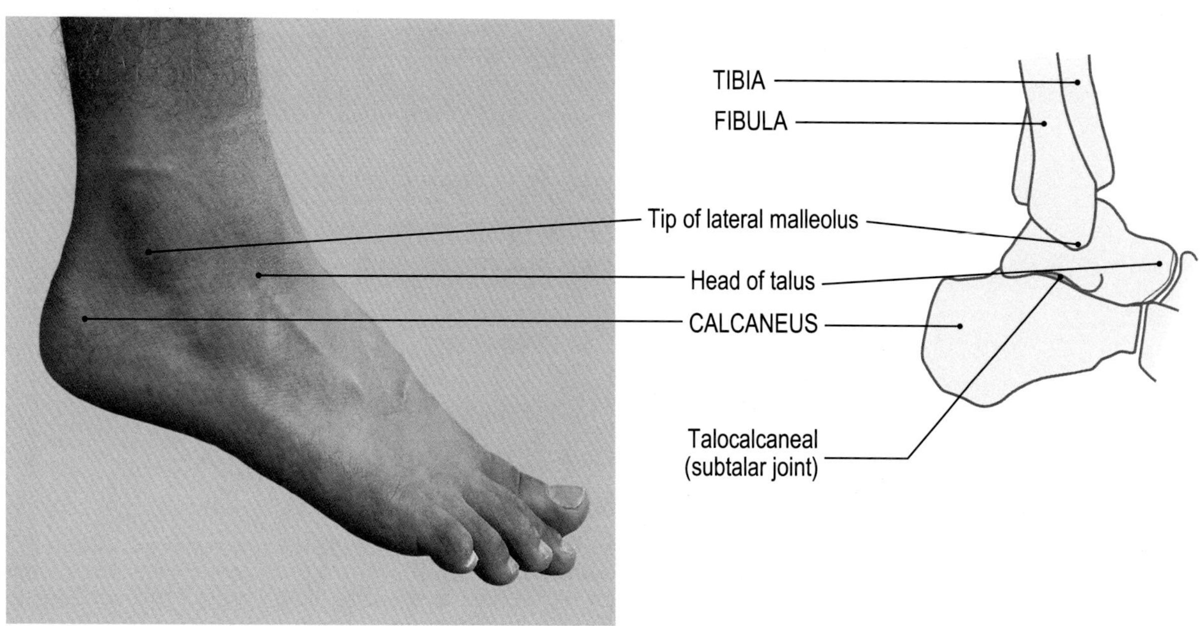

Fig. 3.13 (g, h) The talocalcaneal (subtalar) joint of the right foot (lateral aspect)

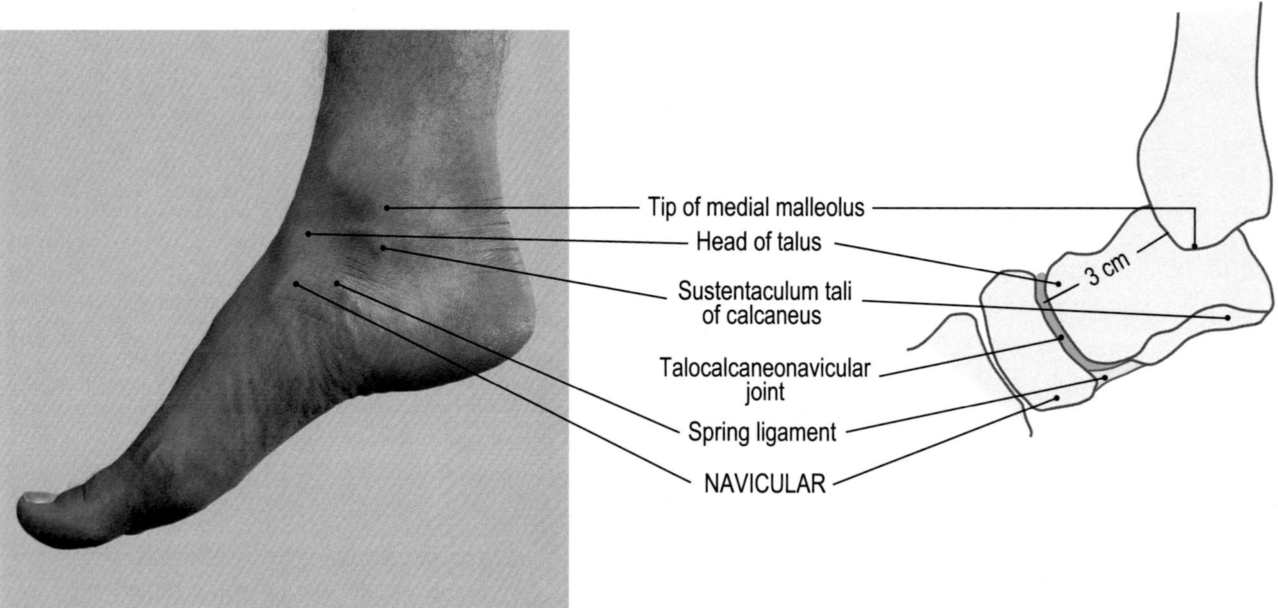

Fig. 3.14 (a, b) The talocalcaneonavicular joint of the right foot (medial aspect)

The talocalcaneonavicular joint (Fig. 3.14a–d)

This is a synovial, modified ball-and-socket joint between the **head of the talus** and a socket comprising the posterior surface of **navicular**, the superior surface of the **sustentaculum tali** of the calcaneus and the 'spring' ligament which joins the two (Fig. 3.14). It is surrounded by a capsule lined with synovial membrane and is supported by the talonavicular ligament dorsally, the medial band of the bifurcate ('Y'-shaped) ligament laterally, the tibionavicular part of the deltoid ligament medially and posteroinferiorly, under the neck, by the anterior section of the interosseous ligament in the sinus tarsi. The plantar calcaneonavicular (spring) ligament is a fibroelastic ligament forming part of the socket and lies below the head of the talus, having articular cartilage on its superior surface.

Palpation: surface marking

- Draw a line, convex distally, transversely across the medial half of the dorsum of the foot at the level of the tubercle of the navicular.
- As with nearly all the joints in the foot, palpation and identification is only possible on the dorsum. The plantar aspect is hidden as it lies deep by many layers of the plantar fascia, many short but powerful muscles and strong, dense ligaments.

Palpation

- The tubercle of the navicular. Palpate the tubercle, which is situated 2.5 cm anteroinferior to the **tip of the medial malleolus**. As it projects slightly backwards, it is in line with the joint.

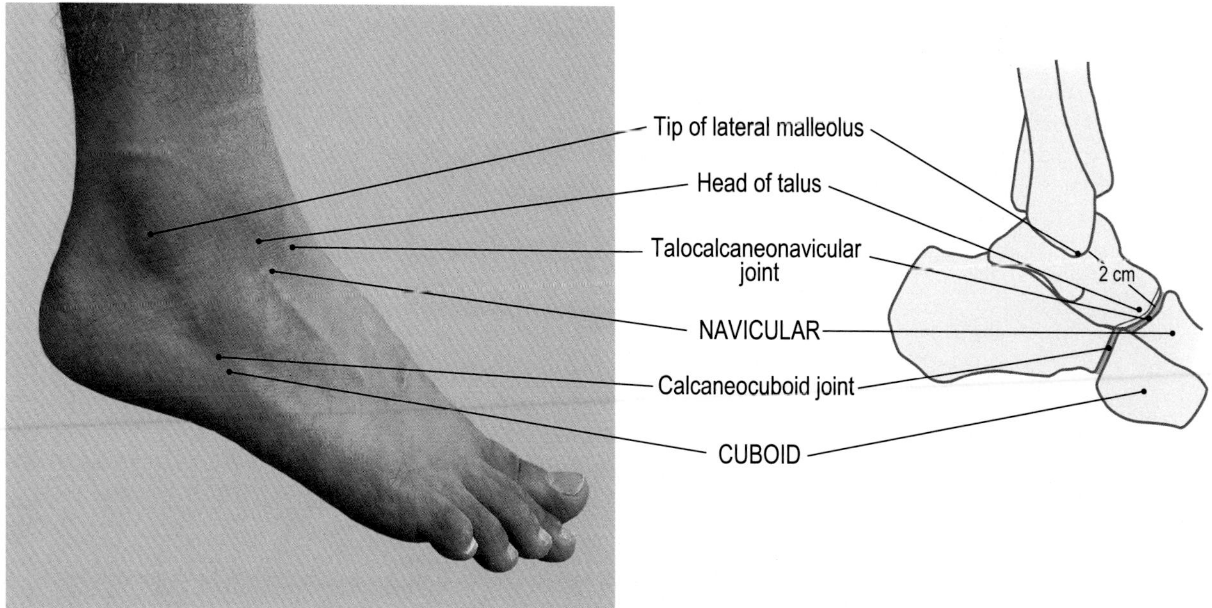

Fig. 3.14 (c, d) The talocalcaneonavicular and calcaneocuboid joints of the right foot (lateral aspect)

- The head of the talus. Trace down the proximal side of the tubercle of the navicular to a small gap underneath, housing the 'spring' ligament.
- The sustentaculum tali of the calcaneus. Palpate the anterior section of the sustentaculum tali posterior to the gap.
- The joint line. Ask the model to hold the foot in slight plantar-flexion with the muscles relaxed. You can now trace the joint across the dorsum of the foot almost to the mid point where the head of the talus and the navicular dip towards the bifurcate ligament.
- Note. The tendons of tibialis anterior and extensor hallucis longus may have to be moved to the side to follow the line clearly.

Accessory movements

Palpation

- Gliding. Stand on the lateral side of the model's foot. With your proximal hand, stabilize the talus from the medial side with your fingers on the plantar and your thumb on the dorsal aspect. With your distal hand, grasp the forefoot as far back-wards as the navicular, again with your fingers on the plantar and thumb on the dorsal aspect. You can now obtain slight up-and-down gliding of the navicular on the head of the talus.
- Rotation of the forefoot on the head of the talus. This is also possible using the same hand position as described above, but this movement normally occurs during inversion and eversion.

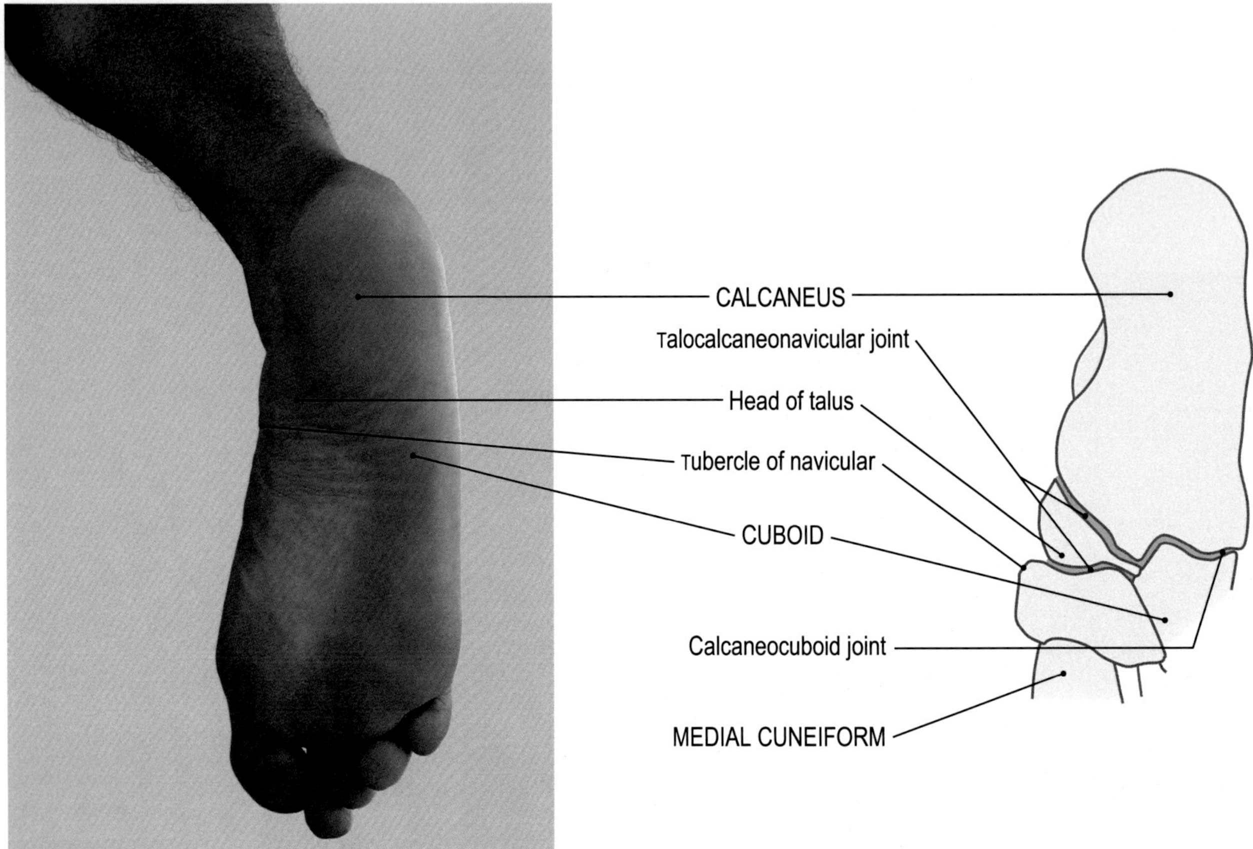

Fig. 3.14 (e, f) The talocalcaneonavicular and calcaneocuboid joint of the right foot (plantar aspect)

The calcaneocuboid joint (Fig. 3.14e, f)

This is a synovial, plane joint between the quadrilateral anterior surface of the calcaneus and the posterior surface of the cuboid. Both surfaces are covered with articular cartilage and the joint is surrounded by a capsule, lined with synovial membrane. It is supported by the lateral portion of the bifurcate ligament medially, by the dorsal calcaneocuboid ligament and by the plantar calcaneocuboid and long plantar ligaments inferiorly.

Palpation: surface marking

- The line of the joint is just proximal to the tubercle of the fifth metatarsal bone on the lateral and dorsal aspect of the base of the foot. It is slightly concave forwards.

Palpation

This joint is difficult to identify, although certain landmarks can be palpated.

- The anterior border of the superior surface of the calcaneus. From the tip of the tubercle of the fifth metatarsal move dorsally 2 cm. Just proximal to your finger, you will feel the anterior border of the superior surface of the calcaneus. This is 2 cm anterior to the tip of the lateral malleolus. Trace the border medially until it dips towards the bifurcate ligament. Trace it laterally to the anterior border of the lateral surface almost down to the tubercle.

Accessory movements

This plane synovial joint allows slight upward movement during eversion and slight downward movement during inversion accompanying the rotation of the navicular on the **head of the talus**. This movement is physiological and its loss would severely interfere with the functional movement of the foot.

Palpation

- Upward and downward movement with rotation of the navicular on the head of the talus. Stand to the right of the model's right foot. With your left hand, stabilize the talus and **calcaneus** by gripping below the two malleoli with your fingers on the inside and your thumb on the outside. With your right hand, grasp the cuboid with your thumb on the dorsum and your index and middle fingers underneath. Now move the cuboid up and down.
- **Note.** Only slight movement will be present.

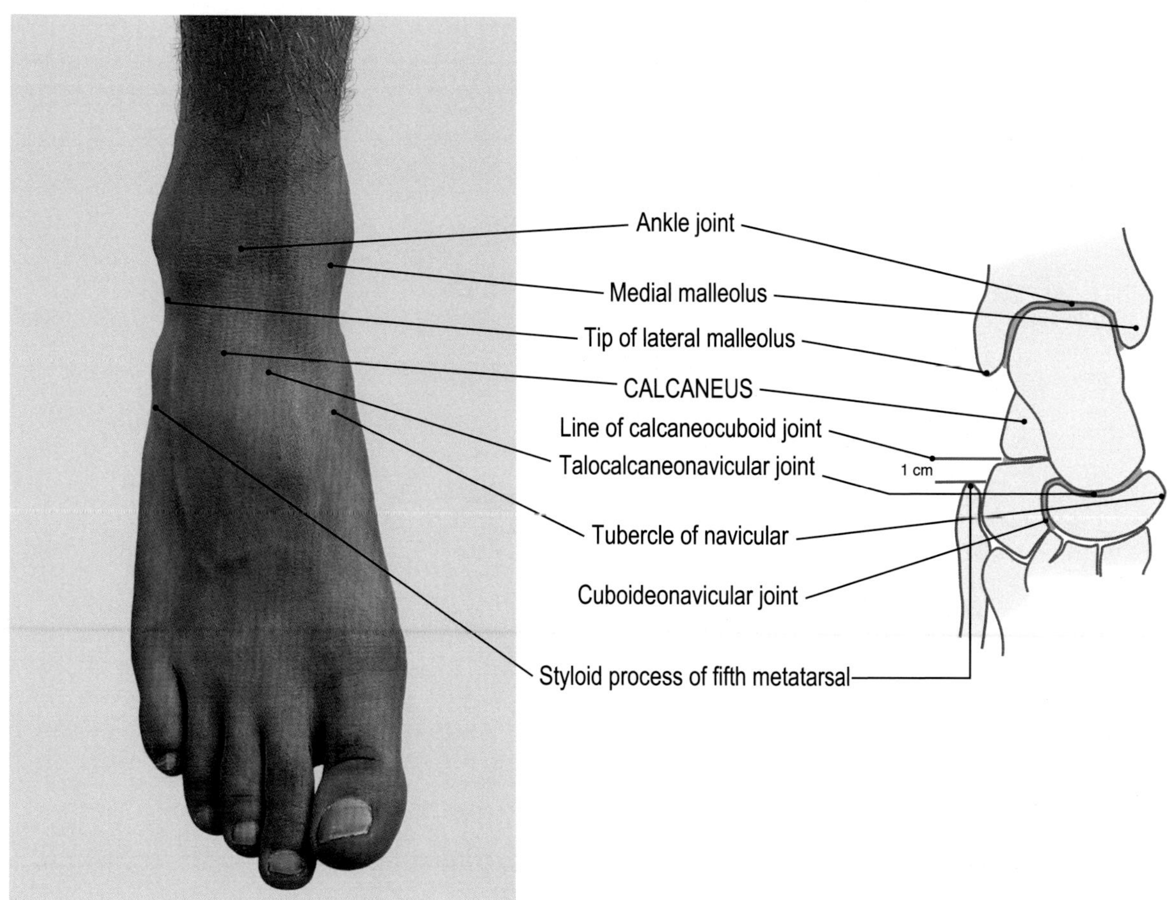

Fig. 3.14 (g, h) The midtarsal joint of the right foot (dorsal aspect)

The cuboideonavicular joint (Fig. 3.14h)

This joint between the navicular and the cuboid is normally a syndesmosis. The articular surfaces are joined entirely by a strong fibrous interosseous ligament and this is further supported by dorsal and plantar ligaments. Sometimes it is replaced by a small synovial joint which is surrounded by a capsule, lined by synovial membrane and supported by dorsal and plantar ligaments.

Palpation: surface marking

- Draw a line 1 cm long running from back to front, 1 cm forward and 1 cm lateral to the lateral side of the head of the talus.

Palpation

- The joint is impossible to palpate.

Accessory movements

- As the function of a syndesmosis is to restrict movement, there is little point in trying to move the joint.

The midtarsal joint (Fig. 3.14g, h)

This is a composite articulation of the talocalcaneonavicular joint medially and the **calcaneocuboid joint** laterally. The two proximal bones are firmly united by the interosseous ligament in the sinus tarsi; the two distal bones are firmly united by the cuboideonavicular syndesmosis. The two joints are therefore considered to move as one unit, particularly in inversion and eversion of the foot.

Palpation: surface marking

- The joint line can be marked across the dorsum of the foot by drawing a line from just proximal to the tuberosity of the navicular medially to a point 1 cm proximal to the tip of the tubercle of the fifth metatarsal laterally (Fig. 3.14g, h).

Palpation

- As in the separate joints above.

Accessory movements

- As in the separate joints above.

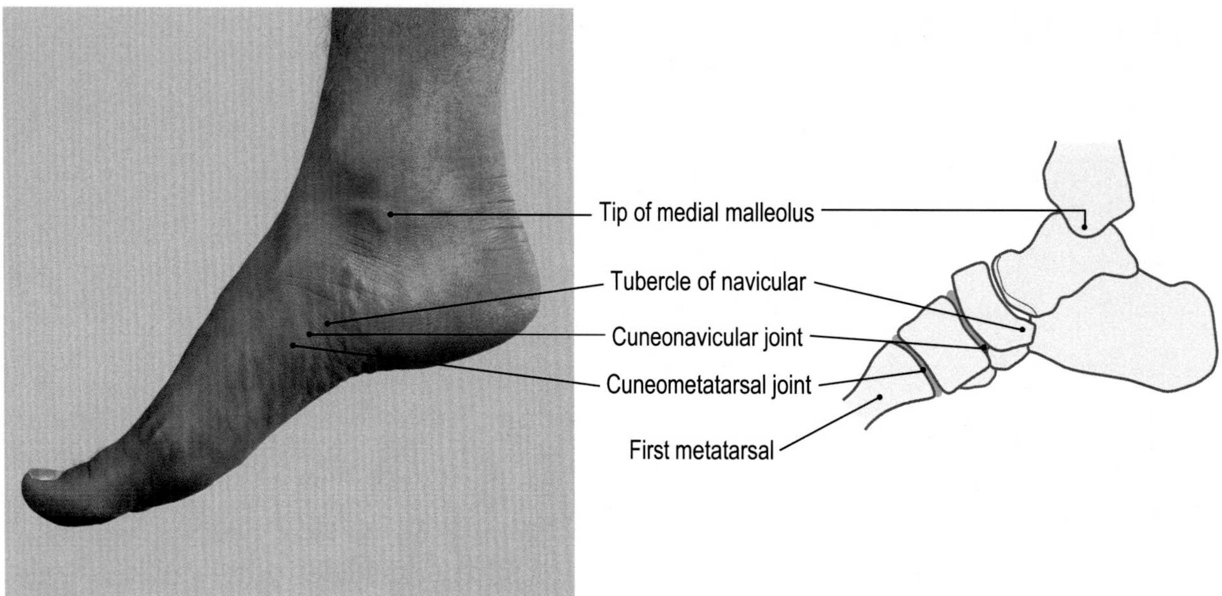

Fig. 3.14 (i, j) The cuneonavicular and cuneometatarsal joints of the right foot (medial aspect)

The cuneonavicular and intercuneiform joints (Figs 3.14i, j and 3.15c, d)

- The three cuneiform bones articulate proximally with the distal surface of the navicular by plane synovial joints. They are surrounded by a common capsule which is lined by synovial membrane and are supported by relatively weak dorsal and stronger plantar ligaments. The cuneiform bones are also bound together distally by interosseous ligaments.

Palpation

- The cuneonavicular joint. You can palpate this joint on its medial and dorsal aspects just distal to the navicular tuberosity and, with care, you can trace it across the foot between the extensor tendons, being slightly concave proximally (Fig. 3.14i, j).
- The joints between the cuneiforms themselves, and between the lateral cuneiform and the cuboid, are extremely difficult to palpate, although the joint lines can be determined by following proximally from the first, second and third metatarsal bones (Fig. 3.15a, b).

Accessory movements

The joints between the navicular and the cuneiforms, as well as those between the cuneiforms themselves, are all plane synovial joints but as they also possess interosseous ligaments which bind the adjacent surfaces together, they possess very little movement.

- Passive movements. Stabilize the most proximal component with the fingers and thumb of one hand. Now glide the distal component up and down with your other hand. The grip is similar to that used on the talocalcaneonavicular joint.
- Note. Although only slight gliding is present at these joints, loss of this movement can lead to complete dysfunction of the foot.

The cuneocuboid joint is a synovial plane joint but is also tightly bound together by an interosseous ligament, becoming, in part, a syndesmosis. Consequently, passive accessory movement between the two bones is virtually impossible.

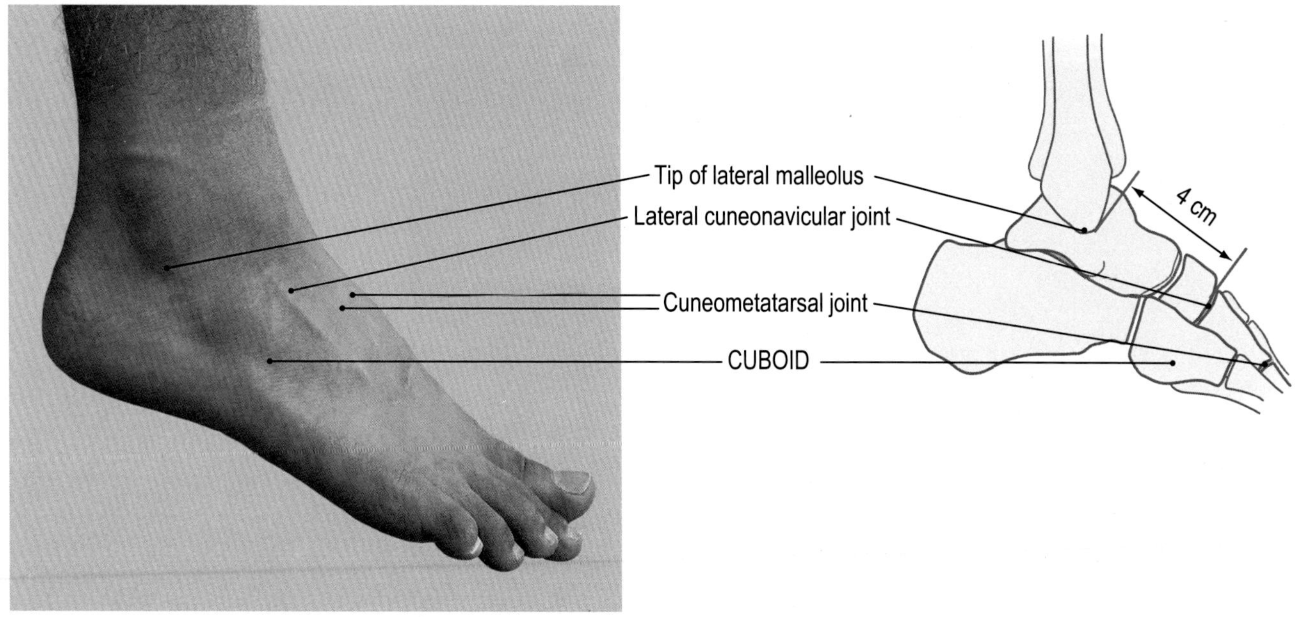

Fig. 3.15 (a, b) The cuneonavicular and cuneometatarsal joints of the right foot (lateral aspect)

The tarsometatarsal joints

The tarsometatarsal joints are between the bases of the metatarsals and the cuneiform and cuboid bones. The first metatarsal articulates with the medial cuneiform bone, the second fits in between the medial and lateral cuneiforms with its base articulating with the middle, shorter, cuneiform, and the third metatarsal articulates with the lateral cuneiform. The fourth and fifth articulate with the cuboid. They are all plane synovial joints surrounded by a capsule which is lined with synovial membrane and supported by dorsal and plantar tarsometatarsal ligaments. There are also two or possibly three interosseous ligaments, two to the base of the second metatarsal as it fits into this mortice and the other between the lateral cuneiform to the tip of fourth metatarsal.

Palpation: surface marking

- The joint between the first metatarsal and the medial cuneiform. This joint can be palpated 2 cm distal to the navicular tuberosity. It can also be identified by following the first metatarsal proximally to where its base is marked by an expanded area. Trace this line on to the dorsum of the foot, where it is crossed by the tendon of extensor hallucis longus (Fig. 3.14i, j).
- The joint between the second metatarsal and the middle cuneiform bone. This joint is extremely difficult to palpate as it is set more proximally between the medial and lateral cuneiforms.
- The joint between the third metatarsal and the lateral cuneiform. Identify this joint by following the line of the metatarsal to its base, which is slightly raised.
- The joints between the fourth and fifth metatarsals and the cuboid. Use the same procedure as above to identify these joints. Their surface is marked by a line running laterally and proximally towards the tip of the tubercle on the fifth metatarsal (Figs 3.15a, b and 3.17a, b).

Accessory movements

Palpation

- Movements of the metatarsal bones. Stand to the right of the model's right foot. With the cleft between your thumb and fingers of your left hand, grip the cuneiform bones. Grip the first metatarsal bone with your right hand. Now produce up-and-down movements. You may be able to obtain a little rotation.
- Note. Little movement at these joints can be obtained when the metatarsals are moved on each other (see intermetatarsal joints, p. 124).

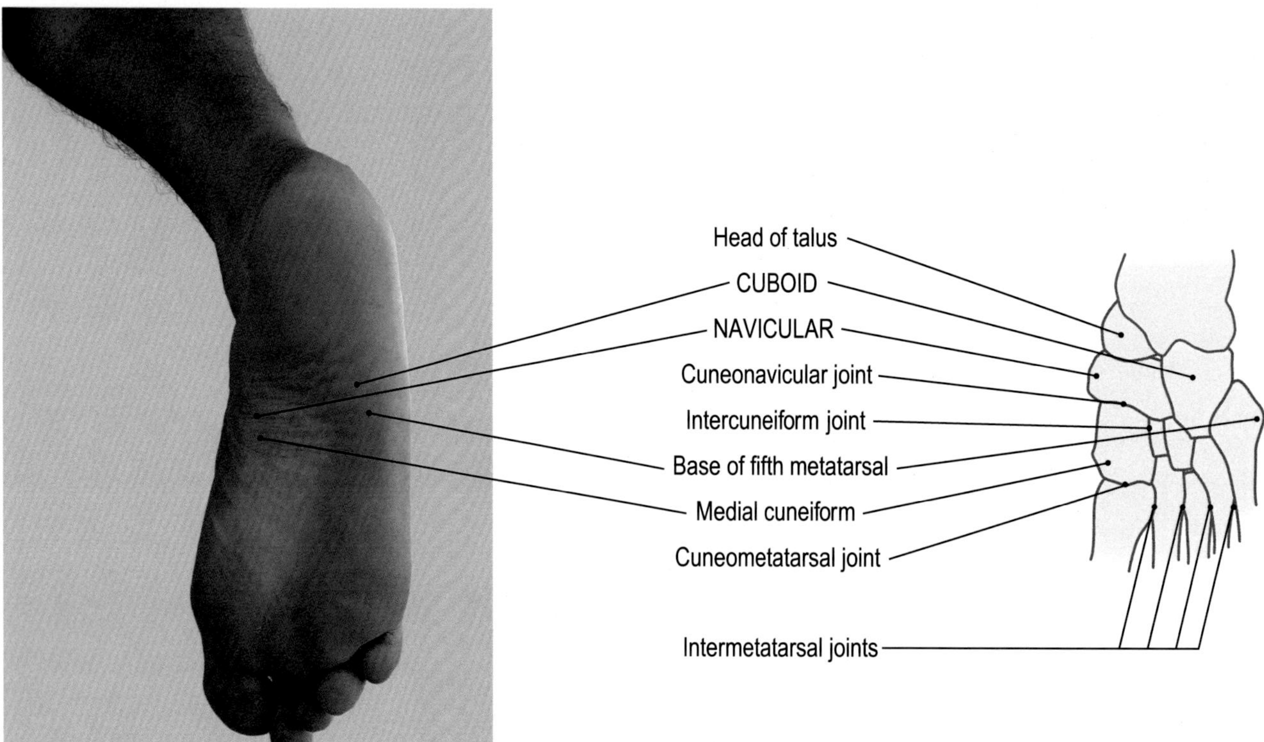

Fig. 3.15 (c, d) Joints of cuneiform bones and metatarsals of the right foot, plantar aspect (not palpable)

The intermetatarsal joints (Fig. 3.15c–f)

These are four small synovial joints between the adjacent sides of the bases of the second to fifth metatarsals. They are surrounded by a capsule lined with synovial membrane and their joint space is continuous with that of the tarsometatarsal joints. The capsule is supported by a dorsal and plantar ligament and an interosseous ligament at its distal end. The base of the first metatarsal is connected to the base of the second by an interosseous ligament only.

Palpation: surface marking

- From a line drawn across the dorsum of the foot from the base of the first metatarsal to the tubercle on the base of the fifth, the joints pass distally for 0.5 cm in line with the spaces between the second to fifth metatarsal.

Palpation

- The intermetatarsal joints. Place your finger between the metatarsals on the dorsum of the foot and draw it proximally. The space between them gradually narrows, with the bones eventually coming into contact with each other. These small plane joints run anteroposteriorly for approximately 0.5 cm, as far proximally as the line drawn across the dorsum of the foot from the base of the first metatarsal and the tubercle on the lateral side of the base of the fifth. That between the second and third metatarsals is slightly smaller due to the arrangement of the cuneiforms (Fig. 3.15e, f).
- The interosseous ligament between the first and second metatarsals can be marked in a similar fashion.

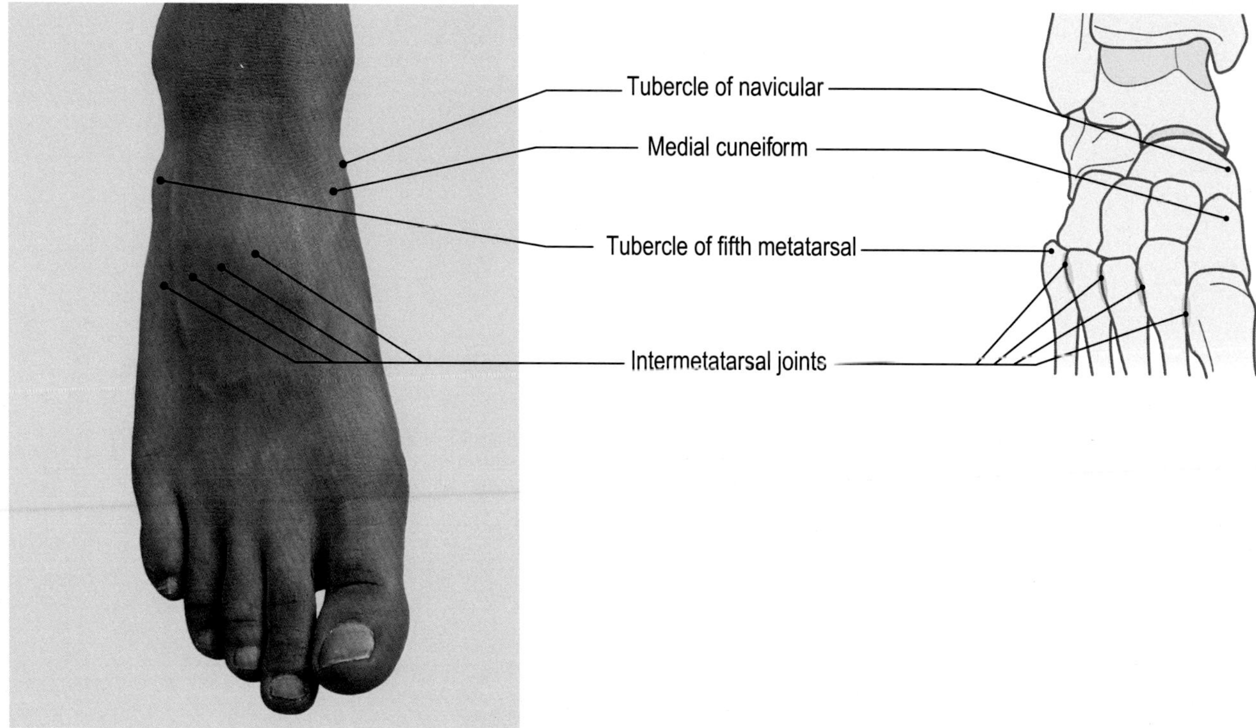

Fig. 3.15 (e, f) The intermetatarsal joints of the right foot (dorsal aspect)

Accessory movements

Movement between the metatarsal bases and either the cuneiforms or the cuboid is virtually non-existent. Only slight movements can be produced, even when the metatarsals are used as levers. Obviously this also results in a slight gliding movement at the intermetatarsal joints.

Palpation

- Gliding movement of the intermetatarsal joints. Stand distal to the model's foot. Grip one metatarsal head between the fingers and thumb of one hand and the adjacent head with the other hand. Both your thumbs should be on the dorsum of the foot. Now apply downward pressure on one metatarsal head and upward pressure on the other. You will producc a small degree of movement at the intermetatarsal joint.
- Note. This small movement between the heads creates an even smaller, but definite, movement between the bases.
- Combined forward and backward movement of all metatarsal bones. Take the lateral metatarsal head in one hand and the metatarsal of the great toe in the other. Apply downward pressure on the medial metatarsal and upward pressure on the lateral metatarsal. This produces a considerable movement between all metatarsal bases.
- Note. Although there is no contact between the two metatarsal heads, they are joined to each other by the powerful deep transverse metatarsal ligament. Occasionally this may become shortened; movement of one metatarsal head against its neighbour will help to mobilize this region.

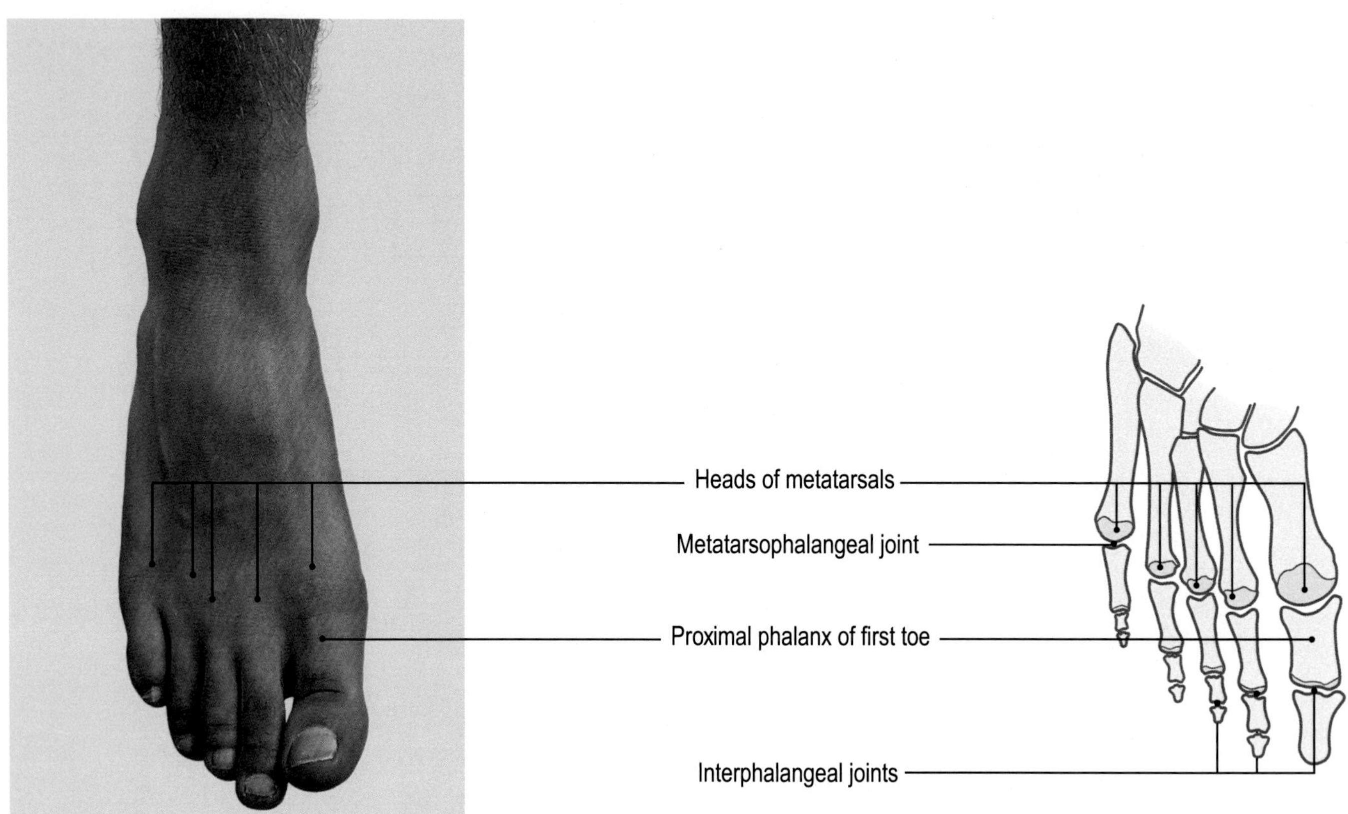

Fig. 3.16 (a, b) The metatarsophalangeal and interphalangeal joints of the right foot (dorsal aspect)

The metatarsophalangeal joints (Figs 3.16 and 3.17)

These joints exist between the smooth, rounded heads of the metatarsal bones and the shallow cavity on the base of the proximal phalanx. They are synovial condyloid joints, surrounded by a fairly loose capsule which is lined with synovial membrane. The articular surface on the head of the metatarsal extends onto its dorsal, distal and particularly plantar surfaces. The capsule is supported by cord-like collateral and strong plantar ligaments. A deep transverse metatarsal ligament joins all the plantar ligaments together, forming a strong link between the heads of the metatarsals while allowing some up-and-down movement to occur between them.

Palpation: surface marking

- Draw a line from just distal to the head of the first metatarsal to just distal to the head of the fifth metatarsal. The line is slightly convex forward at its centre.

Palpation

- The joint space. Grip the **head of the first metatarsal** between your fingers and thumb. Let them slide slightly forwards. You can easily identify the joint space on the medial and dorsal aspect just distal to the head.
- The joint line. The undersurface of the head is masked by a thick pad of fascia, but you should be able to trace the joint line, although with some difficulty.
- The dorsal aspect. Ask the model to flex the lesser toes strongly. Palpate the heads of the metatarsals which protrude on the dorsum of the foot. With care you can palpate the joints just beyond these heads.
- **Note.** The tendons of extensor digitorum longus and brevis may have to be moved to the side.
- The joint of the fifth metatarsal. You can easily palpate this joint on its lateral side just beyond the head.
- The plantar aspect. Ask the model to extend the toes strongly. Now identify the joints from their plantar aspect:

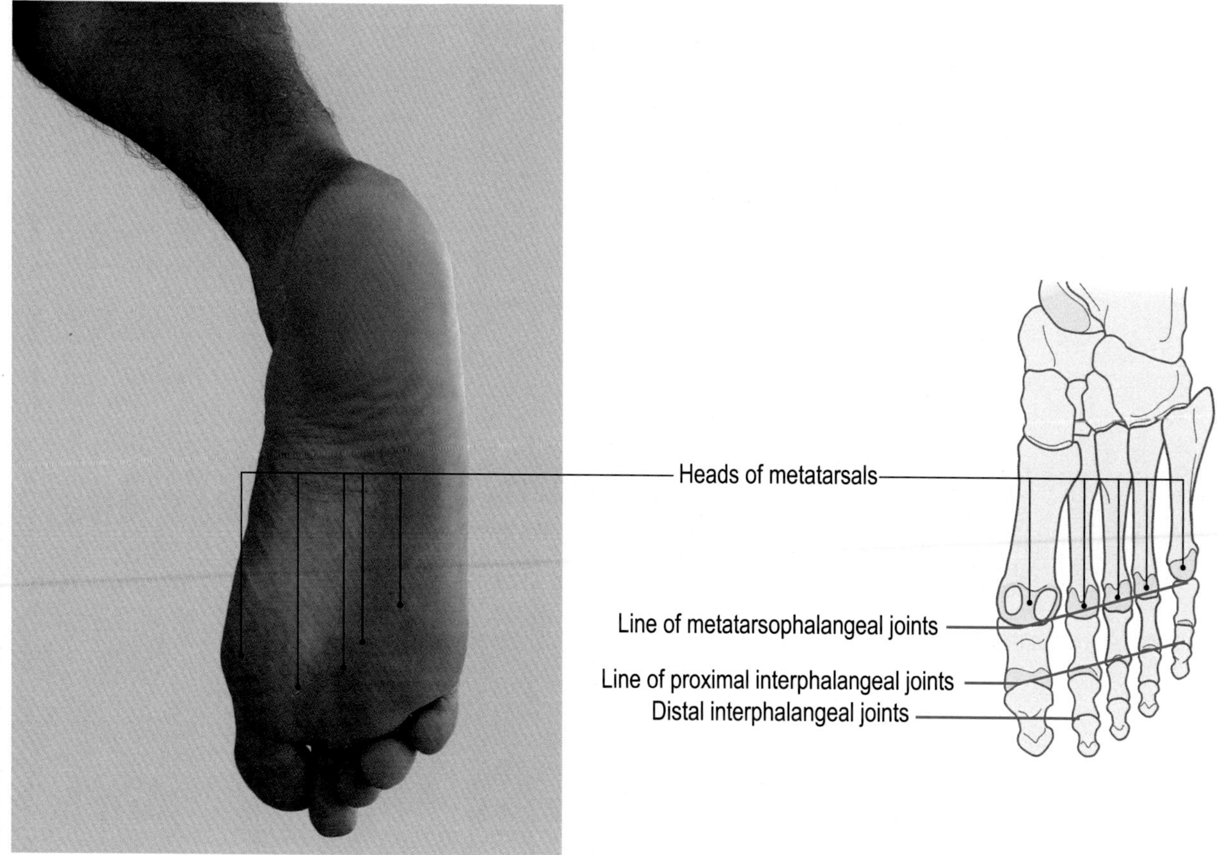

Fig. 3.16 (c, d) The metatarsophalangeal and interphalangeal joints of the right foot (plantar aspect)

they are partially masked by the thick fascia which covers them.

- Gliding. Ask the model to flex and extend the toes rhythmically. Now palpate the proximal phalanges gliding over the heads of the metatarsals.

Accessory movements

Movement at the metatarsophalangeal joints is similar to that at the metacarpophalangeal joints of the hand, although a little more difficult to perform. These movements include rotation and a gliding of the proximal phalanx on the corresponding metatarsal head.

Palpation

- Movements of the toes. Grip the whole toe to be moved between the fingers and thumb of one hand; stabilize the remainder of the foot with the other. Now rotate the toe about its long axis; move it upwards, downwards and from side to side against the metatarsal head.
- Note. As in the case of many of the synovial joints which have comparatively loose capsules, these joints can also be distracted, although not as much as the metacarpophalangeal joints of the hand and certainly not enough to cause the 'popping' sound that can be produced sometimes in the hand.
- Traction. Stabilize the whole foot with one hand and grip the appropriate phalanx with the fingers and thumb of the other. Now just apply a traction force on the phalanx.
- Abduction and adduction. Although abduction and adduction are active movements at these joints, they are often quite difficult to perform actively. You will easily be able to obtain these movements by using the same technique as described above and moving the phalanges from side to side.

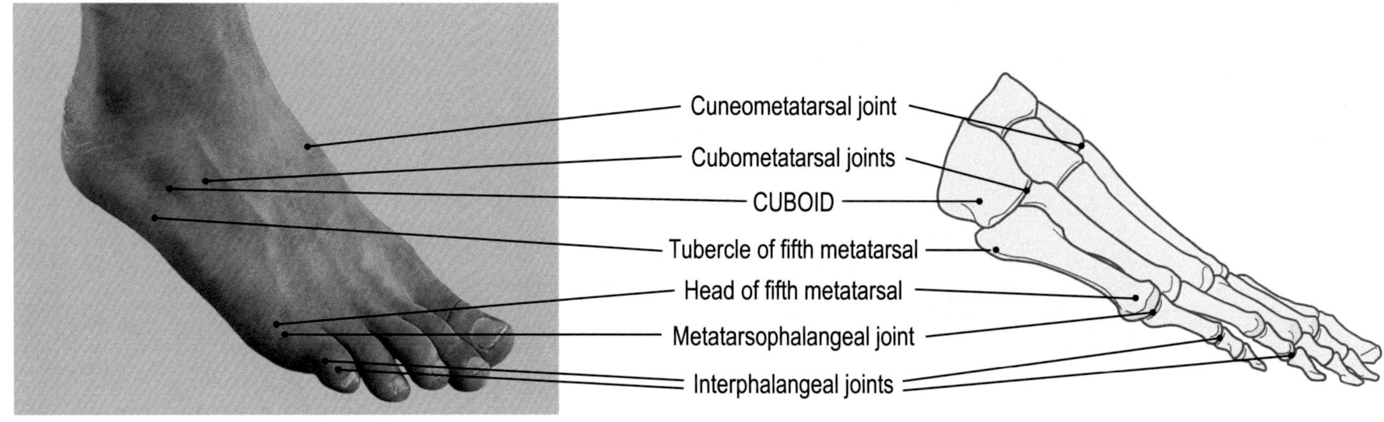

Fig. 3.17 (a, b) The metatarsophalangeal and interphalangeal joints of the right foot (lateral aspect)

The interphalangeal joints (Figs 3.16 and 3.17)

These joints exist between the proximal and middle, and middle and distal phalanges of each of the lesser toes. As there are only two phalanges in the great toe, there is only one interphalangeal joint. These joints are synovial hinge joints surrounded by a capsule which is lined with synovial membrane and supported by strong collateral and thick plantar ligaments. The plantar ligaments are composed of fibrocartilage and form part of the joint capsule.

At the distal end of each distal phalanx the joint surface is replaced with the nail bed.

Palpation

- Dorsal aspect. On the second to fifth toes, the proximal interphalangeal joints are usually flexed so you will find it easy to palpate the head of the proximal phalanx.
- Note. In many subjects the second and third metatarsal head is marked by a small bursa on the dorsal aspect.
- The interphalangeal joints. Identify these joints as a faint horizontal line just beyond this bicondylar head of the proximal phalanx. Palpation is facilitated if you grip the middle phalanx between your finger and thumb and gently move it forwards and backwards.
- Plantar aspect. The joint is difficult to palpate on its plantar aspect. The distal interphalangeal joint is usually hyperextended and, although the joint itself is difficult to feel, the movement available clearly marks its line, particularly when palpated from the plantar aspect (Figs 3.16c, d, and 3.17).
- The interphalangeal joint of the great toe. Ask the model to flex the great toe. Palpate this joint just beyond the head of the proximal phalanx. Palpation is facilitated if you move the distal phalanx forwards and backwards using a similar technique to that described for the lesser toes (Fig. 3.16c, d).

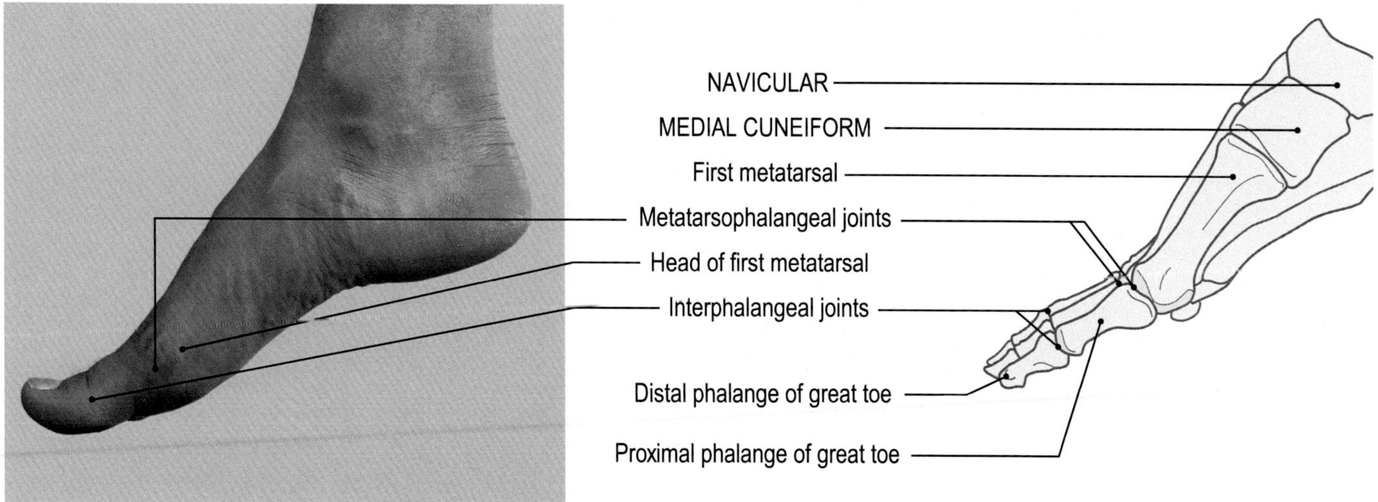

Fig. 3.17 (c, d) The metatarsophalangeal and interphalangeal joints of the right foot (medial aspect)

Accessory movements

The interphalangeal joints are hinge joints. With the joint in slight flexion some side-to-side rocking of the joint can be produced.

- Side-to-side rocking. Grasp the proximal of the two phalanges between the finger and thumb of one hand; use a similar grip for the distal phalanx with your other hand. Now move the distal phalanx from side to side.
- Note 1. The joints of the foot are generally more difficult to mark and palpate. They are, however, all important in the functions of the foot, especially locomotion. Stiffness of just one small joint may lead to severe pain and dysfunction. It is therefore important to be able to locate and mobilize all joints, noting the direction of their articular surfaces and the resultant shape of the part as a whole.
- Note 2. Most feet react favourably to fairly strong manipulative techniques being performed on them, and these combined with the correct strengthening and mobilizing exercises can improve function dramatically.
- Note 3. All the joints of the foot, including the ankle, contribute to the overall position and shape of the foot. This will vary considerably according to its function at the time, i.e. weight-bearing or non-weight-bearing, mobile or stationary. It is therefore important to examine the structure in as many positions as possible.

In the standing position, weight transference through the foot is worthy of close examination. Body weight is transmitted through the tibia to the talus and then via the longitudinal and transverse arches to the ground. The shape and position of the foot depend on where this downward force is applied to the arches and how the weight is distributed through the forefoot and hindfoot to the ground. If the weight is applied too far to the medial side, the medial longitudinal arch becomes flattened, whereas if the weight is applied to the lateral side, the lateral longitudinal arch becomes flattened and the medial arch raised.

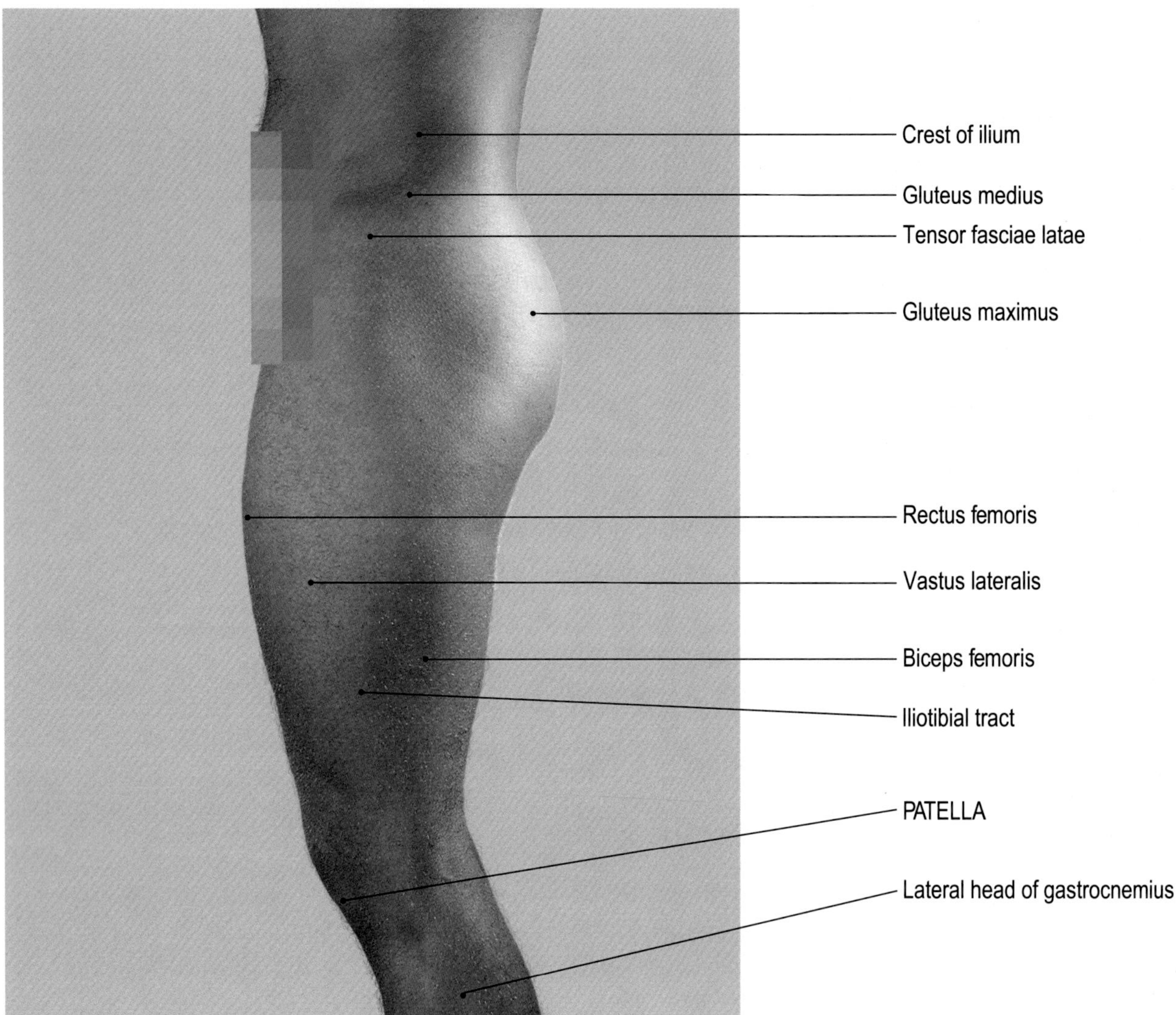

Fig. 3.18 (a) Muscles of the left thigh (lateral aspect)

MUSCLES

The lateral and anterior aspect of the hip

Gluteus medius, gluteus minimus and tensor fasciae latae

Palpation

- Gluteus medius (Fig. 3.18a, b). Locate gluteus medius on the lateral aspect of the ilium. It is situated just anterior and deep to gluteus maximus, between the most lateral part of the iliac crest and the greater trochanter of the femur. Although it is covered by strong, thick fascia you should be able to feel it contracting and relaxing.

Action

- Position 1. The model is in the standing position. Place your fingers just below the level of the lateral side of the crest of the right ilium. Ask the model to raise the left leg from the ground. You will feel the contraction of the muscle preventing the pelvis from dropping to the left side.
- Position 2. The model is in the left-side lying position. Place your fingers just distal to the level of the iliac crest. Ask the model to raise and lower the right leg and palpate the muscle contraction.

Gluteus minimus (Fig. 3.18a, b). Gluteus minimus lies anterior to gluteus medius, covered by tensor fasciae lata.

Action

- The model is in the standing position. Place your fingers just below the anterior section of the iliac crest. Ask the model to medially rotate the lower limb. Palpate the muscle contraction between the anterior section of the iliac crest and the greater trochanter of the femur.
- Note 1. Gluteus medius, minimus and tensor fasciae latae come into action when the lower limb is medially rotated as in the weight-bearing phase of walking when the lower limb is moving into extension, just before the thrust phase produced by gastrocnemius.
- Note 2. It is important to practise the palpation of gluteus maximus, medius, minimus and tensor fasciae latae. Contraction of these muscles can be identified during walking. Much

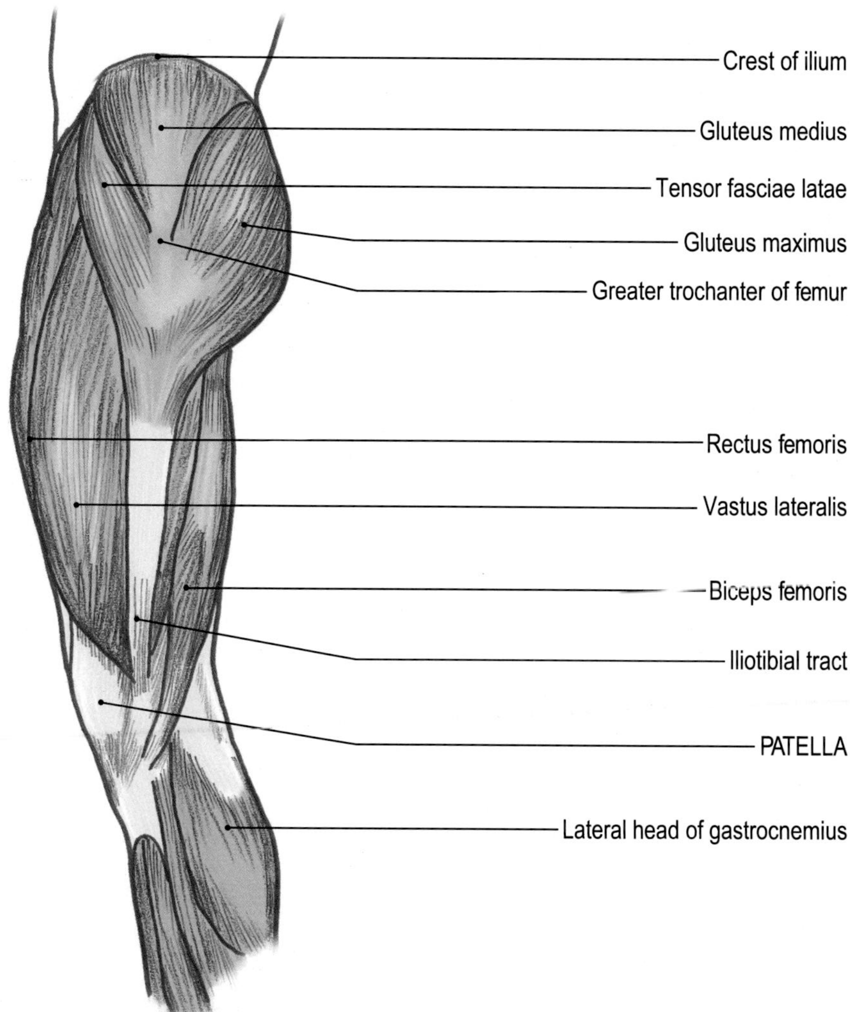

Fig. 3.18 (b) Muscles of the left thigh (lateral aspect)

information can be gained from this region regarding the relationships of the bony structures and the power and timing of muscle contraction. As noted above, the gluteus medius should contract on the weight-bearing limb to prevent the pelvis from dropping to the opposite side when the foot is raised from the ground. Therefore, the distance between the iliac crest and the greater trochanter of the femur, on the weight-bearing limb, should remain the same or even decrease slightly.

- Note 3. It is also worth noting, through palpation of these muscles, that as the weight-bearing limb moves from the flexed to the extended position, the muscles appear to contract in sequence from posterior to anterior. As the heel comes in contact with the ground, the limb is in lateral rotation and the posterior section of gluteus medius and possibly gluteus maximus is contracted. As the hip moves forwards over the foot, the middle of gluteus medius can be felt contracting. As the limb moves into extension and medial rotation, the anterior section of gluteus medius, gluteus minimus and tensor fasciae latae is contracting. During this sequence, the pelvis will rotate forwards around the weight-bearing hip joint towards the weight-bearing side.
- Note 4. Finally, it is worth noting that immediately the limb is weight-bearing, the gluteus medius contracts. Dysfunction of the hip joint may upset the precise firing off of these muscles.

Iliopsoas and pectineus

The front of the hip joint is crossed by iliopsoas and pectineus. The former is a broad tendon and the latter a quadrilateral muscle. Because they are both covered by several layers of fascia, as well as the femoral sheath and its contents, they are difficult to palpate (see Fig. 3.20a, b).

Palpation

- Iliopsoas and pectineus. The model is in supine lying with both the hip and knee supported and flexed to 90°. Place your fingers on the anterior aspect of the hip joint 3.5 cm below the centre of the inguinal ligament. Ask the model to flex and extend the hip joint slowly. Now palpate the contraction of both iliopsoas laterally and pectineus medially.

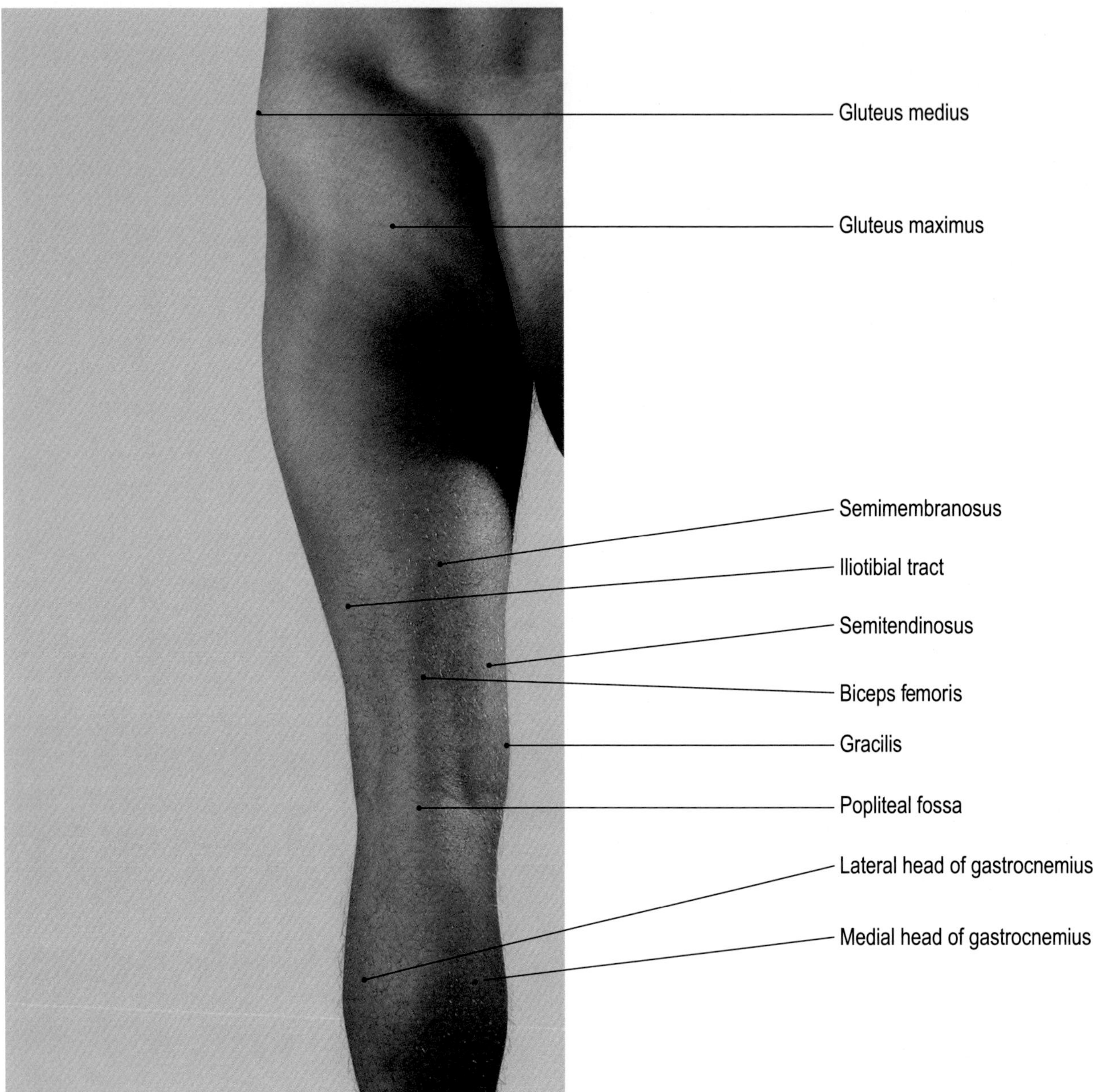

Fig. 3.19 (a) Muscles of the left thigh (posterior aspect)

The posterior aspect of the hip and thigh

Gluteus maximus

The extremely well-developed muscles around the hip joint are the gluteal muscles, especially the **gluteus maximus**, which is important in maintaining the upright posture. It is a large and powerful muscle, giving the gluteal region its rounded shape.

Palpation

- Gluteus maximus (Figs 3.18 and 3.19). The model is in the prone lying position. Ask the model to extend the lower limb. The muscle lies between the posterior part of the iliac crest superiorly, the anal cleft medially and the gluteal fold inferiorly. With care, you can trace its coarse fibres running downwards and laterally towards the greater trochanter of the femur. It is often possible, especially with the hip extended, to trace the more superficial fibres to their attachment into the fascia lata (**iliotibial tract**).

The hamstrings

- Below the gluteal fold the hamstrings are evident. These powerful muscles cover the whole of the back of the thigh.
- **Semitendinosus** and **semimembranosus** pass downwards and medially, with the **biceps** femoris crossing to lie laterally as it passes down to the knee. The muscle bellies of the hamstrings separate approximately two-thirds of the way down the thigh, giving rise to their tendons: semitendinosus and semimembranosus medially and **biceps femoris** laterally (Fig. 3.19).

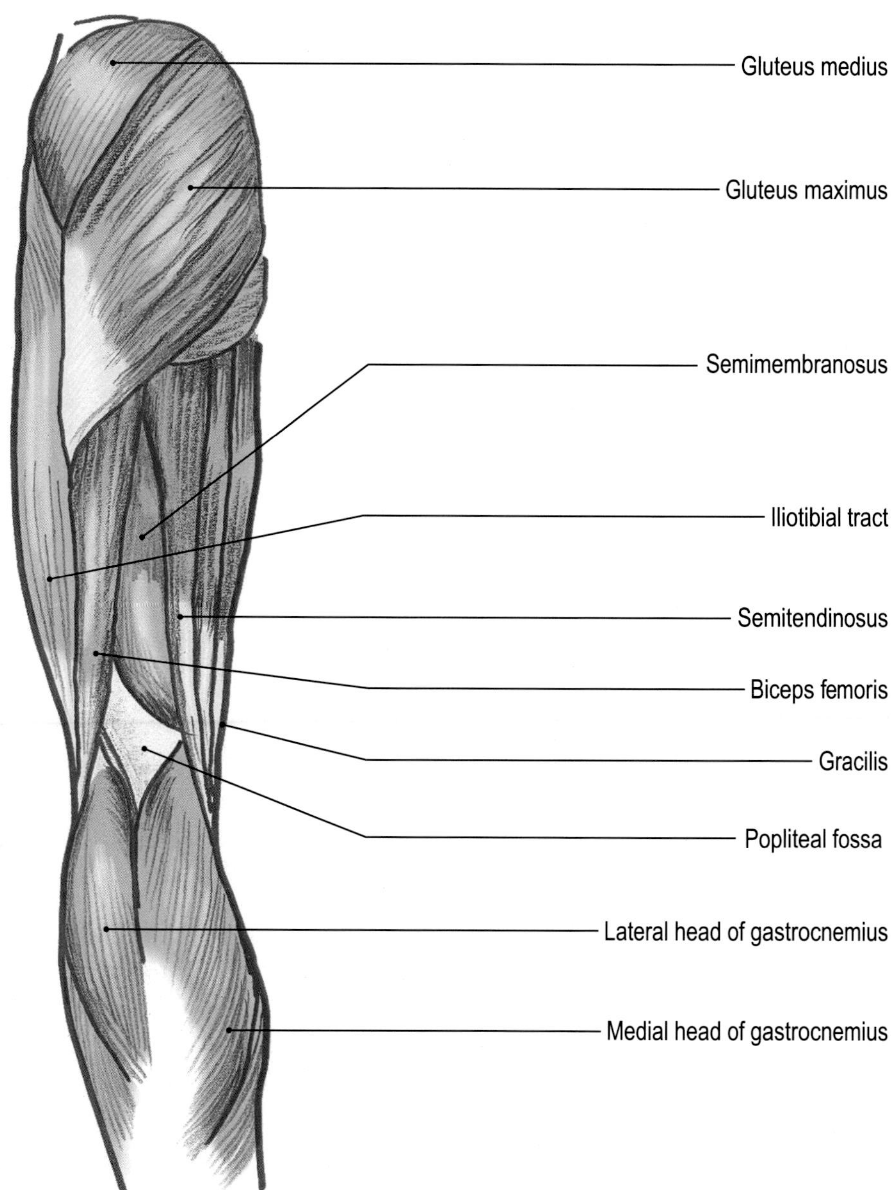

Fig. 3.19 (b) Muscles of the left thigh (posterior aspect)

Palpation

- The tendon of biceps femoris. The model is in the prone lying position. Ask the model to flex the knees and apply resistance to the movement. The tendon of biceps femoris stands clear on the posterolateral side of the knee which you can trace to its insertion to the head of the fibula.
- The belly of biceps femoris (Fig. 3.2). Proximally, you can follow the superficial fusiform muscle belly towards the ischial tuberosity. You can palpate the deeper fibres of biceps femoris on the medial side of the tendon in the upper part of the **popliteal fossa**.
- The tendon of semitendinosus. Palpate the tendon on the posteromedial side of the knee joint as it passes downwards to its attachment on the medial surface of the tibial condyle and shaft.
- The belly of semitendinosus. Proximally, its fusiform muscle belly joins that of biceps femoris near the gluteal fold.
- The tendon of **gracilis**. Identify the slightly thinner tendon of gracilis lying anteromedially. Trace its muscle belly up the medial side of the thigh as far as the body of the pubis. Palpation is easier if you ask the model to flex the knee and apply resistance to the movement.
- Semimembranosus. This muscle lies deep to semitendinosus just above the knee. It is difficult to palpate, even at its distal end, because it attaches, via a broad aponeurosis, to the postero-medial aspect of the medial condyle of the tibia. With the model's knee supported in approximately 60° of flexion, press your fingertips and thumb into the space on either side of the semitendinosus tendon approximately 5 cm above the level of the knee joint. Ask the model to flex and extend the knee. Now palpate the muscle below, contracting and relaxing.

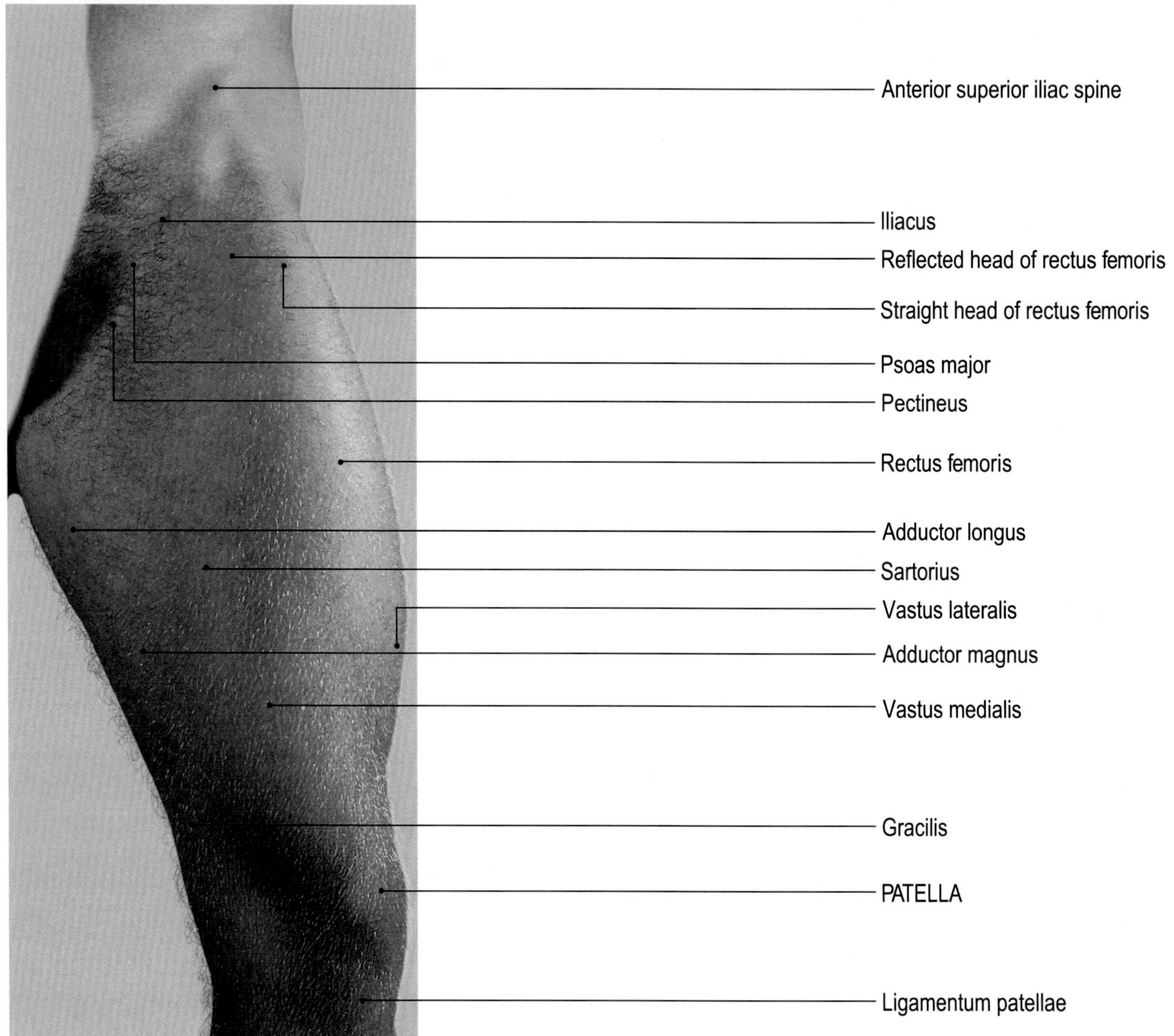

Fig. 3.20 (a) Muscles of the left thigh (medial aspect)

The anterior and medial aspects of the thigh

The adductors and quadriceps femoris

Palpation

- The adductor group of muscles. The model is in the supine lying position. Ask the model to adduct the thigh. The adductor group of muscles now comes into action. You can palpate the following:
  - The tendinous part of **adductor magnus** running down the medial aspect of the thigh from the ischial tuberosity to the **adductor tubercle**.
  - The **adductor longus** lying anteriorly and laterally with adductor brevis and the aponeurotic part of adductor magnus lying more posteriorly.
- **Note.** It is difficult to identify the adductor muscles separately.

The quadriceps muscle forms the great bulk of muscle on the front of the thigh (Fig. 3.20). It comprises **vastus medialis**, **vastus intermedius**, **vastus lateralis** and **rectus femoris**.

Palpation

- Quadriceps femoris. The model is in the sitting position. Ask the model to extend the knee and apply resistance to the movement. You can palpate three of the four bellies of quadriceps femoris.
- The belly of the vastus intermedius. This lies deep to the other three and is difficult to identify separately.
- **Rectus femoris**. The muscle passes straight down the front of the thigh from the anterior inferior iliac spine to the base of the patella. Palpate its proximal and distal tendons and its belly, which appears as a fusiform shape on the front of the thigh.
- The belly of **vastus lateralis** (Fig. 3.18). Palpate this muscle belly halfway down the lateral surface of the thigh, being flattened posteriorly by the fascia lata (iliotibial tract).

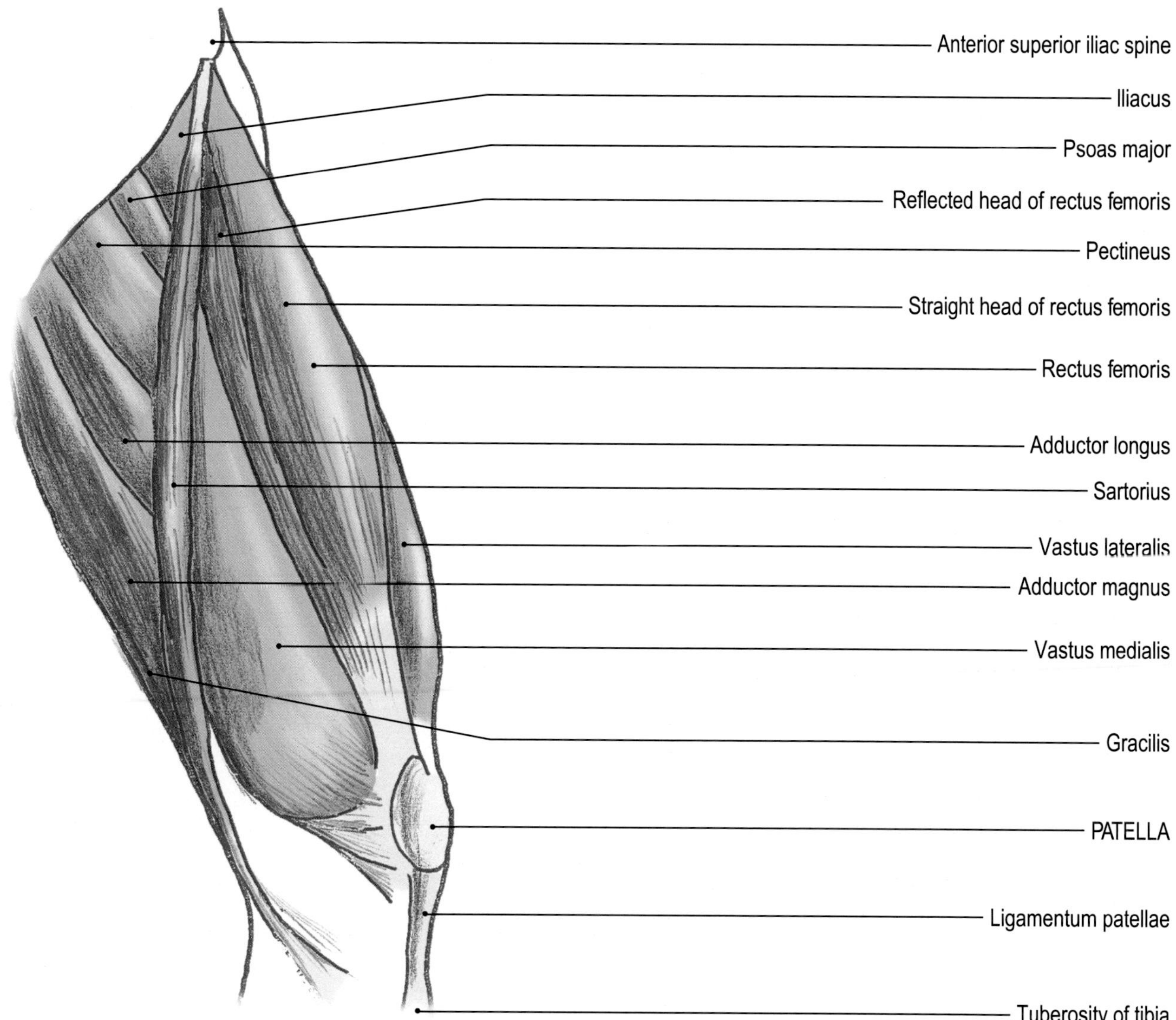

Fig. 3.20 (b) Muscles of the left thigh (medial aspect)

- **Vastus medialis**. Palpate this muscle on the medial side of the thigh just above the level of the patella. Trace its lowest fibres running almost horizontally and laterally to attach to the medial border of the patella.
- **Note.** This muscle varies considerably in size according to its use and is the first part of the quadriceps to show signs of weakness.
- The tendons of quadriceps. Palpate the tendons, particularly those of rectus femoris and vastus intermedius, attaching to the upper border of the patella.
- **Note 1.** There are often small depressions on its medial and lateral edges where it joins the expansion of vastus lateralis and vastus medialis.
- **Note 2.** The patella is a sesamoid bone and lies within the tendon of quadriceps femoris, the ligamentum patellae being a continuation of the quadriceps tendon (Fig. 3.20).
- The **ligamentum patellae**. Palpate this structure, which joins the apex of the patella to the upper part of the tibial tuberosity. It is approximately 5 cm long and 2 cm wide, with its central point level with the knee joint (see p. 107).
- The iliotibial tract (Fig. 3.21a, b). Ask the model to extend the knee fully. Now palpate the strong tendon-like structure lying lateral to the patella and running down to attach to the lateral tibial condyle. This is the lower part of the iliotibial tract. You can trace it superiorly along the lateral side of the thigh to the ilium.
- **Sartorius** (Fig. 3.20). The model is in the supine lying position. Ask the model to flex, laterally rotate and abduct the hip whilst also flexing the knee. Apply resistance to the movement at the heel. You can now palpate the long strap-like muscle crossing the thigh from the **anterior superior iliac spine** above to the medial condyle of the tibia below.
- **Note.** Its upper third appears to stand away from the groin region.
- 'Tailor sitting'. The model is in the sitting position with the knees extended. Ask the model to flex both knees and hips simultaneously. This produces the 'tailor sitting' position. Sartorius [*sartor* (L) = tailor] can be observed and palpated during this action.

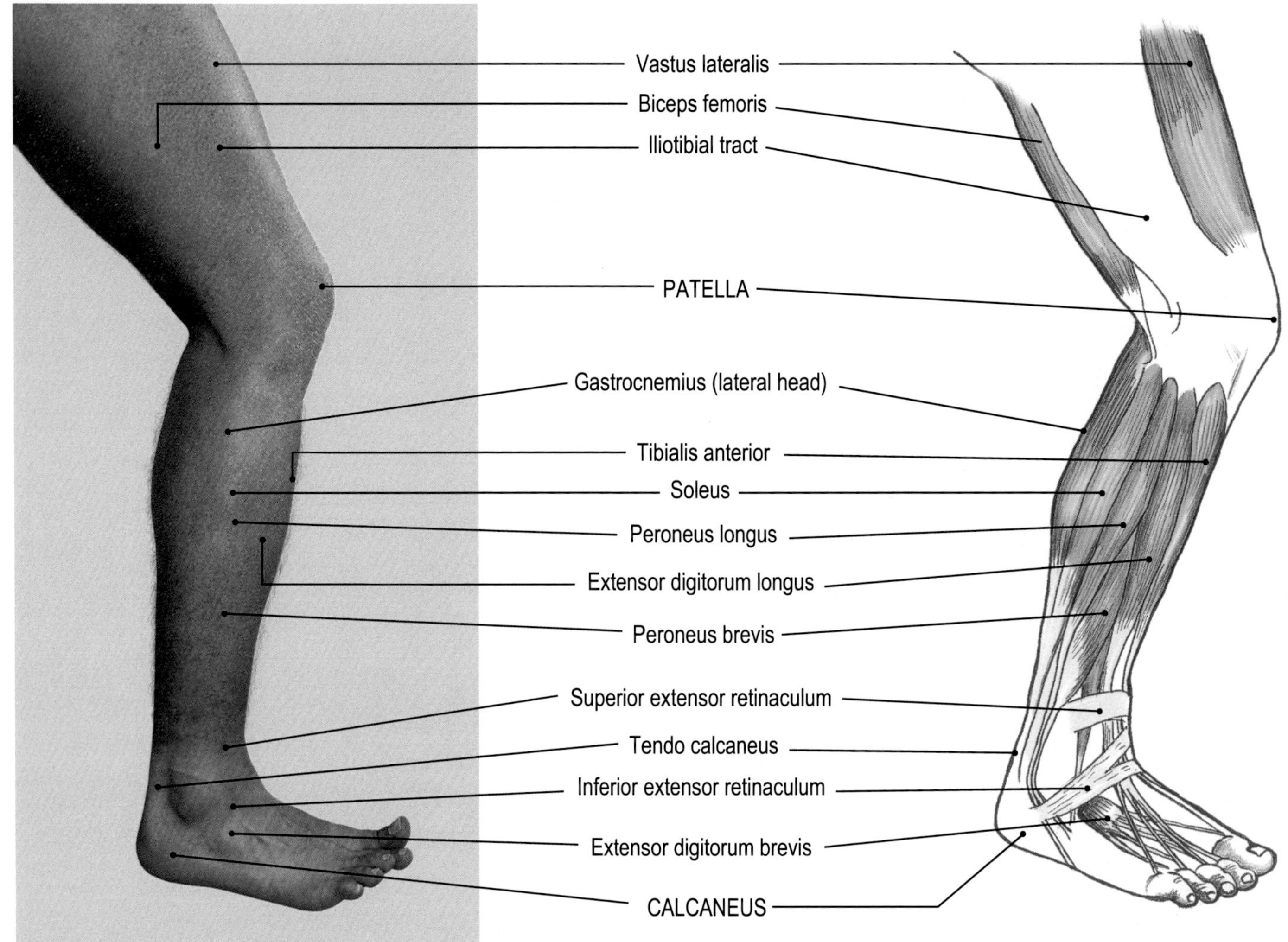

Fig. 3.21 (a, b) Muscles of the right leg (lateral aspect)

The anterior and lateral aspects of the leg and foot

The muscles in the anterior compartment of the leg are somewhat easier to identify than those in the corresponding aspect of the forearm. Even so, differentiation is easiest where the tendons pass over the front of the ankle joint. Consequently, palpation should begin here.

Palpation

- Tibialis anterior. The model is in the supine lying position with the foot dorsiflexed. Find the most medial tendon, that of **tibialis anterior** (Fig. 3.21). Although it lies deep to the **superior** and **inferior extensor retinacula**, you will find it easy to feel. Distally, trace it to its insertion on the medial cuneiform and base of the first metatarsal bones.
- **Note.** Proximally, the strong tendon gives way to a firm but narrow muscle which fills the space lateral to the anterior border of the tibia. The muscle is contained within strong fascia and becomes particularly hard on contraction. There is often a narrow space between the muscle and the tibia anteriorly.
- **Extensor hallucis longus** (Fig. 3.21c, d). Palpate the tendon which lies lateral to tibialis anterior. It stands clear of the joint and you can trace it across the medial side of the foot to the great toe. Ask the model to extend the toe and follow the tendon to its insertion into the base of the distal phalanx. Proximally, the tendon is soon lost between the other muscles. If you trace the line of the tendon to the middle of the fibula, however, you can feel the muscle contracting deep to extensor digitorum longus.

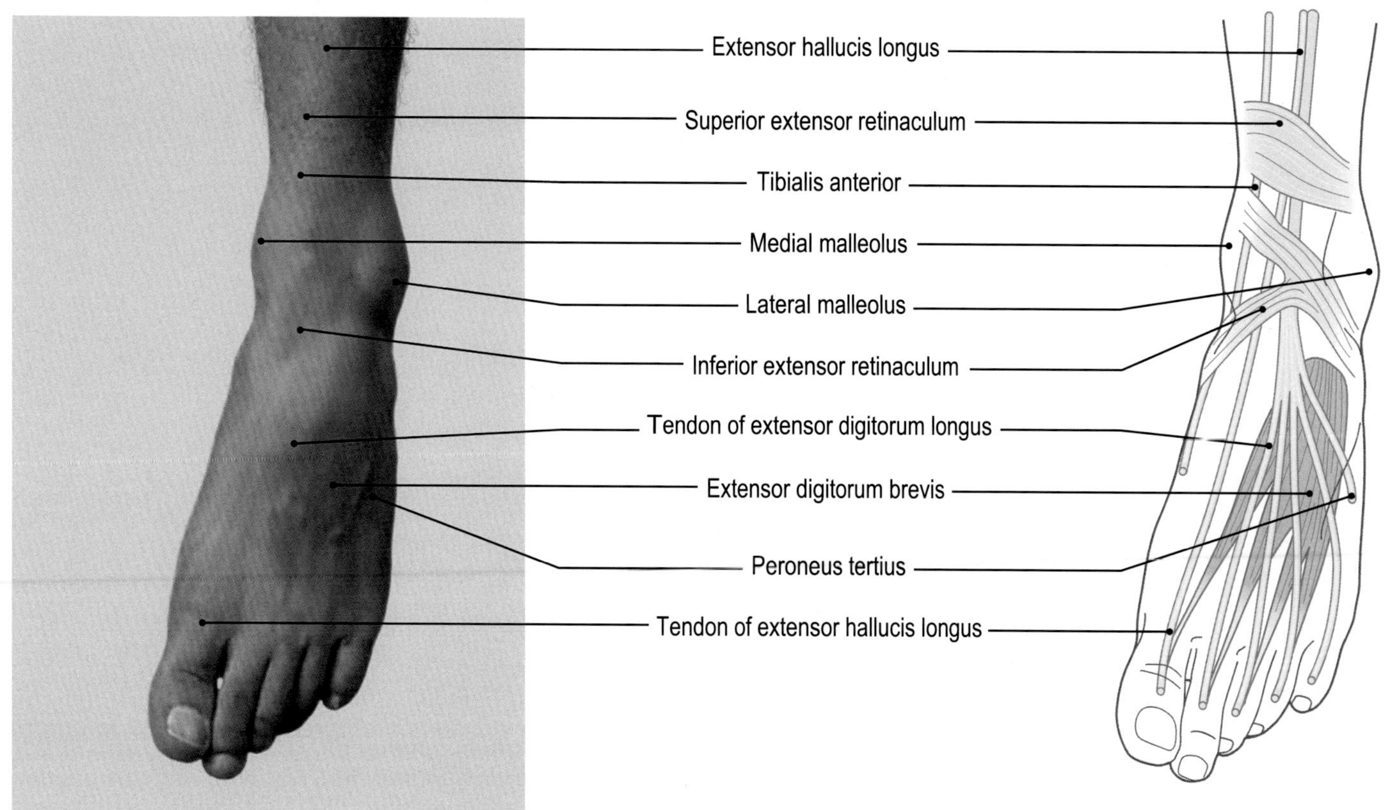

Fig. 3.21 (c, d) Tendons and muscles of the left foot (dorsal aspect)

- Extensor digitorum longus (Fig. 3.21a–d). Identify the tendon where it lies lateral to the tendon of extensor hallucis longus. Palpate the tendon immediately distal to the ankle where it divides into four separate tendons. Trace these to the dorsal surface of the lateral four toes.
- Note. Occasionally, when the toes are flexed at the metatarsophalangeal joint, you can feel the tendons as they 'bowstring' across the joint. Proximally, the tendon soon becomes muscular, extending superiorly as far as the superior tibiofibular joint, lying between tibialis anterior medially and the fibula laterally.

Peroneus tertius

Although this small muscle is named as one of the peroneal muscles, peroneus tertius is considered to be part of the extensor digitorum longus, in fact its fifth tendon. This is because it arises from thc lower third of the fibula in line with, and passes under, the superior extensor retinaculum and through the loop of the inferior retinaculum, with, and lateral to, the extensor digitorum longus. Unlike extensor digitorum longus, however, it does not insert into the digits but into the medial side of the dorsal surface of the base of the fifth metatarsal. In a small percentage of subjects the muscle is absent.

Palpation

- Peroneus tertius. From the base of the fifth metatarsal, draw a line from its medial side towards the lower quarter of the shaft of the fibula. Ask the model to evert the foot. You will find it easier to palpate the tendon along this line.
- Extensor digitorum brevis (Fig. 3.21). Identify this muscle as a large swelling some 2 cm anterior to the lateral malleolus on the dorsolateral aspect of the foot. Palpate the four narrow tendons, leaving its distal aspect passing towards the medial four toes. In the second, third and fourth toes the tendons join those of extensor digitorum longus, while in the great toe the tendon passes to the lateral side of the proximal phalanx.

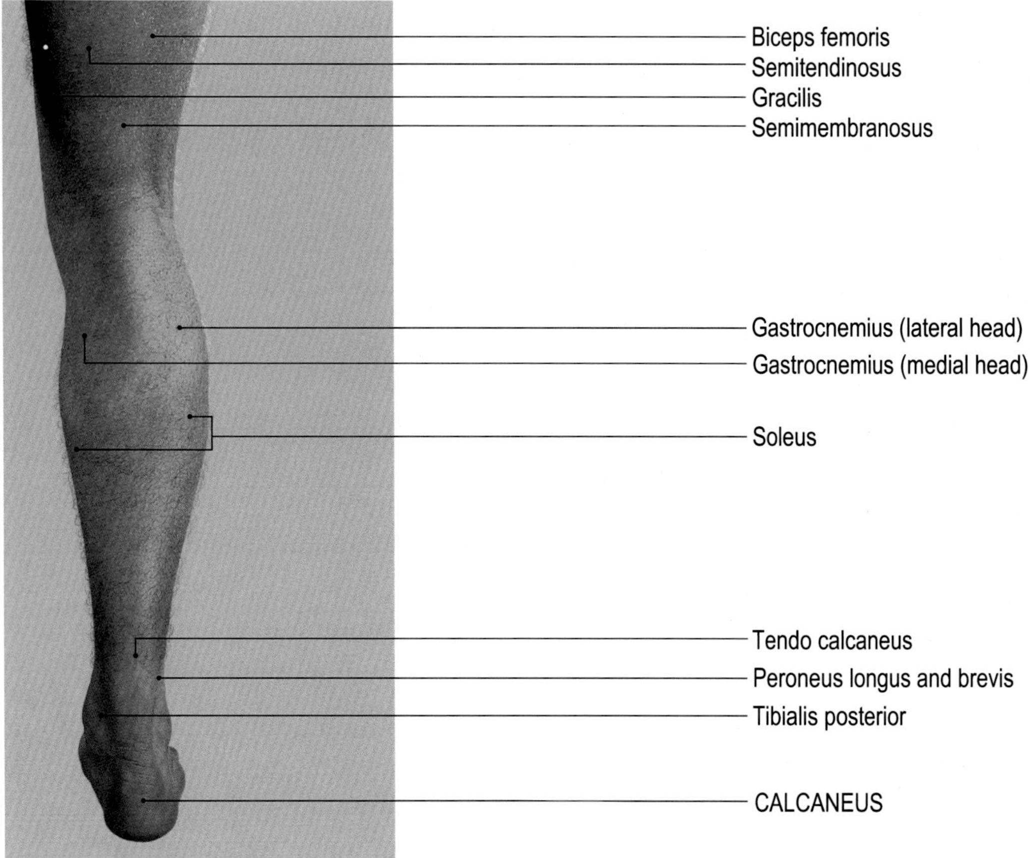

Fig. 3.22 (a) Muscles of the right leg and foot (posterior aspect)

The posterior and plantar aspects of the leg and foot

Palpation

- Popliteus. This muscle lies deep within the **popliteal fossa** high up on the posterolateral aspect of the knee joint. You can, however, palpate its tendon as it passes below the lateral epicondyle of the femur. The model is sitting with the knee flexed to 90°. Place the tips of your fingers on the lateral surface of the femoral condyle just below and in front of the lateral epicondyle. Ask the model to rotate the leg medially at the knee joint. Now palpate the tendon of popliteus as it runs forwards, in a groove, towards its femoral attachment.
- **Note.** The belly of popliteus is difficult to palpate as it lies deep within the popliteal fossa.

Triceps surae (calf)

The posterior aspect of the leg is dominated by the calf muscles: **gastrocnemius** and **soleus**. Gastrocnemius is more superficial; soleus is deep. Together they are attached distally by the tendo calcaneus to the posterior surface of the **calcaneus**. The two muscles, however, arise from different bones. Gastrocnemius arises from the femur: its medial head from the upper part of the medial condyle and its lateral head from just above the lateral epicondyle. Soleus – whose name is believed to derive from a flat fish, the sole – arises below the knee joint from the posterior surfaces of the tibia, fibula and interosseous membrane.

Plantaris, when present, passes lateral to medial, from the upper part of the lateral condyle of the femur downwards, between gastrocnemius and soleus, to attach to the medial side of the tendo calcaneus.

Palpation

- The tendo calcaneus. The model is in the standing position. Begin at the posterior aspect of the heel, where you can easily palpate the broad tendo calcaneus, which attaches to the calcaneus. Follow the tendon upwards for some 8 cm as it narrows to a width of approximately 1 cm, after which it rapidly widens into an aponeurosis about 8 cm wide.
- The muscle fibres of gastrocnemius. Palpate these fibres attaching to the superficial surface of the aponeurosis.
- The bellies of gastrocnemius (Fig. 3.22). Palpate the two large bellies. The medial and longer belly stretches to the medial femoral condyle; the lateral belly stretches to the lateral femoral condyle. The two bellies are separated by a faint vertical line which you can easily palpate in a well-developed calf.

Soleus lies deep to gastrocnemius. Its fibres contribute to the deep surface of the **tendo calcaneus**. Its upper attachment is to the posterior aspect of the tibia (soleal line) and to the head and shaft of the fibula. The muscle belly is broad and thick.

Palpation

- Soleus (Fig. 3.22). As soleus is primarily a postural muscle, preventing the tibia from tilting forwards in the standing position, you will find it is easier to palpate when the model is in standing. First locate the broad aponeurosis of the tendo calcaneus where it joins the muscle fibres of gastrocnemius. Now run your fingers to the outer borders. Immediately adjacent is the muscle belly of soleus, bulging either side and deep to the aponeurosis.
- Gastrocnemius. Ask the model to raise the heel. Palpate the contracting muscle fibres of gastrocnemius.
- Soleus. The model is in the supine lying with the hip and knee flexed. Now ask the model to plantarflex the foot

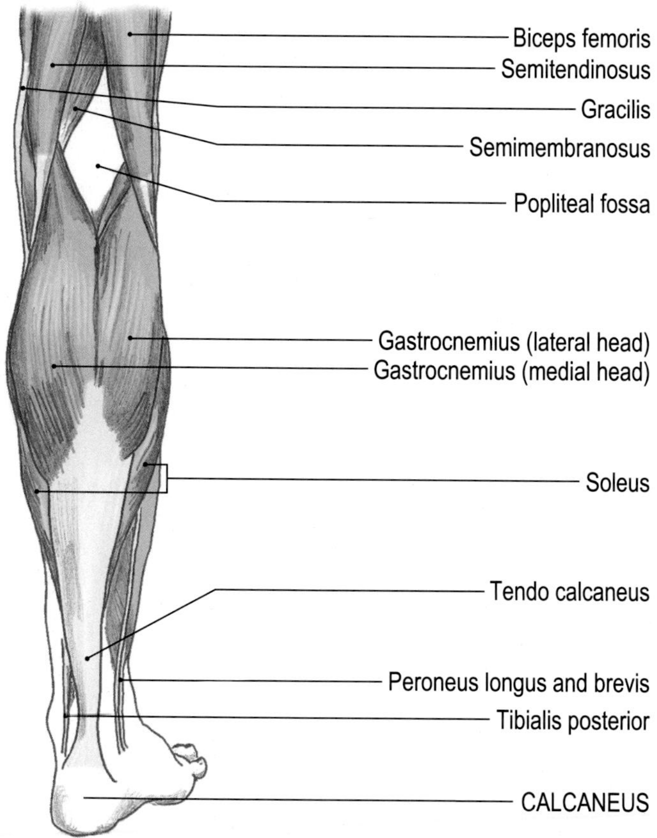

Fig. 3.22 (b) Muscles of the right leg and foot (posterior aspect)

Palpate the contraction of soleus while gastrocnemius remains relaxed.

- **Note.** This muscle remains relaxed because the upper (femoral) and lower (calcaneal) attachments of gastrocnemius are brought closer together, shortening the muscle and essentially preventing it from contracting. This is known as 'muscle insufficiency'.

Tibialis posterior

This muscle is situated deep in the posterior aspect of the leg. It attaches, proximally, to the lateral section of the posterior surface of the tibia, the interosseous membrane and the medial section of the posterior surface of the fibula and the covering fascia. After passing downwards and medially it forms a tendon, which passes, in conjunction with that of flexor digitorum longus, in a groove behind the medial malleolus. The tendon then passes forwards and downwards to attach to the medial and undersurface of the tubercle of the navicular. From here, fibrous slips pass under the foot to attach to the plantar surface of many other bones.

Palpation

As this muscle is situated deep in the calf it is impossible to palpate except for its tendon running from behind the medial malleolus to the navicular.

For palpation in this region, the model is in the supine lying position.

- The tendon of tibialis posterior. Ask the model to invert and plantarflex the foot. The tendon can be easily identified running from the posterior part of the medial malleolus to the navicular.

The peronei: peroneus longus and brevis

These muscles are situated on the lateral aspect of the leg.

The upper attachment of peroneus longus is from the head and upper two-thirds of the lateral surface of the fibula. The upper attachment of peroneus brevis is to the lower two-thirds of the lateral surface of the fibula. The upper part overlaps, anteriorly, the lower third of the origin of peroneus longus. Each muscle also attaches to the surrounding intermuscular septa. Both tendons pass vertically downward to pass behind the lateral malleolus in a common sheath. Peroneus longus then passes forward to groove the under part of the peroneal trochlea (tubercle), being held in place by a fibrous sheath. The tendon then passes to the lateral side of the cuboid bone, grooving its lateral border. It changes direction to pass medially and forwards under the foot, finally attaching to the lateral side of the base of the first metacarpal and adjacent part of the medial cuneiform bone.

The tendon of peroneus brevis also passes behind the lateral malleolus downwards and forwards, grooving the upper part of the peroneal trochlea, being held in place by fibrous tissue. It finally attaches to the lateral side of the tubercle on the base of the fifth metatarsal.

Palpation

- The tendons of peroneus longus and brevis. Locate the posterior part of the lateral malleolus. Ask the model to evert the foot. You will easily be able to locate both tendons. Continue to trace downwards where the tendons can be identified, not quite as easily, passing forwards and downwards. Note that peroneus longus lies posterior and passes below the peroneal trochanter to the lateral side of the cuboid while peroneus brevis passes above the peroneal trochlea forwards and downwards to attach to the tubercle of the fifth metatarsal.
- The muscle bellies of peroneus longus and brevis. Now trace up the tendons to the lateral side of the fibula, where you can identify the bellies of both muscles.
- **Note.** The tendon of the peroneus longus cannot be palpated as it passes under the foot.

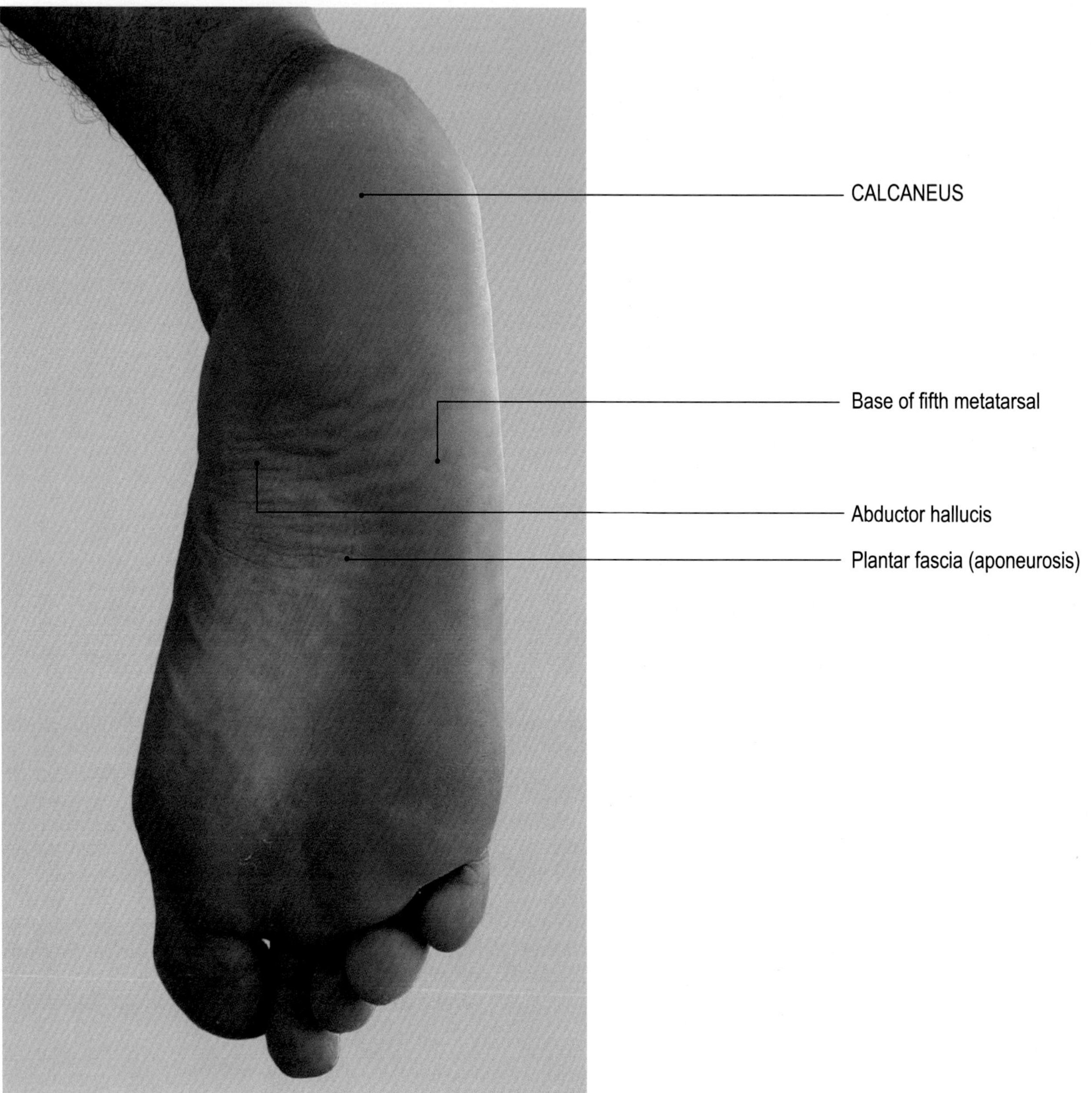

Fig. 3.23 (a) Abductor hallucis

The plantar muscles (Fig. 3.23)

The plantar surface of the foot is covered centrally by a thick dense layer of fascia known as the plantar aponeurosis. This is triangular in shape. It is narrower posteriorly, where it attaches to the calcaneus, and broader anteriorly, where it splits to attach to either side of the proximal phalanx of each toe. It gives the central portion of the plantar aspect of the foot a pale appearance. The heel, lateral border and under the metatarsal heads are darker and covered with harder skin as a result of weight-bearing.

The plantar muscles are arranged in four layers deep to the plantar fascia and are relatively easily recognized on dissection. The deepest muscles are the shortest, whereas those just deep to the plantar aponeurosis are the longest. All of these muscles, except abductor hallucis, are impossible to palpate due to the thickness and tension of the fascia.

Palpation

- Abductor hallucis 1. Only abductor hallucis is easily recognizable on the medial side of the foot. Some subjects may be able to abduct the great toe. In this case, you can palpate the belly of abductor hallucis along the medial border of the foot. The broad fusiform-shaped muscle belly passes forwards from the medial tubercle of the calcaneus, continuing as a tendon to the medial side of the proximal phalanx of the great toe.
- Abductor hallucis 2. If abduction of the great toe proves difficult, ask the model to shorten the foot whilst in standing and

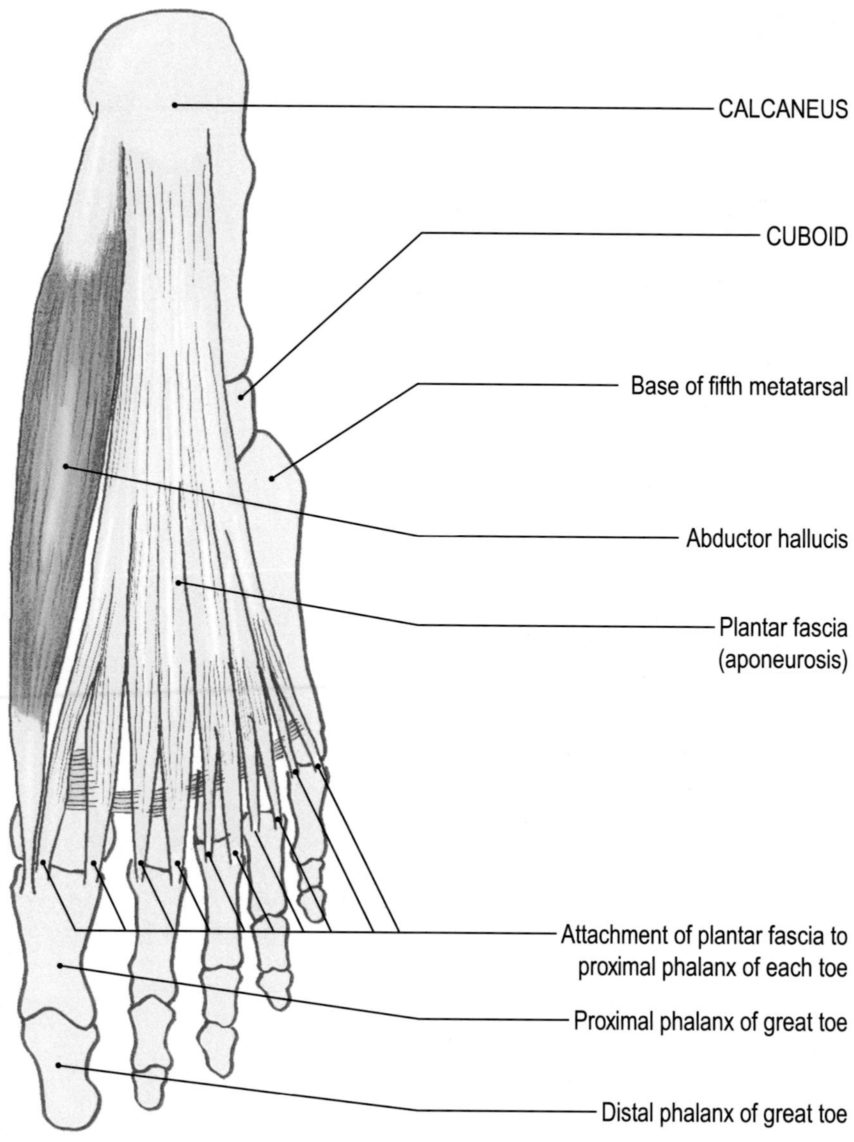

Fig. 3.23 (b) Abductor hallucis and plantar fascia of the right foot (plantar aspect)

weight-bearing position. This produces a powerful contraction of the muscle which you can palpate.

- Note. This is most probably the muscle's main functional activity.
- Abductor hallucis 3. Palpate the bulk of the muscle in its posterior section, with the relatively thick tendon distinct in its anterior half inserting into the medial side of the base of the proximal phalanx of the great toe. Ask the model to extend the toe. Now palpate the medial edge of the plantar fascia as it is being stretched.
- Note 1. The use and type of footwear, if any, habitually worn, together with the activities and weight of the subject, will influence the structure and appearance of the foot. There is usually a thickening of the fascia and hardening of the skin over weight-bearing areas. These are normally over the heel, lateral border of the foot and heads of the metatarsals, particularly the first and fifth.
- Note 2. The amount of the sole of the foot which is in contact with the supporting surface is inversely proportional to the height of the plantar arches. The medial side of the foot is rarely in contact with the ground, except in subjects who have extremely flat feet. Anteriorly, the metatarsal heads are normally in contact with the ground. They may show a downward convexity which produces areas of hardened skin (callus) under the second, third and fourth metatarsal heads.

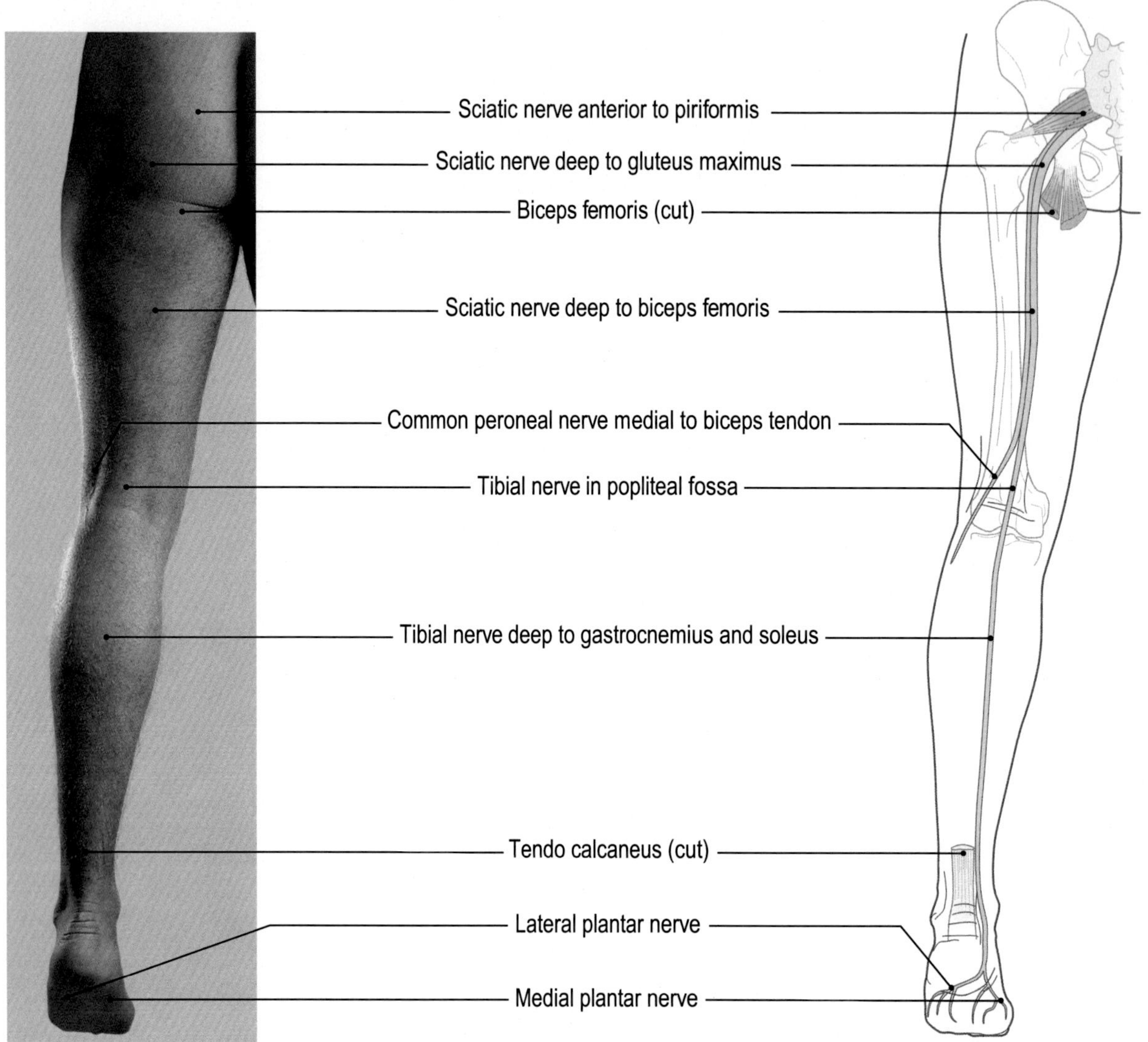

Fig. 3.24 (a, b) The sciatic nerve and branches in the left lower limb (posterior view)

NERVES (FIG. 3.24)

The nerves of the lower limb are normally deep within the tissues and are thus extremely difficult to palpate. Nevertheless, it is important to be aware of their location and to be able to palpate those that venture close to the surface.

The whole of the lower limb is supplied from the lumbar, sacral and coccygeal plexi. The lumbar plexus derives its fibres from T12, L1, L2, L3 and L4 roots. The sacral (lumbosacral) plexus derives its fibres from L4, L5, S1, S2, S3 and S4. The coccygeal (sacral) plexus derives its fibres from S4 and S5. These form a complex arrangement of nerves, most of which are not palpable, but nevertheless remain essential knowledge for the practitioner.

The nerves of the lumbar plexus lie deep within the abdominal cavity, passing into the pelvis, medial to the ilia. They pass into the thigh, mainly above the superior pubic ramus, supplying the muscles on the anterior and medial aspects of the thigh. They also supply the skin covering these areas. It is virtually impossible to palpate any of these nerves.

Palpation: surface marking

The **sciatic nerve** derives its fibres from the anterior primary rami of L4 and L5 through the lumbosacral trunk, and S1, S2 and S3. It is formed **in front of piriformis** in the posterior part of the pelvis. It emerges from the pelvis through the sciatic notch below piriformis and **deep to the gluteus maximus**. It is the largest peripheral nerve in the body.

- The sciatic nerve. Trace its course as it runs vertically down the back of the thigh, deep to biceps **femoris**, having emerged from below piriformis approximately halfway between the greater trochanter of the femur and the ischial tuberosity. About two-thirds of the way down the thigh, it splits into its terminal branches: the **tibial** and **common peroneal nerves** (Fig. 3.24a–d).
- **Note.** Although it is difficult to palpate the nerve directly, pressure applied over the area of its course can cause considerable discomfort.
- The tibial nerve (Fig. 3.24a, b) continues through the popliteal fossa to enter the calf **deep to gastrocnemius** and **soleus**

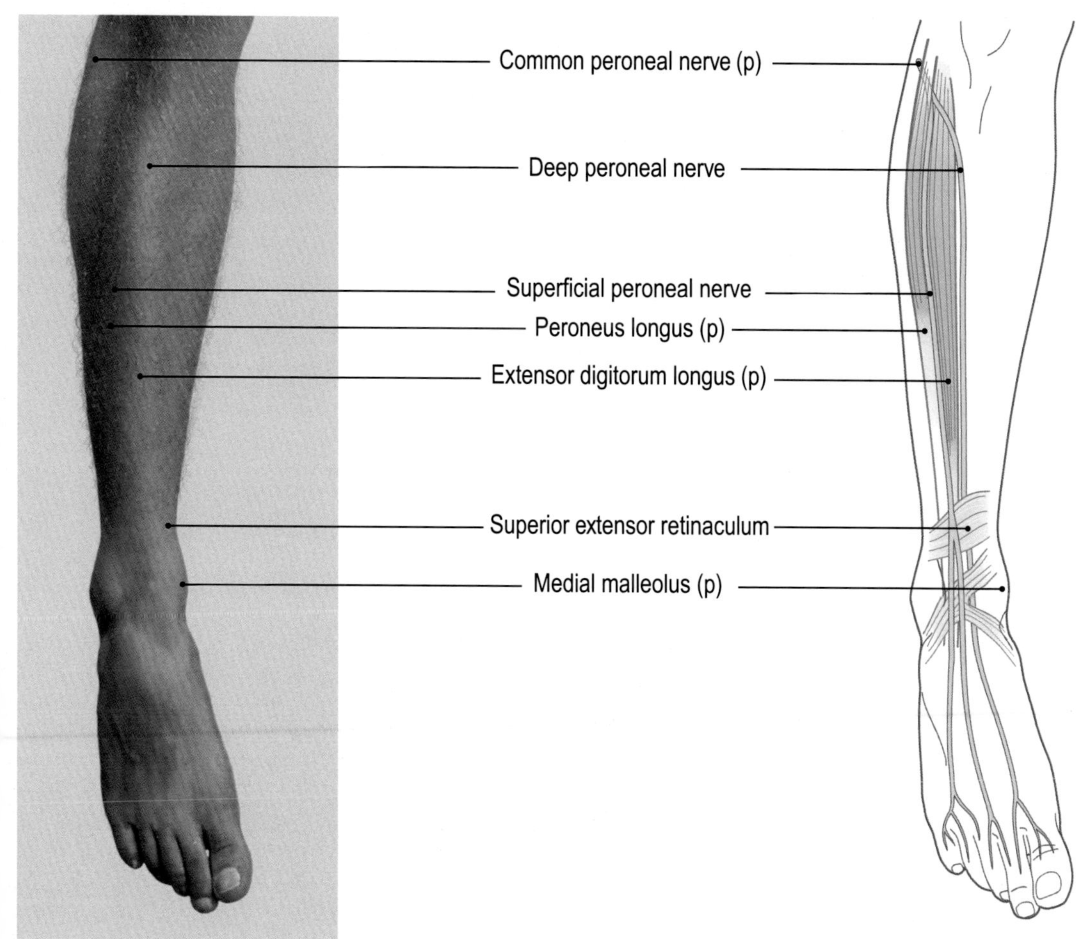

Fig. 3.24 (c, d) Branches of the common peroneal nerve of the right leg, anterior aspect (p, palpable)

where it lies between superficial and deep groups of muscles.

- Note. The tibial nerve is difficult to palpate in this region, although an unpleasant sensation can be produced if you apply excessive pressure. In the lower third of the leg the tibial nerve becomes medial to the tendo calcaneus and continues to the space behind the medial malleolus where you can palpate it. Trace it proximally into the leg and distally into the foot, where it almost immediately divides into the medial and lateral plantar nerves. These terminal branches soon become too deep to be palpated.
- The common peroneal nerve, the lateral terminal branch of the sciatic nerve, enters the popliteal fossa. It passes down the medial side of the tendon of biceps femoris. Here you can palpate it passing behind the head of the fibula and as it winds forwards around the neck (Fig. 3.24). It then splits into superficial and deep branches.
- The common peroneal nerve. The model is in the prone lying position. Ask the model to semiflex the knee. Now locate the tendon of biceps femoris as it passes down to the head of the fibula, posterolateral to the knee. You will find the common peroneal nerve below the level of the knee joint, just medial and deep to the tendon of biceps femoris, passing behind the head of the fibula and winding forwards around the neck (Fig. 3.24). It is easier to palpate posteriorly but more difficult anteriorly as it becomes covered by peroneus longus and tibialis anterior.
- The deep peroneal nerve. This nerve lies deep within the anterior compartment of the leg and is impossible to palpate until it crosses the anterior aspect of the ankle joint between the tendons of extensor hallucis longus and extensor digitorum longus. First find the anterior tibial pulse on the front of the ankle joint between extensor hallucis longus and extensor digitorum longus. The nerve runs just lateral to this, but it is difficult to find as it lies deep to the superior extensor retinaculum.
- The superficial peroneal nerve. You can palpate this nerve passing over the anterolateral aspect of the ankle, just medial to the anterior border of the lateral malleolus. Trace it proximally for approximately 5 cm to where it emerges from between peroneus brevis and extensor digitorum longus. Trace it distally on to the lateral side of the dorsum of the foot, dividing into fine terminal cutaneous branches (Fig. 3.24c, d).

Although the nerves to the skin are not palpable, the areas supplied are normally superficial to the muscles lying deep below. For further information, refer to *Anatomy and Human Movement* (Palastanga et al 2002).

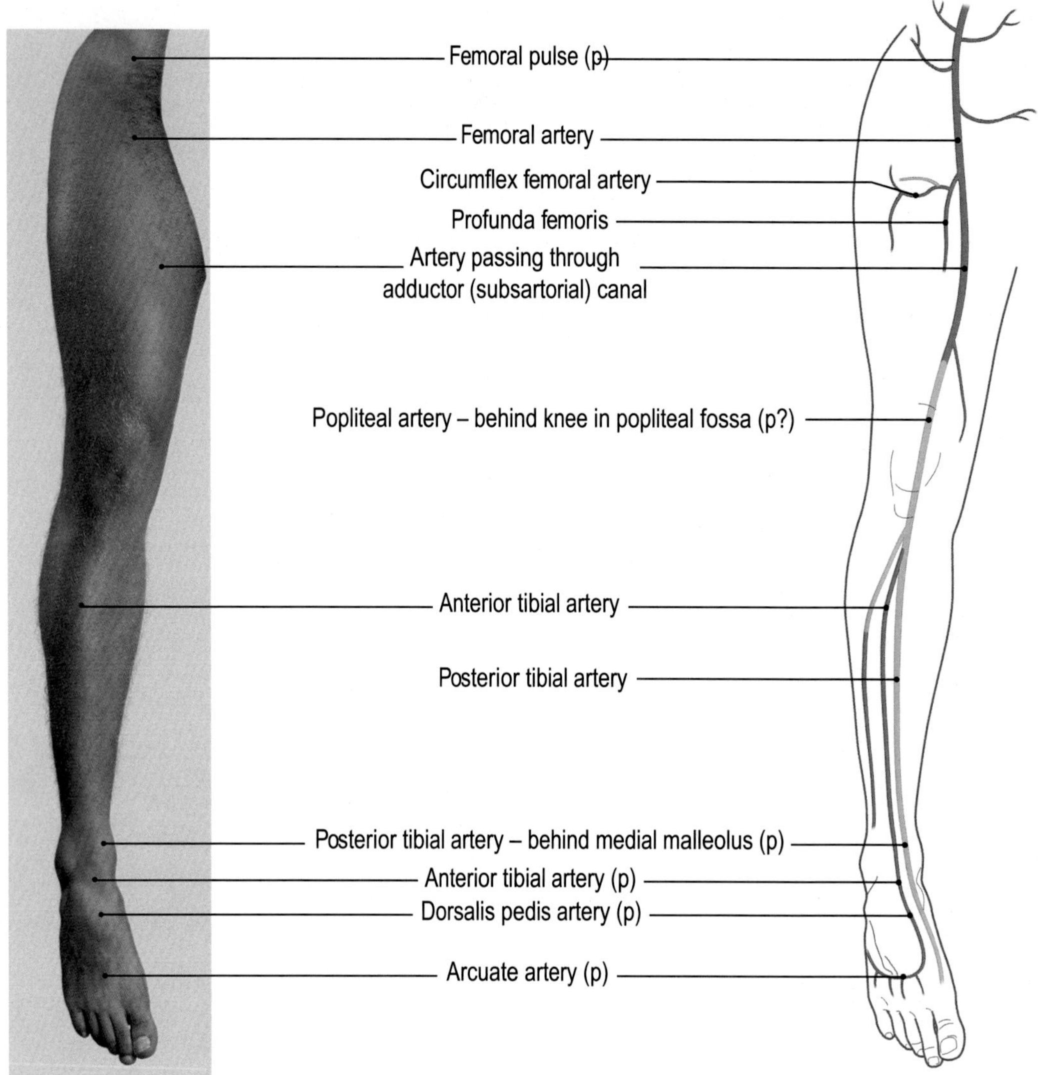

Fig. 3.25 (a, b) The arteries of the right lower limb, anterior aspect (p, palpable)

ARTERIES (FIG. 3.25)

As in the upper limb, most of the large arteries are located deep within the tissues and are normally difficult to palpate.

Palpation

- The **pulsation** of the **femoral artery**. The model is in the supine lying position. Palpate this artery in the groin just below the mid point (halfway between the anterior superior iliac spines and the pubic tubercle) below the inguinal ligament directly anterior to the head of the femur at the hip joint. Above, the vessel lies within the abdomen and below it is hidden by fascia as it lies in the femoral triangle on the proximal anteromedial aspect of the thigh.
- The popliteal artery. Just above the knee the femoral artery passes through the opening in adductor magnus (adductor hiatus) lying deep to sartorius in the **adductor (subsartorial) canal** to enter the popliteal fossa, becoming the **popliteal artery**. By applying deep, but sensitive pressure, you can palpate this artery as it crosses the back of the knee joint. You will find it easier to identify if tension of the superficial tissues is reduced by asking the model to bend the knee to about 45°.
- **Note.** Success in palpation is largely dependent on the amount of fat within the fossa and, in reality, it is extremely difficult to find. This is, therefore, a good region in which to practise the careful use of the fingers in palpation of pulses.

As the popliteal artery enters the calf, it divides into the anterior and posterior tibial arteries. The **anterior tibial artery** passes over the main section of the interosseous membrane and below the most superior fibres (see p. 109), into the anterior

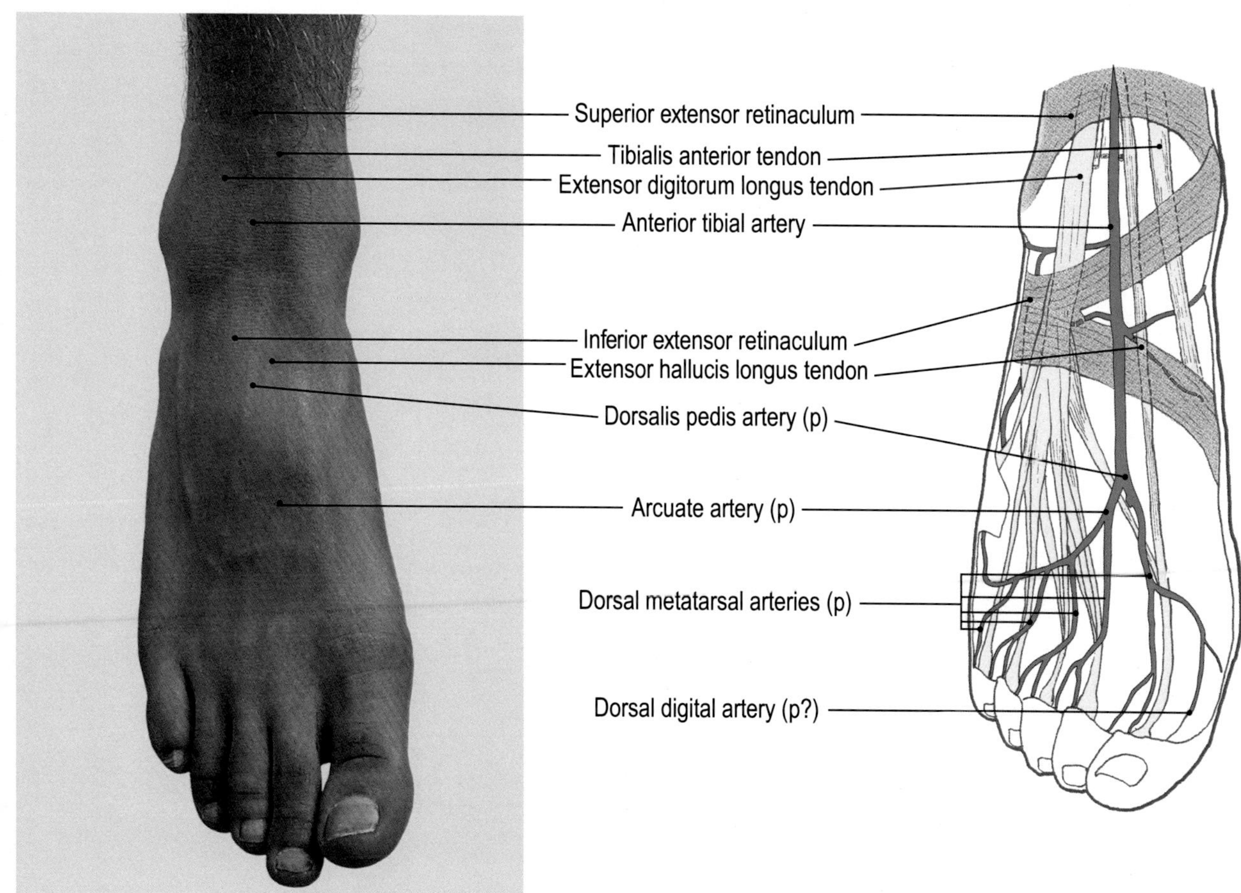

Fig. 3.25 (c, d) The arteries of the right foot, dorsal aspect (p, palpable)

compartment of the leg, deep to the anterior tibial muscles. The **posterior tibial artery** passes down the back of the leg deep to gastrocnemius, soleus and plantaris (triceps surae).

- The **anterior tibial artery**. Palpate this artery as it crosses the anteromedial aspect of the ankle joint between the tendons of extensor hallucis longus and extensor digitorum longus where it lies medial to the deep branch of the common peroneal nerve. With care, you can trace it down to the space between the first and second metatarsals where it passes into the plantar aspect of the foot between the two bones.
- The dorsalis pedis artery (Fig. 3.25a–d). Beyond the extensor retinaculum the anterior tibial artery is called the dorsalis pedis and is commonly the point at which the arterial supply is checked. You must be careful not to palpate too distally as the artery will have already passed through to the plantar aspect of the foot.
- The **arcuate artery**. This is a continuation of the dorsalis pedis artery. You will be able to palpate this artery on the dorsum of the metatarsals if there is a good blood supply to the foot.
- The posterior tibial artery (Fig. 3.25a, b). This artery crosses the ankle joint **behind the medial malleolus** between the tendons of flexor digitorum longus and flexor hallucis longus, medial to the posterior tibial nerve. Although it is quite clear as it crosses the ankle joint, it is difficult to trace into the medial side of the foot and the lower part of the leg.

It is important to practise finding these arterial pulses, as they give a good indication of the competence of the blood supply to the lower limb.

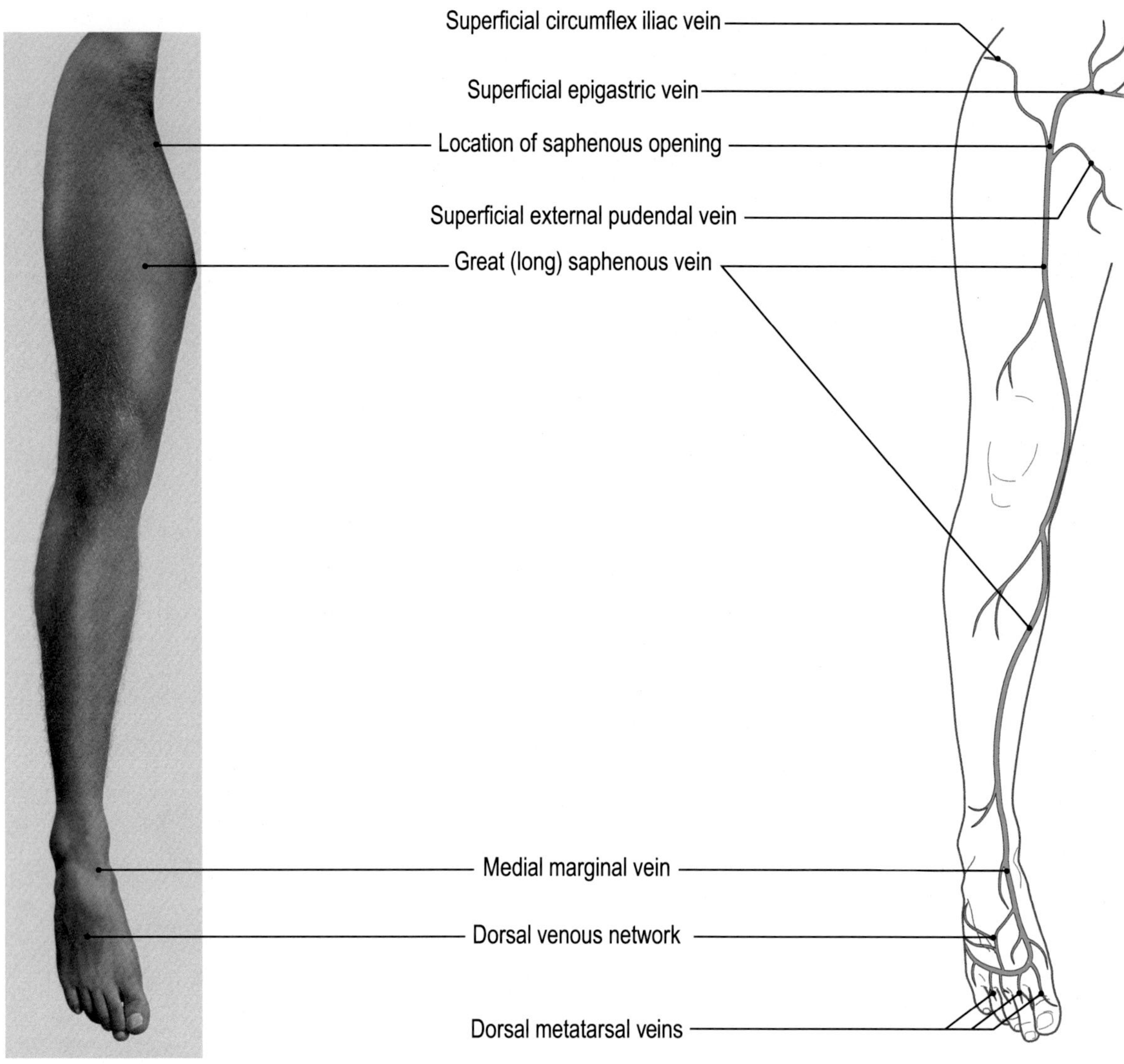

Fig. 3.26 (a, b) The veins of the right lower limb (anterior view)

VEINS (FIG. 3.26)

The arrangement of veins in the lower limb is similar to that in the upper limb (see p. 66–68) There are two main systems: deep, accompanying the arteries; and superficial, contained within the superficial fascia. All veins of the lower limb possess valves which facilitate central venous return. The valves in the communicating vessels normally only permit blood to flow from the superficial to the deep system.

The deep veins

The smaller arteries are normally accompanied by two small veins (venae comitantes), one on either side of the artery. The larger arteries are usually accompanied by a single large vein of approximately the same diameter as the artery. None of the deep veins can be palpated.

The superficial veins

In normal subjects most veins are difficult to see or palpate, except in the distal part of the leg and on the dorsum of the foot.

Palpation

- The network of veins on the dorsum of the foot. The model is in the standing position. Note that the **network of vessels** on the dorsum of the foot appear blue and raised. You may have difficulty palpating them. One vein on either side of the network appears to be slightly larger than the rest; these are termed **marginal veins**.

The **great** or **long saphenous vein** (Fig. 3.26a, b) begins on the medial side of the dorsal venous network as a continuation of the **medial marginal vein**. It passes proximally in front of the medial malleolus, along the medial side of the calf and crosses the knee joint just posterior to the medial condyles of both the tibia and femur. The vein then ascends on the medial side of the thigh to join the deep system (femoral vein) after passing through the **saphenous opening** which lies below the mid point of the inguinal ligament immediately medial to the pulsations of the femoral artery (see Fig. 3.25a, b).

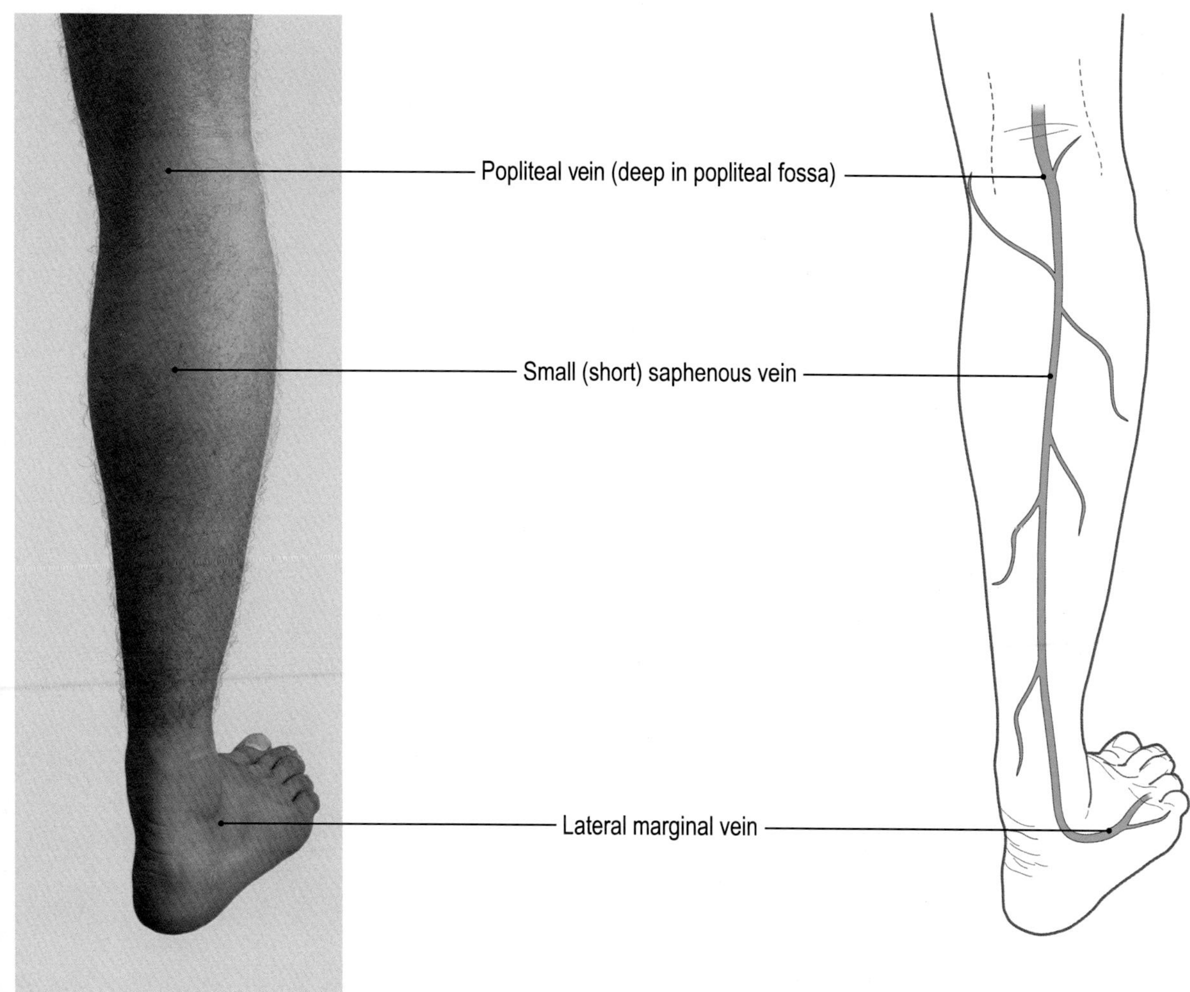

Fig. 3.26 (c, d) The veins of the right leg (posterior view)

Palpation

- The great (long) saphenous vein. You will normally only be able to palpate the lower part of the vein as it lies deep within the superficial fascia. The model is in the standing position. Find the medial marginal vein (the major vessel on the medial aspect of the dorsum of the foot). Brushing the skin surface with your fingertips, move up anterior to the medial malleolus. Above this level, you can feel the vein passing up the medial aspect of the calf. Trace it posteromedial to the knee. Here, it soon disappears as it enters the thigh. In some individuals it can be seen in the thigh as a bluish line running upwards towards the mid point of the groin.

The small (short) saphenous vein. Beginning on the lateral side of the dorsal venous network as a continuation of the lateral marginal vein, the **small** or **short saphenous vein** passes behind the lateral malleolus and up the lateral side of the tendo calcaneus to the posterior aspect of the calf. It pierces the deep fascia in the lower part of the popliteal fossa to join the deep popliteal vein (Fig. 3.26c, d).

Palpation

- The small (short) saphenous vein. The lateral marginal vein is a little more difficult to recognize than the medial. You can trace it along the lateral side of the dorsum of the foot, but its continuation is difficult to palpate behind the lateral malleolus. The section between the lateral malleolus and the popliteal fossa may be difficult to palpate. After a long period of standing, however, it usually becomes quite visible and therefore more easily palpable.
- **Note.** In some individuals, particularly in elderly subjects, a network of vessels can be palpated on the medial side of the leg and thigh, which roughly follow the course of the great saphenous vein. Most of these join with the great saphenous vein along its length.

The head and neck 4

Contents

At the end of this chapter you should be able to:

1. Find, recognize and name the constituent components of the external surface of the skull, noting their size and position.
2. Palpate many of the bony features, being able to relate one to another.
3. Locate, name and palpate the bony and cartilaginous structures at the front of the neck.
4. Recognize and palpate bony landmarks of the cervical spine.
5. Name all the joints of the skull, recognizing the bones which form them.
6. Palpate and trace the lines of the sutures and joints of the skull and cervical spine, where possible, indicating their bony landmarks and surface markings.
7. Describe or carry out any accessory movements possible, noting the ranges in which they are most evident.
8. Note the range of movement of the cervical spine and indicate the factors limiting the movement.
9. Give the class and type of each of the joints.
10. Name and demonstrate the action of all the muscles palpable in the head and neck.
11. Draw the shape of the muscle on the surface and palpate its contraction.
12. Name all the main cutaneous nerves supplying the head and neck, giving their distribution.
13. Name the main arteries of the head and neck, giving their course and distribution.
14. Name the main veins of the head and neck, noting their drainage areas and course.

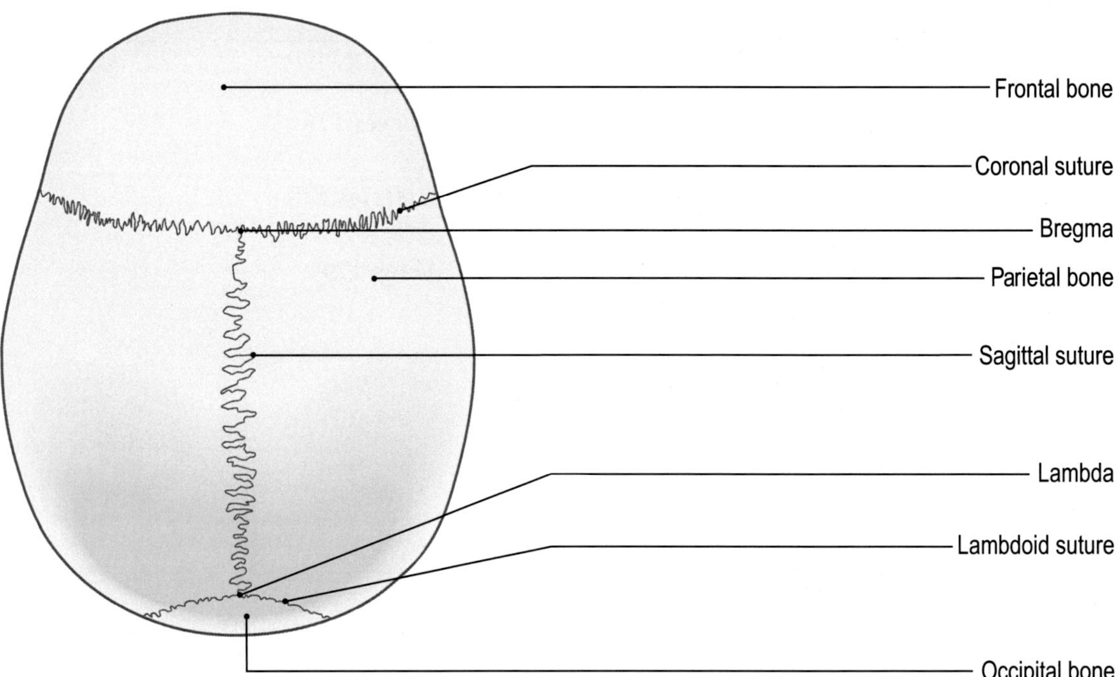

Fig. 4.1 (a) The skull (superior aspect)

BONES

The skull

Superior aspect (Fig. 4.1a)

The skull, viewed from above, is shaped like a flattened egg. It is broader across the posterior dimension and narrower across the anterior dimension. Its length, from front to back, is normally almost twice its breadth from side to side.

It comprises the **frontal, two parietal** [*paries* (L) = a wall] and part of the occipital [*occipitum* (L) = the back of the head] bones. Viewed from above, the frontal bone makes up the anterior section, forming approximately one-third. The two parietal bones form most of the posterior two-thirds. The occipital bone fits into just the central posterior part of the skull.

The frontal bone joins the anterior borders of the two parietal bones at the **coronal** [*corona* (L) = crown] **suture** which runs transversely across the skull. The intersection of all three bones is known as '**bregma**' [*brechein* (Gk) = to moisten, the most humid and delicate part of the infant's brain]. The two parietal bones join at the **sagittal** [*sagitta* (L) = an arrow, the direction in which an arrow would pass through the body] **suture**, which runs anteroposteriorly along the centre of the skull.

The posterior borders of both parietal bones meet the anterior border of the squamous part of the occipital bone at the **lambdoid** [*lambda* = the Greek letter 'L'] **sutures**. The point at which all three bones meet is termed '**lambda**'.

Palpation

The skull is covered, superiorly, by a fibromuscular sheet (aponeurosis) from the eyebrows anteriorly to the **external occipital protuberance** and the superior nuchal lines posteriorly. This is thick and adherent to the skin covering the skull but only attached to the pericranium by areolar tissue. This gives it a certain amount of freedom to move over the skull. It is continuous laterally with the temporal and zygomatic fascia.

Due to this arrangement and the fact that there is normally a covering of hair, palpation of the bones, sutures and landmarks of the skull requires a slightly different technique if exact location is required. Use all the fingertips of both hands to locate and mark the structures, using a gentle forward and backward motion, moving the aponeurosis on the underlying bone.

For palpation in this region, the model is in the sitting position.

- The sagital suture. Place your fingers anterior and posterior to the vertex of the skull. On pressing the tips in and moving them from side to side, the sagittal suture can be palpated, particularly posteriorly.
- The point of lambda. Halfway between the vertex and the external occipital protuberance a hollow can be felt with two sutures running downwards and laterally in front of the occipital bone. This is the point 'lambda'.
- The point of bregma. Moving approximately 5 cm forwards from the vertex there is another palpable slight hollow with

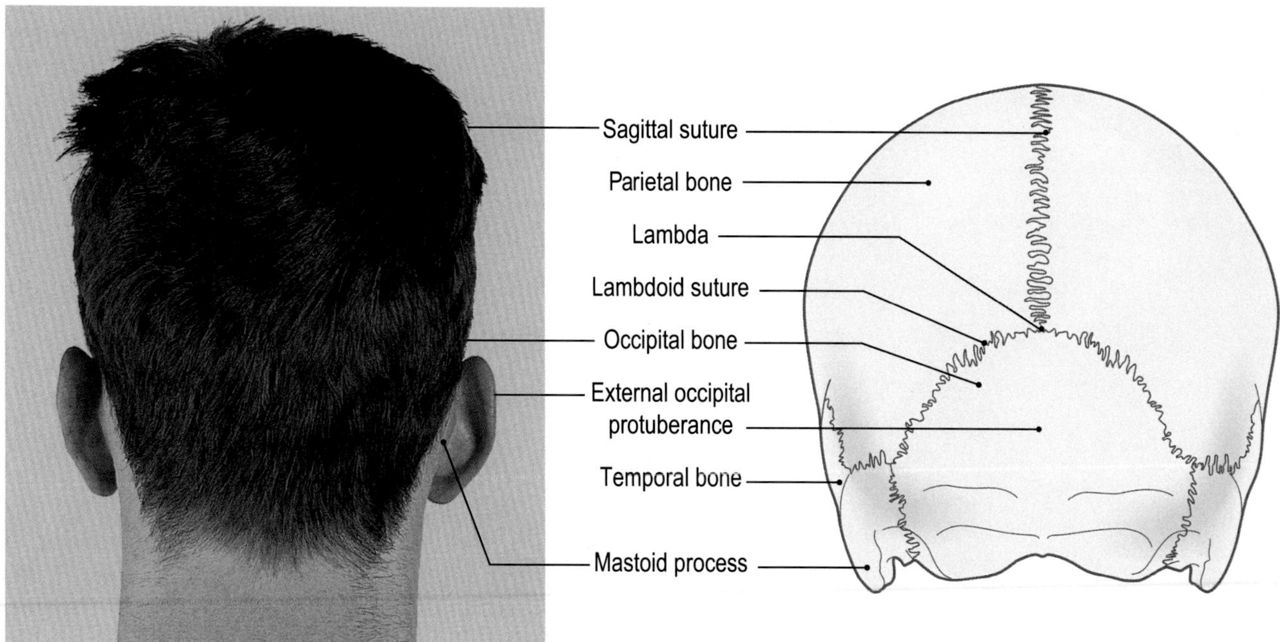

Fig. 4.1 (b, c) The skull (posterior aspect)

the coronal suture running laterally to either side. This point is termed 'bregma'.

- The frontal bone (forehead). In front of the coronal suture the frontal bone can be palpated, sometimes with a central raised line where the two bones have fused.
- The parietal bones. Either side of the sagittal suture, behind the frontal bones and in front of the occipital bone, are the two large plates of the parietal bones.

Posterior aspect (Fig. 4.1b, c)

The posteroinferior part of the skull consists mainly of the occipital bone. On either side it joins the **temporal bones**, each of which has a large downward-projecting prominence termed the **mastoid** [*mastos* (Gk) = a breast, *oeides* (Gk) = shape] **process**. Superiorly the occipital bone joins the two parietal bones forming the vault of the skull. Its anterior portion forms the base of the skull, surrounding the foramen magnum and projecting forwards as the basilar section.

Posteriorly, at its apex, the occipital bone fits between the two parietal bones at the point lambda. Running downwards and laterally from this point, the two lambdoid sutures divide the occiput from the two parietal bones. The bone presents a large tuberosity, about 5 cm below the point lambda, termed the external occipital protuberance, with superior, middle and inferior nuchal lines radiating laterally. The external occipital protuberance varies considerably in its size, being very prominent in some and almost non-existent in others.

Palpation

- The external occipital protuberance. The most prominent bony feature of the posterior aspect of the skull is the external occipital protuberance situated just below its centre. It varies in size and shape between individuals, being large and prominent in some and difficult to find in others.
- The superior nuchal lines of the occipital bone. Radiating laterally and upwards from the external occipital protuberance are the two superior nuchal lines. (Nuchal: believed to come from Arabic '*nugraph*' = the back of the neck.) These are palpable in their central section on most subjects, but are difficult to trace for more than a few centimetres laterally.
- The sagital suture. Approximately 5 cm above the external occipital protuberance the sagittal suture meets two occipitoparietal sutures. In the young child this is the region of the posterior fontanelle [*fons* (L) = small fountain or spring], which in the adult becomes the lambda.
- The occipital bone. Inferiorly the occipital bone can be traced forwards under the skull, but is soon lost in the deep hollow at the level of the tubercle of the first cervical vertebra.
- The mastoid process of the temporal bone. Moving to either side, just behind the pinna of each car, the mastoid process of the temporal bone can be palpated. It is pointed at its inferior aspect where the sternocleidomastoid muscle attaches.

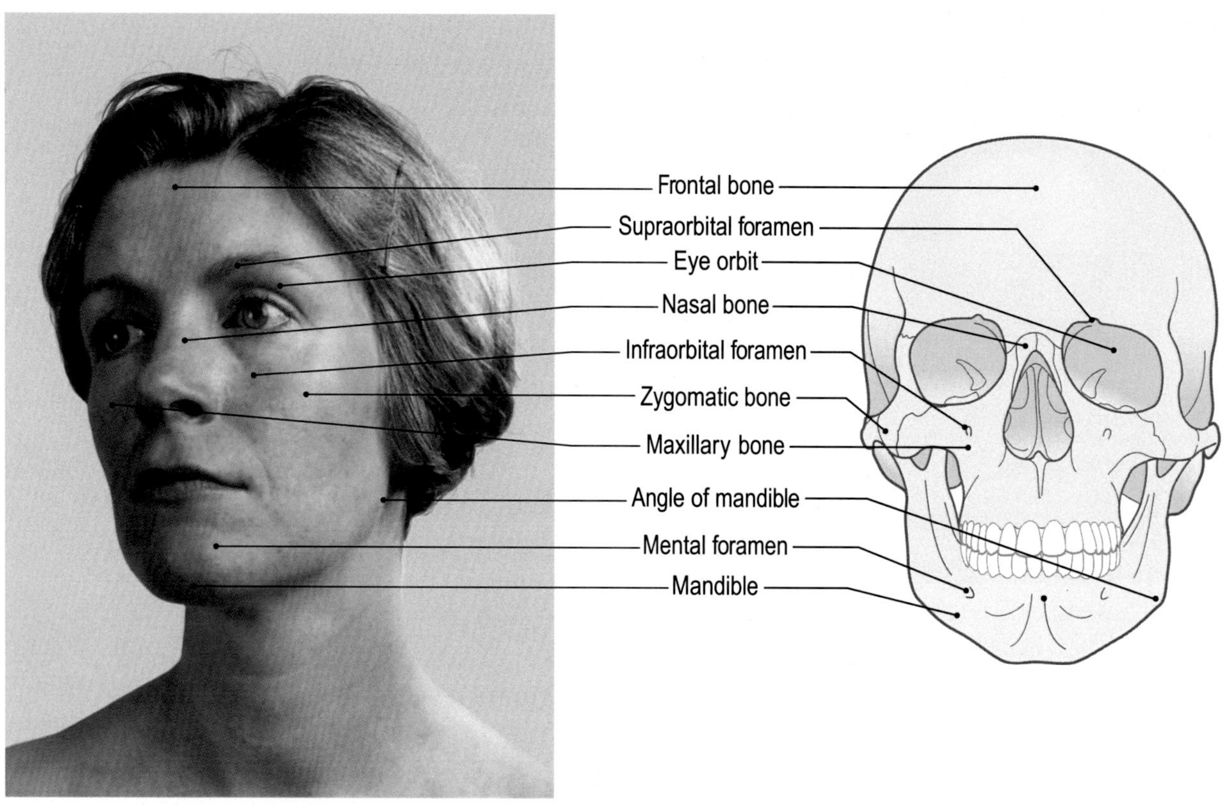

Fig. 4.2 (a, b) The skull (anterior aspect)

Anterior aspect (Fig. 4.2a, b)

Each eye orbit is formed superiorly by the frontal bone (which forms the forehead), laterally by the zygomatic bone, medially by the nasal bone and inferiorly by the maxilla. The upper teeth are associated with the maxilla, while the lower teeth are located in the superior border of the mandible.

Palpation

- The eye orbit. Deep to the eyebrow the upper rim of the eye orbit can be palpated, being slightly notched at its centre where it is crossed by the supraorbital artery. The whole margin of the orbit is subcutaneous and can thus readily be palpated.
- The two nasal bones. These can be palpated centrally, projecting forwards and continuing as a cartilage down to the centre of the nose.
- The upper part of the maxilla. Below this, the upper part of the maxilla can be palpated, investing the upper teeth.

Lateral aspect (Fig. 4.2c, d)

The temporal [*tempus* (L) = time (pertaining to the passing of time and the greying of the temples)] bone forms the central area on the side of the skull. Posteriorly it articulates with the occipital bone, superiorly with the parietal bone and anteriorly, with the sphenoid [*sphen* (Gk) = a wedge] and zygomatic [*zygoma* (Gk) = a yoke or bar] bones.

The anterior section of the lateral aspect consists of the frontal bone and the maxilla, with the lateral part of the ethmoid [*ethmos* (Gk) = a sieve] just projecting between the sphenoid and frontal bones. Inferiorly the mandible [*mando* (L) = I chew] articulates by its condyle with the undersurface of the temporal bone just anterior to the external auditory meatus [*meatus* (L) = a passage].

Palpation

- The external auditory meatus. This is an obvious landmark on the lateral side of the head. The little finger can be pressed

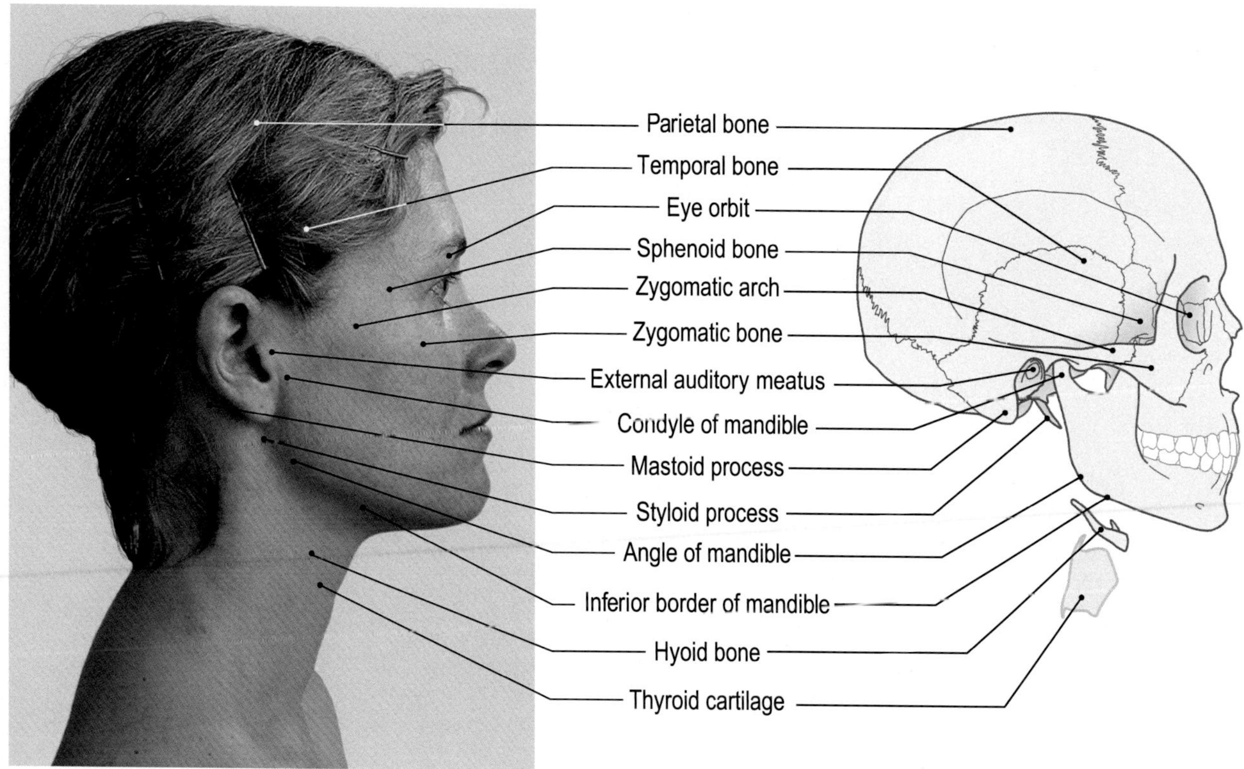

Fig. 4.2 (c, d) The skull (lateral aspect)

deep into this opening to be surrounded by its bony walls. The pinna lies around three sides, while the tragus is the pointed area of soft tissue overlapping the meatus from the front.

- The **zygomatic arch**. Running horizontally forwards just anterior to the tragus [*tragos* (Gk) and *tregus* (L) = a goat (possibly pertaining to the shape of a goat's beard)], a bony bridge can be palpated. This is the zygomatic arch. It forms the point of the cheek at the front where it joins the zygomatic bone (Fig. 4.2c, d). The arch is formed partly from the temporal and partly from the zygomatic bones.
- The condyle of the mandible. Below the posterior part of the zygomatic arch anterior to the tragus a small tubercle can be palpated. This is the most lateral part of the condyle of the mandible. If the model opens the mouth, this bony prominence can be felt, first rotating then moving forwards and downwards over the articular eminence of the temporal bone.
- The **angle of the mandible**. Some 7 cm directly below the condyle of the mandible, the angle of the mandible can be identified, being more prominent in men than in women as it is slightly everted.
- The **inferior border of the mandible**. This can be traced forward to a raised vertical line centrally at the front, where it joins the bone of the opposite side.
- The mental tubercle. A small tubercle (the mental tubercle) can be palpated on the inferior border either side of this line.
- The anterior and lateral surfaces of the mandible. These are subcutaneous and can be traced posteriorly as far as the angle where they are hidden by the powerful muscles of mastication. The lower border is thickened all round, giving a concave appearance to the anterior surface.
- The maxilla. Below the zygomatic bone the maxilla can be palpated, with the teeth and gums easily identifiable through the flesh of the cheek and the upper lip.

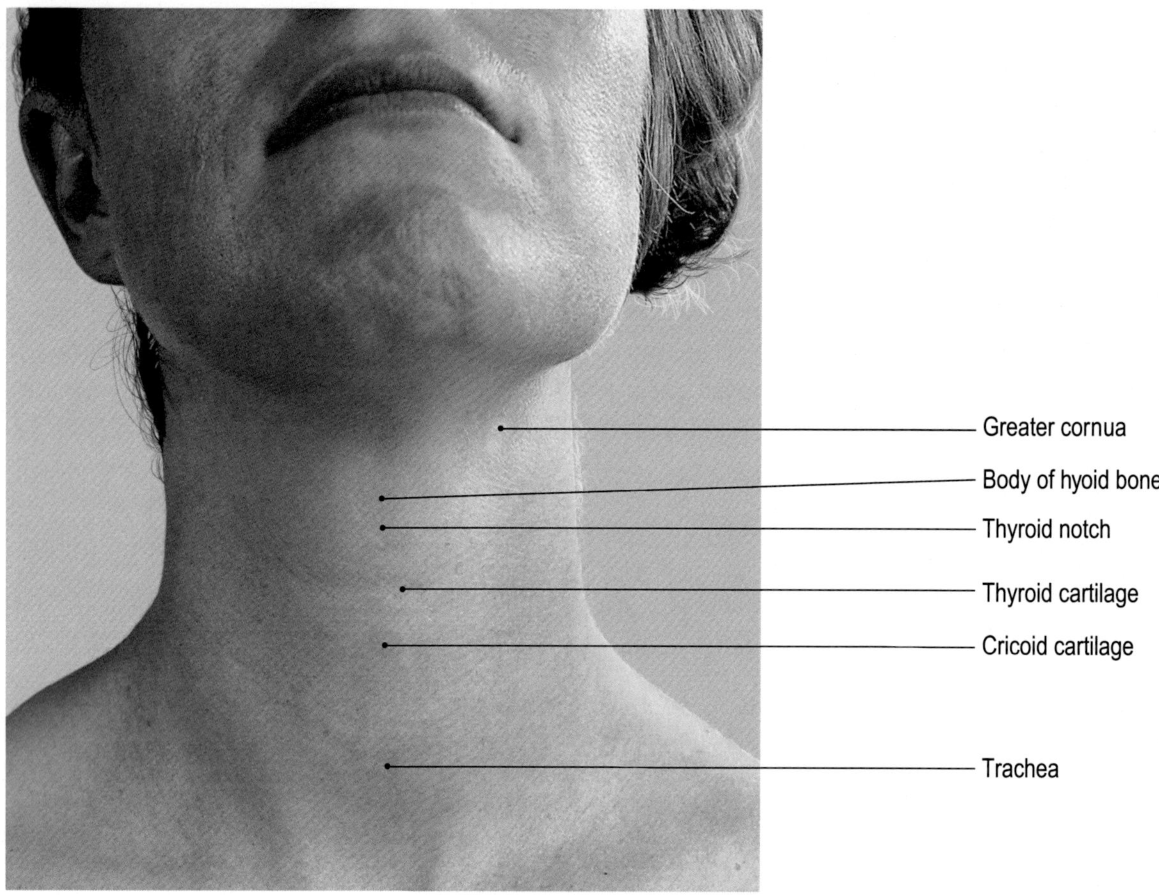

Fig. 4.3 (a) The neck (anterior aspect)

The neck

Anterior aspect (Fig. 4.3a, b)

A series of midline structures run down the anterior aspect of the neck. These are part of the respiratory tract. Just below the mandible is the small horseshoe-shaped **hyoid bone** [*hyoeides* (Gk) = U-shaped, i.e. shaped like the Greek letter ipsilon]. Below, the **thyroid** [*thyreos* (Gk) = a shield] cartilage is formed from two cartilaginous plates which are fused anteriorly to form the 'Adam's apple' (prominent in the male) and the **thyroid notch**.

Behind the sternal notch lie the upper rings of the trachea [*trachys* (Gk) = uneven]. Interestingly, Aristotle mistakenly thought that this structure was an uneven surfaced artery. Between the upper ring and the thyroid cartilage lies the thicker and stronger signet-shaped ring of the **cricoid cartilage** [*krikos* (Gk) = a ring].

The larynx, formed mainly from the thyroid and cricoid cartilages, lies centrally at a level with the third to the sixth vertebral bodies and between the two sternomastoid muscles which converge from above downwards.

The mandible, hyoid bone, thyroid and cricoid cartilages, and the upper part of the trachea are all linked by muscle and ligaments. They provide the tube for air to enter the lungs: 'the windpipe'.

Palpation

It is quite unpleasant, and often frightening, to have these structures palpated by another person. It is therefore advisable to perform the palpation on yourself.

- The hyoid bone. Place the fingers and thumb of one hand on either side of the mandible halfway along its inferior border. Then slide your fingers and thumb down on to the sides of the throat. Some 3–5 cm below the mandible, you will feel the hyoid bone lying almost horizontal. It will appear as a horseshoe-shaped structure, rounded and thicker anteriorly and

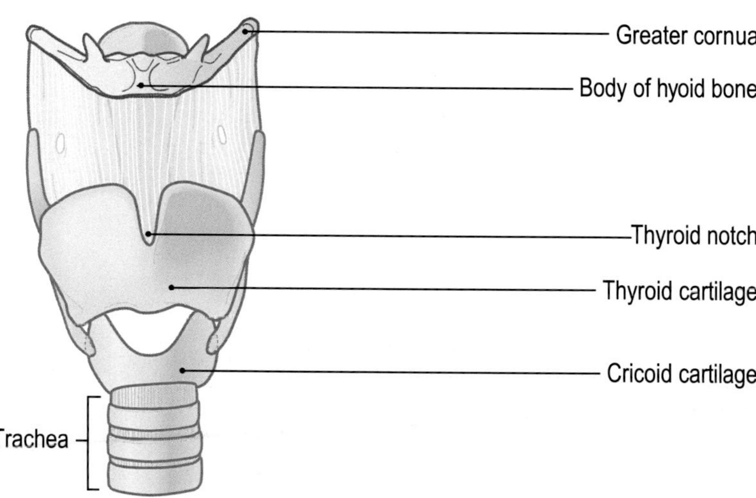

Fig. 4.3 (b) Bones of the neck (anterior aspect)

becoming pointed on either side posteriorly as it curves upwards slightly. This is the greater wing (*cornua*). Gentle pressure applied to either side will confirm its bony consistency.

- The laminae of the thyroid cartilage. Continue down the sides of the neck from the hyoid. After crossing a small space (felt as a depression), you will encounter the broad flat lamina of the thyroid cartilage on either side. Each lamina is angled medially so that they meet in the midline anteriorly.
- The larynx. A marked projection (the laryngeal prominence), more pronounced in men, can be felt superiorly in the midline. This projection is commonly referred to as the 'Adam's apple'.
- The thyroid notch. Now place your finger on the anterosuperior aspect of this prominence. You will identify a small space, concave upwards: this is the thyroid notch.
- The cricoid cartilage. Trace down the sides of the thyroid cartilage for about 4 cm to a line just above the level of the medial ends of the clavicles. Here, after crossing another small space, you will palpate a further ring-shaped structure. This is the cricoid cartilage which presents with a small tubercle at its centre.
- The trachea. Below the cricoid cartilage and deep in the suprasternal (jugular) notch you can palpate the cartilaginous rings of the upper part of the trachea.
- **Note.** Each of the structures identified above can be taken between the finger and thumb of the same hand and carefully moved from side to side for a distance of about 1 cm. Too much side movement can, however, lead to tenderness in this part of the neck. During swallowing, each of the structures rises and then falls approximately 1 cm.
- The sternocleidomastoid muscle. This muscle can be felt on either side of these central structures. This is facilitated if the model adopts the supine lying position. Ask the model to raise the head from a pillow. These muscles are widely spaced at the level of the hyoid bone but become much closer together as they approach the level of the clavicles.

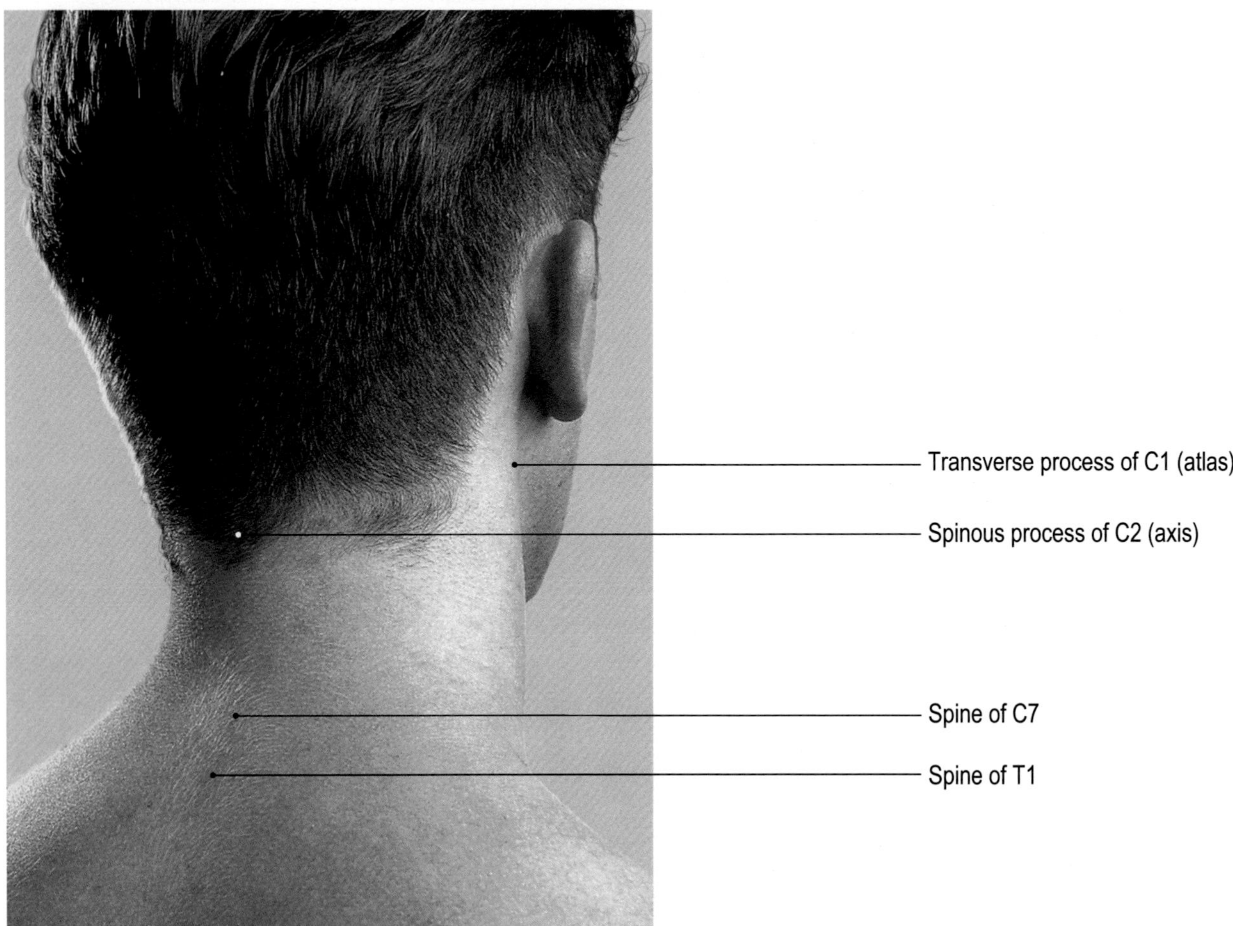

Fig. 4.4 (a) The neck (posterior aspect)

Posterior aspect (Fig. 4.4)

There are seven cervical vertebrae. Except for C1 (the atlas [derived from *atlao* (Gk) = I sustain]), C2 (the axis [*axis* (L) = a pivot or axle]) and C7, they all exhibit similar characteristics: small oval bodies, large vertebral canal, long laminae, a bifid spine and a broad transverse process with a foramen transversarium.

C1 does not possess a body, but has two lateral masses to support the weight of the head transferred via the occipital condyles. It has a posterior tubercle instead of a spine and its transverse processes are wide and relatively pointed.

C2 has a tooth-like process projecting superiorly from its body, the dens or odontoid [*ódous* (Gk) = tooth) peg, a large prominent spine and small transverse processes. The seventh cervical vertebra is noted for its long non-bifid spine (vertebra prominens).

Palpation

For palpation of the neck, the model is in the prone lying position with the forehead resting on the backs of the hands on a pillow to facilitate maximum relaxation. The chin should be tucked in slightly and the neck straight.

- The external occipital protruberance. Begin the palpation by finding the external occipital protuberance, with the raised crescentic superior nuchal lines curving laterally.
- The external occipital crest. Running inferiorly and under the back of the skull from the protuberance, you can palpate the external occipital crest It ends at a deep hollow which is level with the tubercle of the atlas (not palpable). The hollow is bounded below by the large prominence of the spine of the

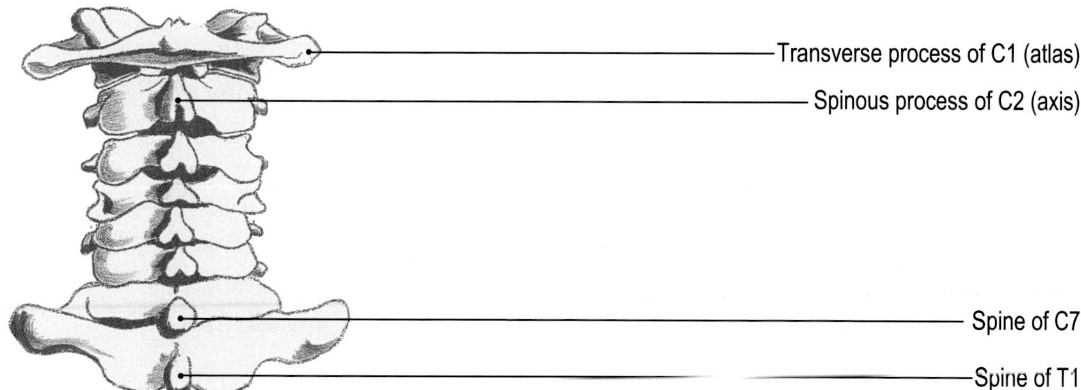

Fig. 4.4 (b) Bones of the neck (posterior aspect)

axis. This is approximately 3 cm below the external occipital protuberance.

- The spine of the axis. This is easy to find and can be used for identification and location of other bony features.
- The spines of C3–C4. Below, the spines of C3, C4 and C5 are closely packed together due to the curvature of the spine at this point. The spine of C3 lies close under the spine of C2 and is therefore difficult to palpate. The spine of C4 is often mistaken for that of C3.
- The spine of C5. Just above the spine of C6, that of C5 is identifiable, being very close to that of C4.
- The spines of C5–T1. Progress to the lower part of the cervical spine where you will feel two, clearly prominent, spinous processes. They are close together and rigid to the touch. The lower of the two is the spine of T1; that just above is the spine of C7. The spine of C6 stands out clearly above that of C7 and can at times be mistaken for it.
- The spine of C7. Differentiation between the spines of C6 and C7 is achieved by asking the model to extend the head and neck while keeping your finger on the spine of C6. This spine tends to move forward, causing it to disappear from beneath the palpating finger, while the spine of C7 remains stationary.
- **Note.** It would be expected that flexion of the neck would improve identification. Unfortunately, except for the spines of C7 and T1, this is not the case as the tightening ligamentum nuchae hides the spines. The spines of C3, C4, C5 and C6, although difficult to identify separately, appear broad due to their bifid nature (Fig. 4.4).

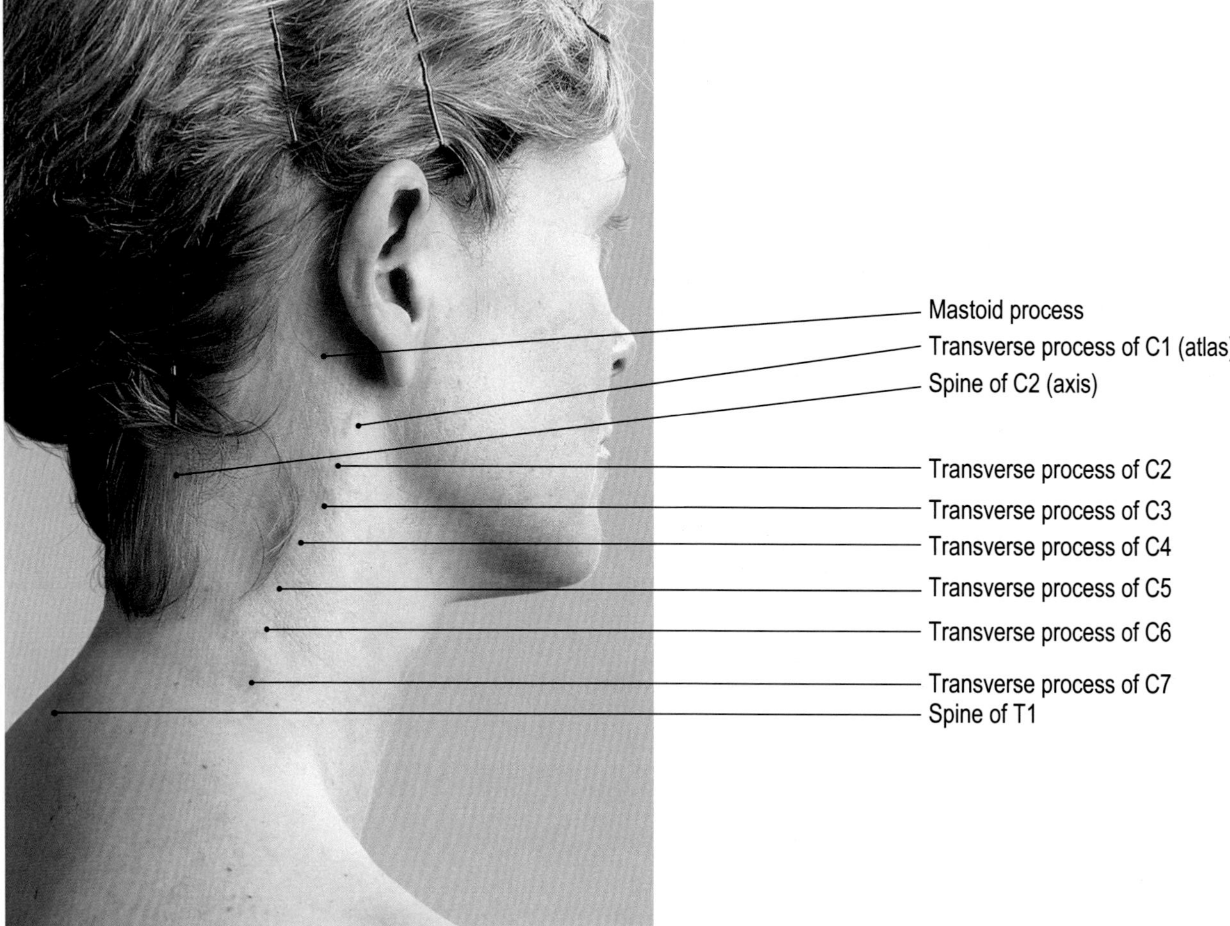

Fig. 4.5 (a) The neck (lateral aspect)

Lateral aspect (Fig. 4.5)

Palpation

- The transverse processes of the cervical vertebrae. Although the transverse processes of the cervical vertebrae appear to project well out to the side, they are in fact quite difficult to palpate and identify.
- The tip of the transverse process of C1. It is possible to palpate the tip of the transverse process of C1 between the angle of the mandible and the tip of the mastoid process. In some subjects, the transverse process of C1 is not only palpable but also visible, as a small prominence. In others, it is difficult to identify even on deep palpation.
- Note. This region can be quite tender if too much pressure is applied and care must be taken to avoid the long and narrow styloid process just deep and anterior to the mastoid process.
- The transverse processes of C2–T1. The other transverse processes, with the exception of C2, present a double point laterally, the anterior and posterior tubercles, but owing to muscle attachments and fascial coverings they are not easy to distinguish. You can identify the line of the transverse processes from the back by easing your fingers into the side of the neck some 2 cm anterior to the tips of the spines. With care, you will be able to palpate the lower articular pillar of the vertebra above, lying medial to each posterior tubercle. This is at the inferior limit of the facet (zygapophyseal) joint. Pressure on

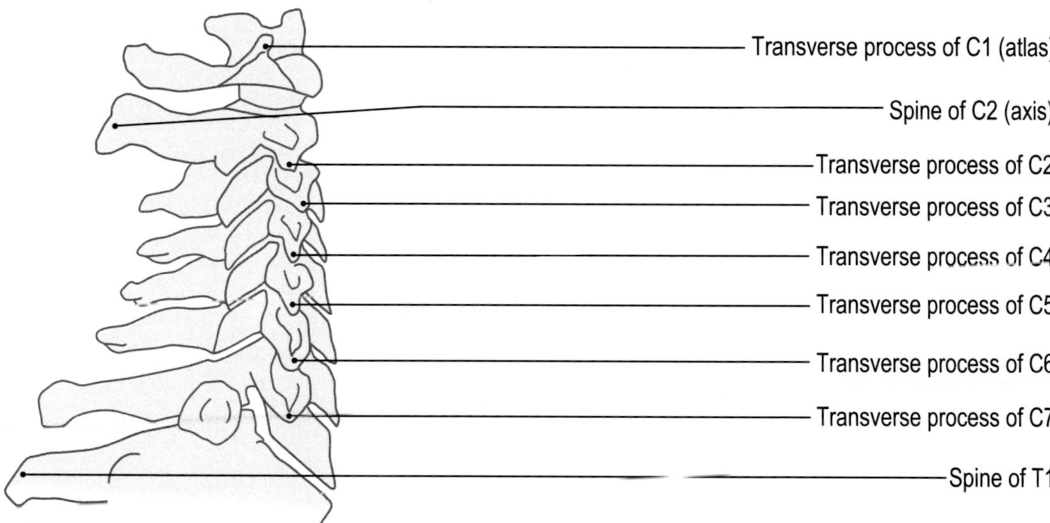

Fig. 4.5 (b) Bones of the neck (lateral aspect)

this tubercle will produce compression of the facet joint, whereas pressure just below the tubercle will produce an anterior movement of the lower articular pillar and slight gapping of the joint surfaces.

- The transverse processes – general. Normally the thick muscles covering the transverse processes need to be moved aside to facilitate palpation. More 'feel' of the transverse processes is possible if you ask the model to adopt a supine position. Stand at the head of the plinth, facing the model's feet, and cradle the occiput in both hands. With the fingers of either hand resting on the posterolateral part of the neck, move the head from side to side. Apply gentle pressure to the transverse process with your fingers on the opposite side to that being examined. This opens up the side of interest with the space between the transverse processes increasing, facilitating their identification.
- The facet joints. The facet joints of this side are also being gapped, causing a greater convexity to the side being examined. You will notice that slight rotation to the opposite side occurs during this movement (see Fig. 4.7a, b). This technique can be used from C1 to T1.
- The transverse processes – anterior aspect. In the lower section of the neck, you can palpate these transverse processes from the front, although it is slightly uncomfortable. Occasionally, the costal element (the anterior segment of the transverse process) of C7 projects more anterolaterally than usual and can be palpated 2 cm above and 2 cm lateral to the medial end of the clavicle. This is often referred to as a 'cervical rib'.

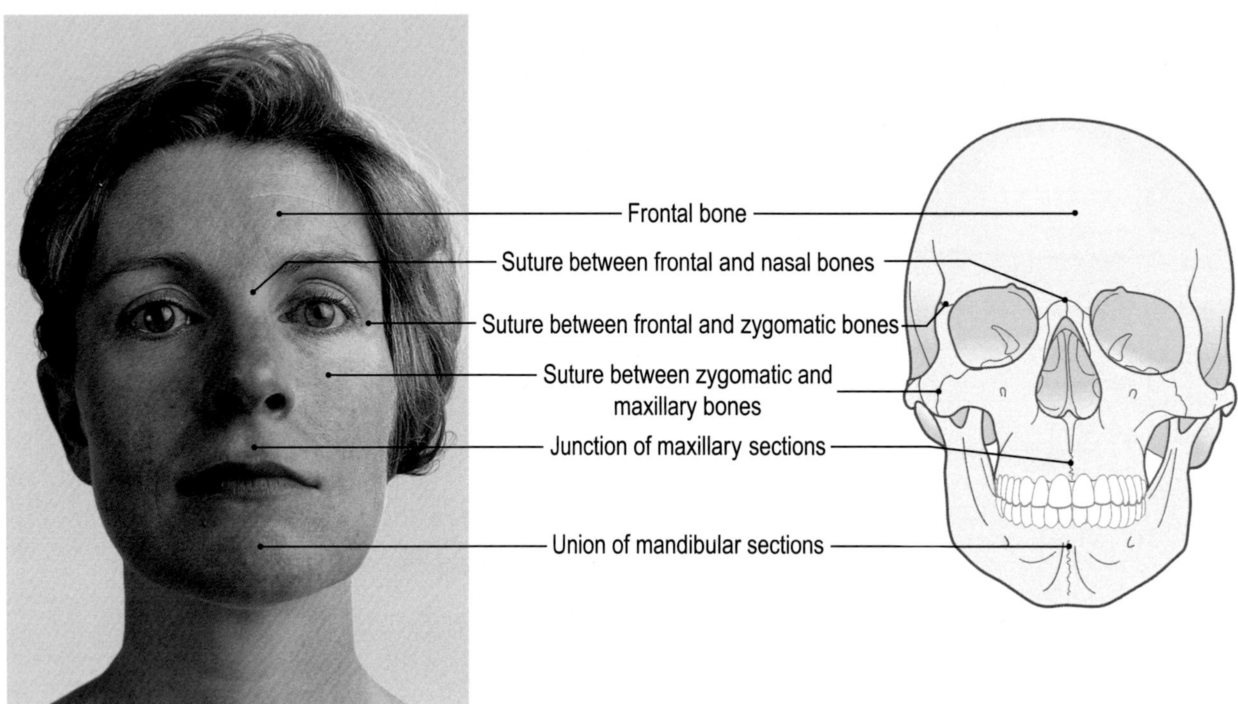

Fig. 4.6 (a, b) The joints of the head (anterior aspect)

JOINTS

The skull (Fig. 4.6)

Most of the plates of bone which contribute to the vault of the skull are united by fibrous joints in the form of sutures. These are often visible on the surface and were described and palpated in the section on bones (see p. 150–153). Other suture lines which can be palpated are those between the parietal and temporal bones, between the temporal and zygomatic bones and between the two halves of the mandibles.

Palpation

- The first suture of the temporal bone. This lies at the upper edge of the squamous portion of the temporal bone. It arches convexly upwards from the depression just lateral to the eye orbit to just anterior to the upper part of the pinna of the ear. Ask the model to clench the teeth and palpate the temporalis muscle contracting above the zygomatic arch (see p. 153). At the curved upper part of this muscle, the line of the suture can be identified.
- The second suture of the temporal bone. This can be palpated approximately halfway along the zygomatic arch. Run your finger anteroposteriorly where the suture can be felt as a raised ridge crossing the arch vertically.
- The suture of the mandible. This can be palpated between the two halves of the mandible, running vertically downwards from the centre of the lower lip to the inferior border between the two mental tubercles. It is often marked by a sharp ridge.

Accessory movements of the joints of the skull

In the unborn child and infant these plates of bone can allow considerable movement and, on occasions, even override each other. There is slight movement throughout childhood and early adult life, but from the twenties through to middle age there is gradual fusion of the various sutures, beginning with the sagittal

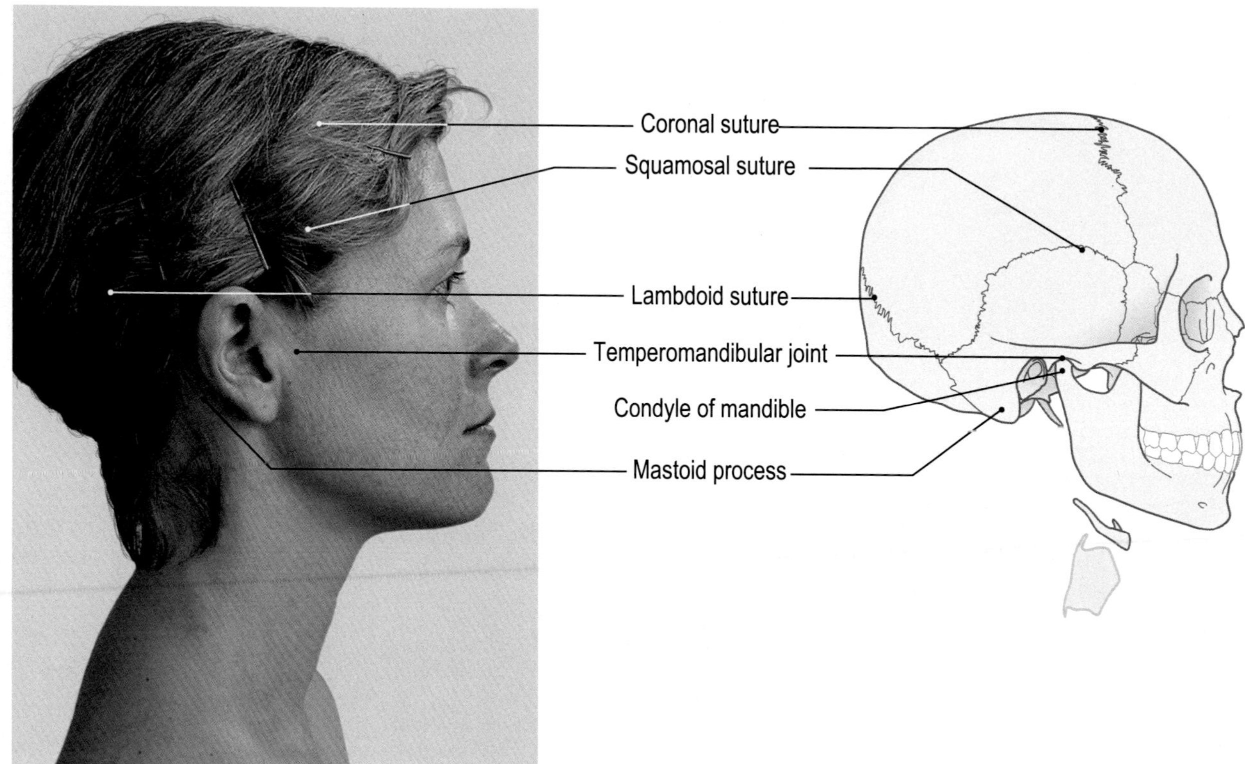

Fig. 4.6 (c, d) The joints of the head (lateral aspect)

suture (Palastanga et al 2002). Some authorities believe that the movement of one plate of bone on another influences the structures below and can be used as a therapeutic technique.

The temporomandibular joint (Fig. 4.6c, d)

This is a bicondylar articulation taking place between the mandibular fossae of the temporal bone and the condylar processes of the mandible, the two joints being linked by the mandible.

Palpation: surface marking

- The joint line. From the tragus of the ear, trace forwards under the posterior section of the zygomatic arch for 2 cm, where a small tubercle on the condyle of the mandible can be palpated. The line of the joint lies just above this tubercle, running forwards for approximately 2 cm concave downwards posteriorly and convex downwards anteriorly. Ask the model to open the mouth; the joint line then becomes clearer as the condyle first rotates and then moves forward on the undersurface of the temporal bone.

Accessory movements

This joint is capable of many physiological movements, mainly involved in mastication. Its only true accessory movement, however, is distraction.

Palpation on movement

- Distraction. This can be produced by placing the thumbs in the mouth on the lower molar teeth on both sides, with the fingers of each hand supporting the underside of the mandible from outside. Downward pressure is then applied to the teeth via the thumbs, using the fingers to hold the anterior part of the mandible stationary. This creates the necessary leverage to pull the condyles away from the temporal bone. Complete relaxation of the muscles of mastication is essential for any gapping to occur.

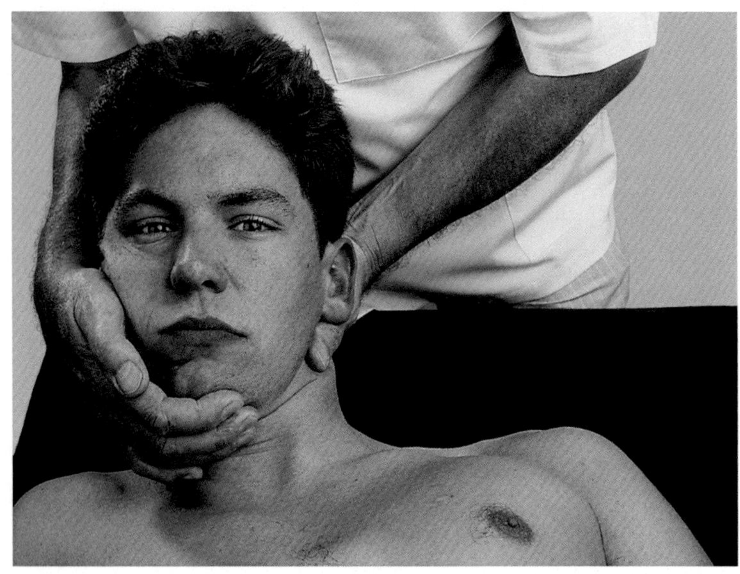

Fig. 4.7 (a) Right lateral movement of the cervical spine

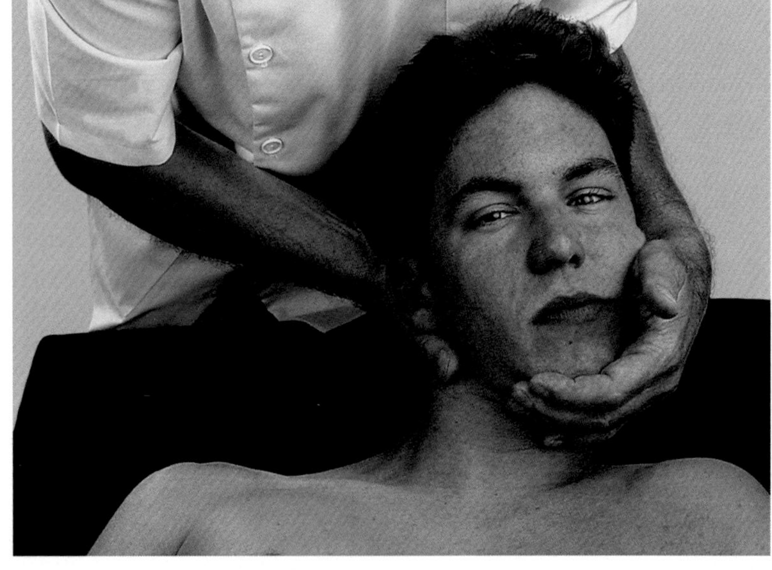

Fig. 4.7 (b) Left lateral movement of the cervical spine

The cervical spine (Figs 4.7 and 4.8)

With the exception of the joints between the occiput and C1, and C1 and C2, the cervical vertebrae articulate by a series of fibrous discs centrally, synovial zygapophyseal joints between the articular processes laterally, and synovial uncovertebral joints between the lateral margins of adjacent vertebral bodies.

The occipital condyles either side of the foramen magnum articulate with the facets on the superior surface of the lateral masses of the atlas (C1) as a bicondylar joint. The atlas articulates with the axis (C2) via plane joints either side of the dens and a single central pivot joint between the dens and the anterior arch of the atlas, in front, and with the transverse ligament, behind. All of these are synovial joints.

Palpation

It is difficult to palpate any joints in the cervical region owing to their depth and location. Movements of many can be achieved by pressure on the bones that take part, but actual joint lines are normally impossible to determine and feel.

- Joint lines. Find the articular pillars of C2–C7 lying 2 cm lateral to the spines (see p. 164). With deep but sensitive palpation, the lines of the lower zygapophyseal joints can just be detected level with the tip of the spinous process of the same vertebra.

Accessory movements

- Traction on the cervical spine (C2–C7), either mechanically or manually, is a true accessory movement, as it is a movement that the subject cannot perform alone. It can be carried out in extension, flexion, rotation or any combination of these, depending on the results required. It produces parting of the surfaces of the zygapophyseal and central joints with a stretching of the disc, the surrounding ligaments and muscles. There will be a decrease in the pressure within the disc, and an

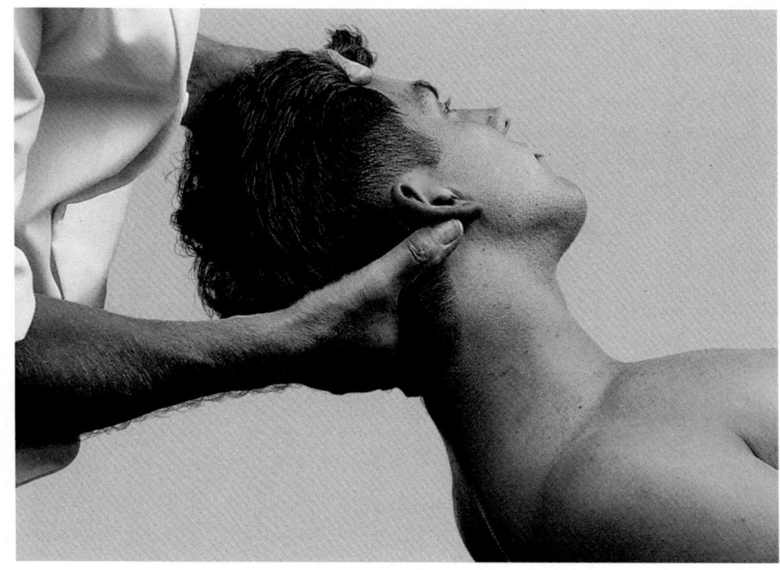

Fig. 4.7 (c) Anterior movement of the cervical spine

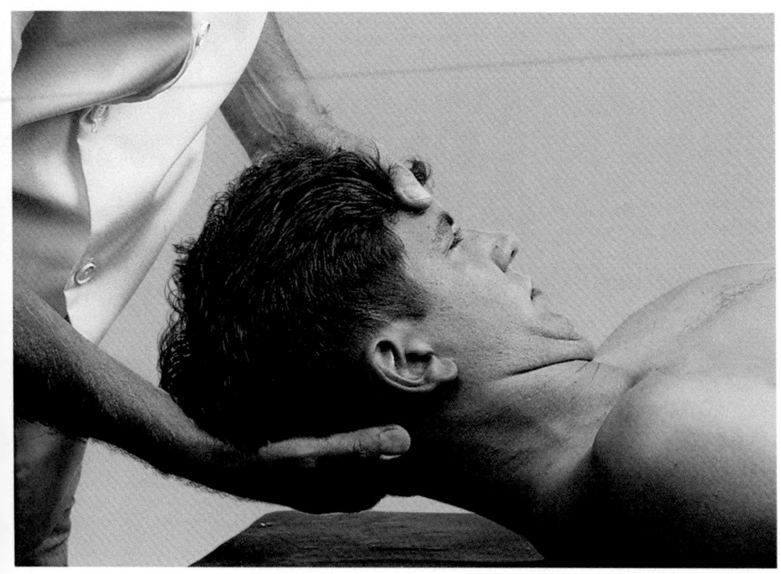

Fig. 4.7 (d) Posterior movement of the cervical spine

increase in the size, particularly in flexion, of the intervertebral foramen, through which the cervical nerves emerge.

- Traction on the joints between the occiput, C1 and C2. This is best obtained when the neck is slightly extended. Its use, however, is normally restricted as it can produce undesirable and dangerous effects, due to the complex nature of these joints, particularly concerning the ligaments around the dens. The ligaments remain taut in all movements, thereby maintaining the relationship of the dens with the atlas and occiput. Accessory movement, necessary for gliding to occur, is only possible because of the precise curvatures of the articular surfaces.
- Sideways movement of the neck. The model is in the supine lying position in which a sideways movement of the whole neck can be achieved. Hold the head between both hands and move it from side to side while maintaining its longitudinal position (Fig. 4.7a, b).
- Forwards and backwards movement. A similar movement forwards and backwards can also be achieved. Place one hand over the forehead and the other hand behind the occiput. Move the head forwards and backwards, again maintaining its longitudinal position (Fig. 4.7c, d).
- Localization of the side-to-side movement. Using a sagittal axis, passing through the nose, the side-to-side movement can be localized to the joints between the condyles of the occipital bone and the lateral masses of the atlas.
- Localized forwards and backwards movement. Using a frontal axis through the centre of the skull, localized forward and backward gliding can also be achieved (Fig. 4.7c, d).

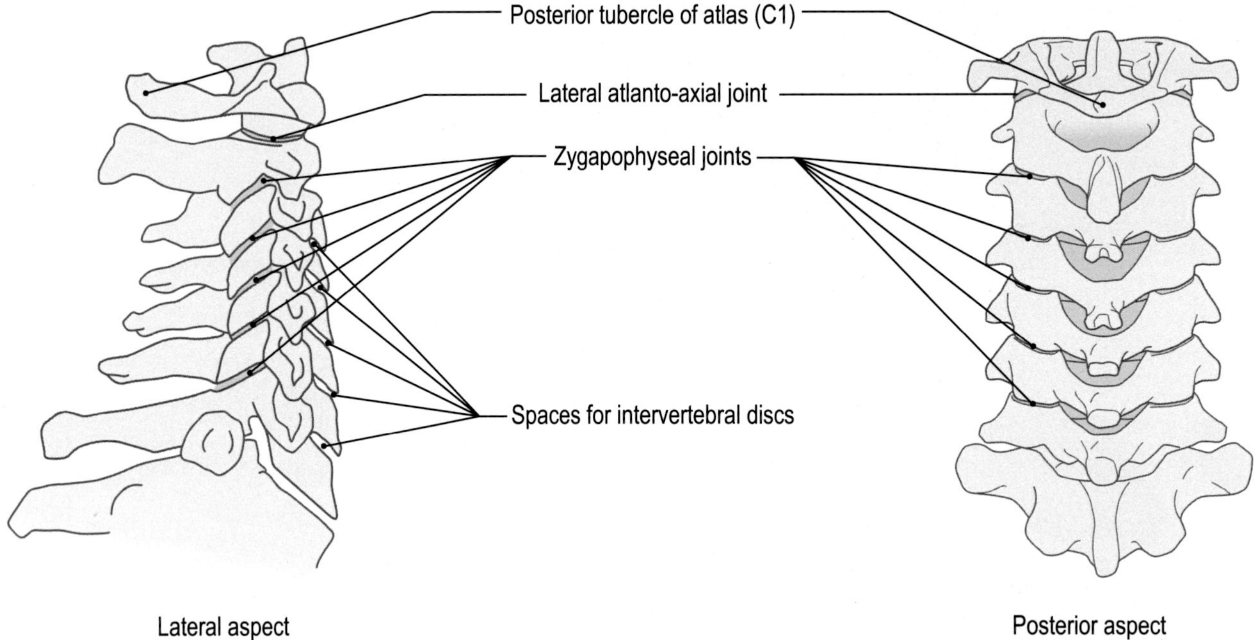

Fig. 4.8 (a, b) Joints of the cervical spine

Other movements of the cervical vertebrae, often considered to be accessory movements, are very similar to normal physiological movements. Nevertheless, certain elements are exaggerated and therefore worthy of note.

- Forward gliding of a vertebra on its neighbour. The model is in the prone lying position. In this position, forward gliding of a whole vertebra on its neighbour can be achieved by pressure applied with your thumbs on the tip of the spinous process. Movement is greatest around C4 and least between C7 and T1. Pressure on the spine of C2 produces no movement between C1 and C2, as the dens is in contact with the anterior arch of C1; however, slight forward gliding will be achieved between the occiput and C1, due to the two bones moving together.
- Forward gliding of the inferior articular surface. Pressure on the inferior articular pillar of C3–C7 produces a forward gliding of the inferior articular surface and a slight gapping of the superior **zygapophyseal joint** in a rotation-type movement.
- Forward gliding of the lateral mass. If a similar pressure is applied to the posterior aspect of the transverse process of C1, similar gliding of the lateral mass of that side against the occipital condyle and upper facet of C2 occurs.
- Side-to-side movement of the vertebrae. The model is in the supine lying position. Side-to-side movement of the vertebrae can be produced in this position. Cradle the head in your palms, as described on p. 163. Using your fingers of one side, apply pressure to the transverse process of the chosen vertebra. Your fingers of the opposite side will then feel the transverse

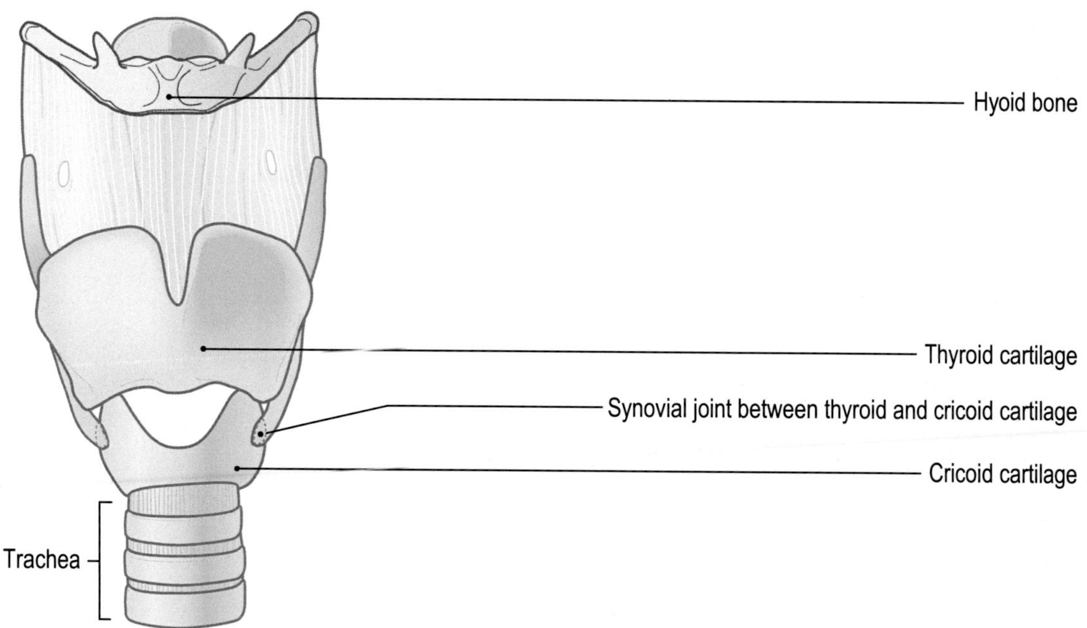

Fig. 4.8 (c) Anterior structures of the neck

processes opening up, as an accompaniment to the gapping of the zygapophyseal joint.

- Rotation of one vertebra on another. This can be taken to its limit if you carefully fix the lower vertebrae with your fingers and thumb and rotate the head with your other hand. These movements can be produced between any two cervical vertebrae, and even to some extent between the occiput and C1, producing gapping of their surfaces.
- **Note.** Most accessory movements of the cervical spine are difficult to perform without a great deal of knowledge and practice. It can be highly dangerous for an unskilled therapist to employ these procedures in this area, and it is recommended that the student must be carefully monitored by an experienced practitioner, who should test for contraindications prior to any movement being performed.

For further information, it is suggested that the reader consults the literature on manipulation and mobilization (Grieve 1986, Maitland 1991).

Anterior aspect of the neck

The **hyoid bone** and the **thyroid** and **cricoid cartilages** can all be moved from side to side approximately 1 cm using the finger and thumb alternately. They are linked by muscle and ligaments to the mandible and temporal bone above and the upper **trachea** below.

Between the inferior cornua of the thyroid cartilage and the arch of the cricoid cartilage are **small synovial joints** which can be located just above the posterior projections of the cricoid cartilage. These possess a capsule and can, at times, give pain and distress when they become inflamed or degenerated.

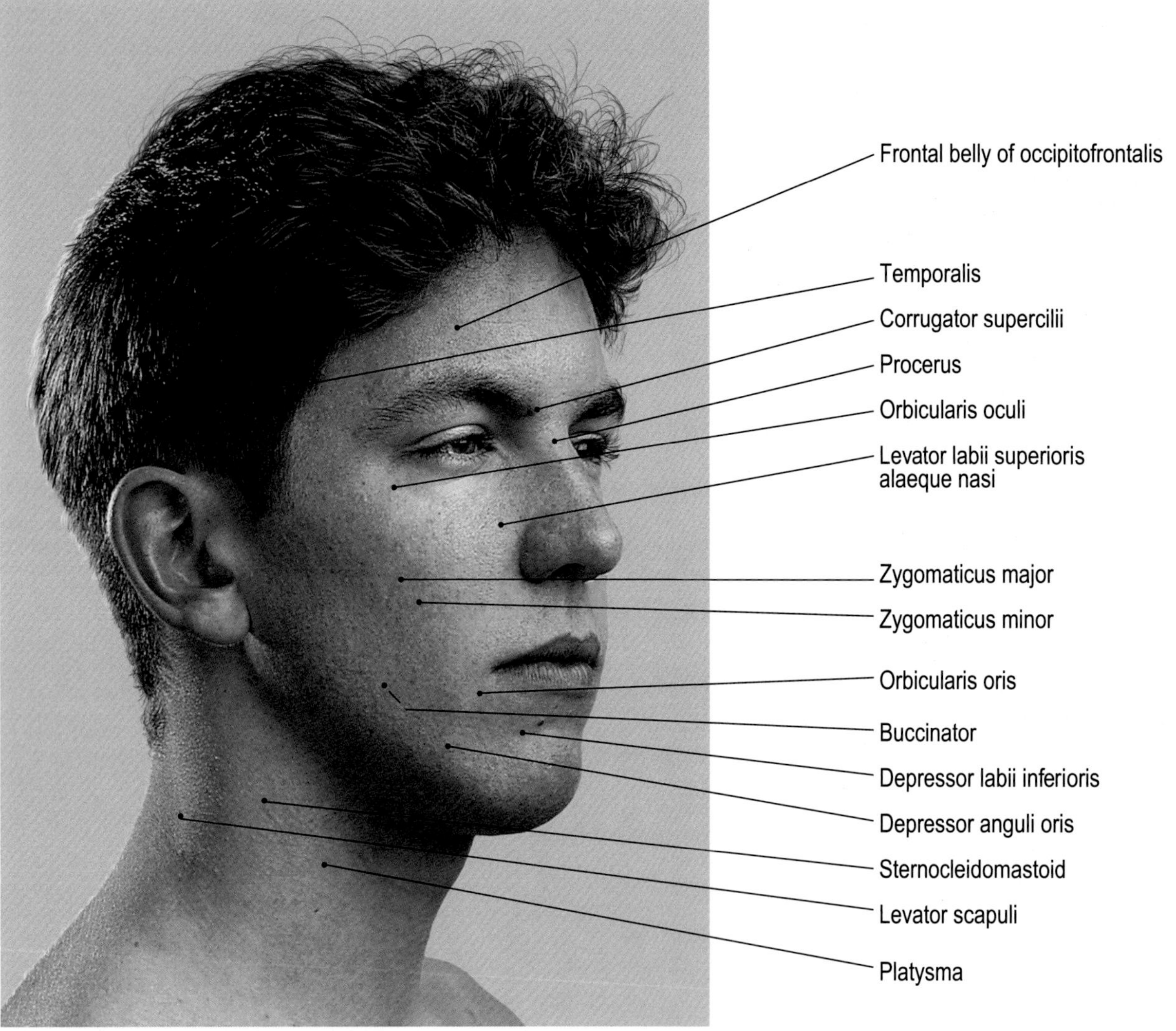

Fig. 4.9 (a) Muscles of the head and neck (lateral aspect)

MUSCLES

Muscles of facial expression (Figs 4.9–4.11)

The muscles associated with the skull are mainly situated anteriorly, where they produce facial expressions, and laterally, where they produce the movements of mastication. The muscles are, however, very difficult to palpate unless they are contracting. Most muscles of the face arise from broad bony and fibrous attachments and pass to the fascia deep to the skin.

Their attachments at both ends are normally highly complex, sending fibres to blend with surrounding muscles, thus influencing the action which produces the many expressions possible in the human face. Because of this complexity only the basic attachments will be given in this text, but enough to demonstrate the action of the muscle.

Palpation

For palpation in this region, the model is in the sitting position.

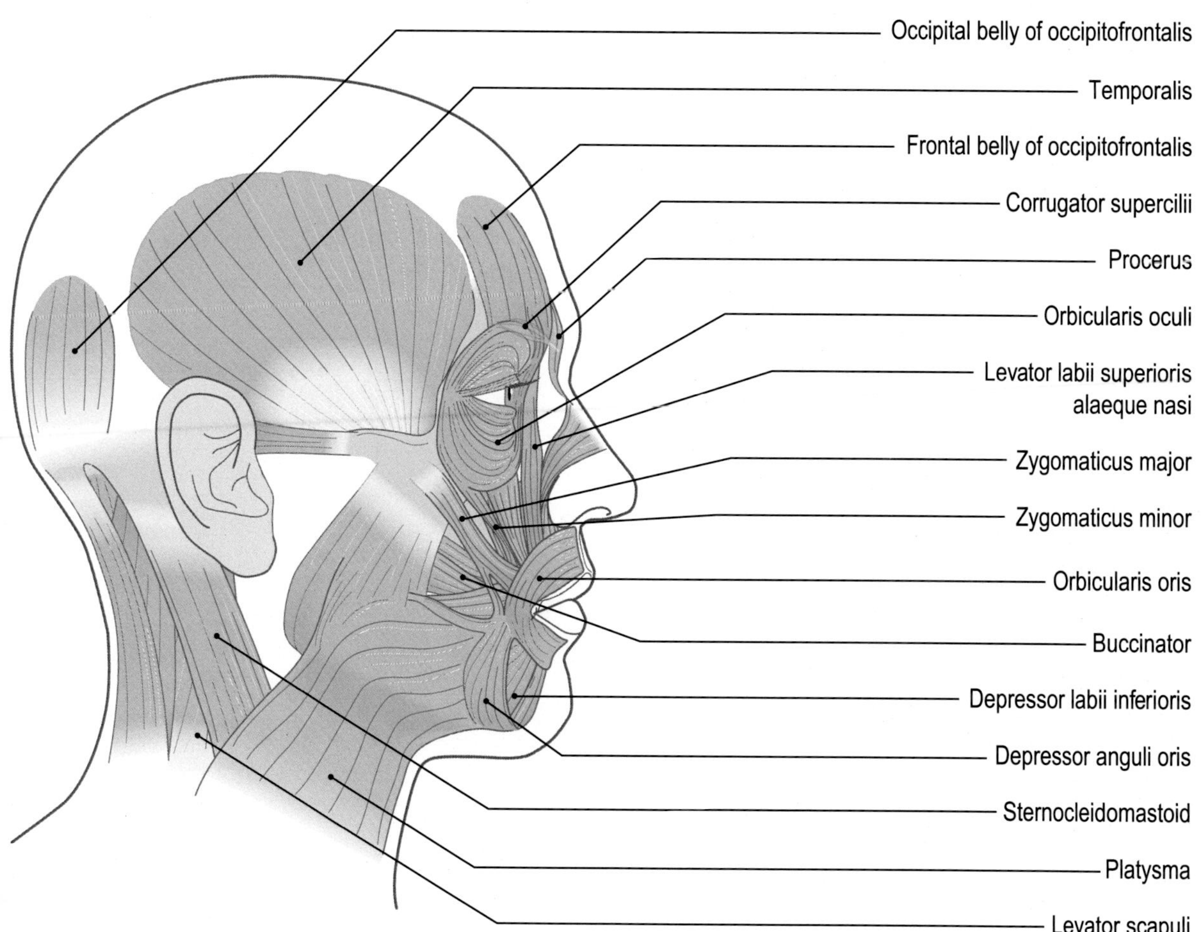

Fig. 4.9 (b) Muscles of the head and neck (lateral aspect)

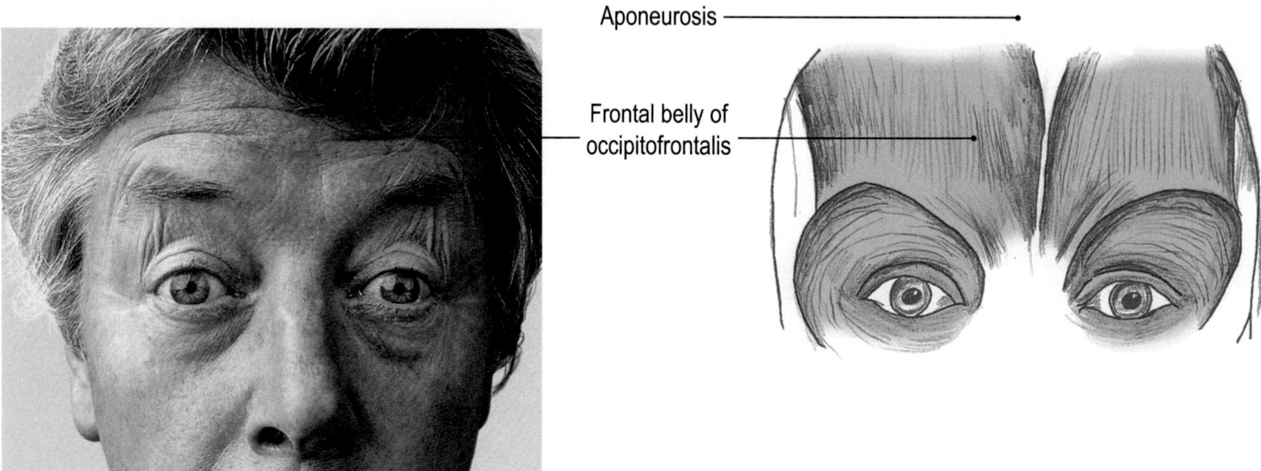

Fig. 4.10 (a, b) Muscles raising the eyebrows (surprise). Frontal belly attaches to the fascia over the upper eye orbit. Posterior belly attaches to the lateral two-thirds of the superior nuchal line. Both bellies attach superiorly to the aponeurosis covering the scalp

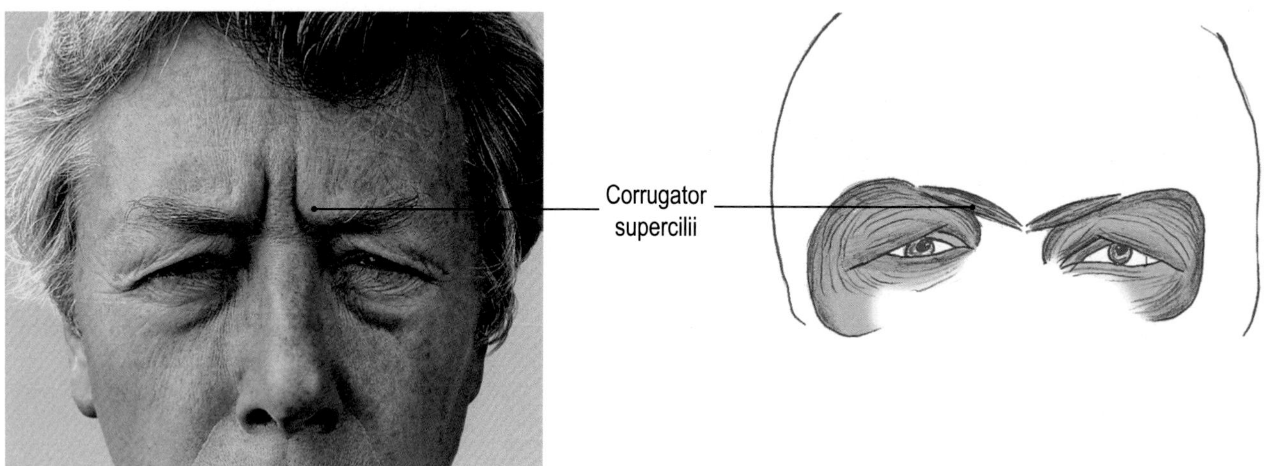

Fig. 4.10 (c, d) Muscles drawing the eyebrows together (frowning). Medially attaches to bone at the medial end of the superciliary arch. Laterally attaches to the skin over mid point of the eye orbit

- The muscle bellies of occipitofrontalis (Figs 4.9 and 4.10a, b). These attach superiorly via a fibrous aponeurotic sheet which passes over the scalp. Anteriorly the muscle attaches to the upper margin of the fascia over the eye orbit and posteriorly to the superior nuchal line. Ask the model to raise and lower the eyebrow several times. The scalp can be felt moving forwards and backwards, with the posterior and anterior bellies contracting alternately.
- Corrugator supercilii (Fig. 4.10c, d). This muscle can be palpated above the nose at the medial end of the eyebrow. Ask the model to frown and palpate the short almost vertical ridges that are produced as the muscle contracts.

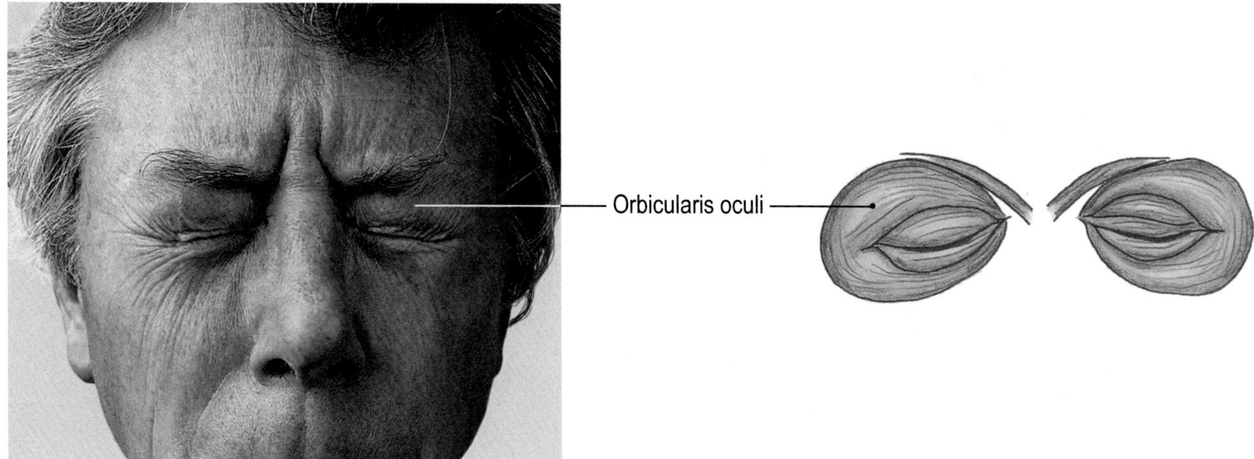

Fig. 4.10 (e, f) Muscles closing the eyes. Elliptical muscle attaching to the bone surrounding the eye orbit

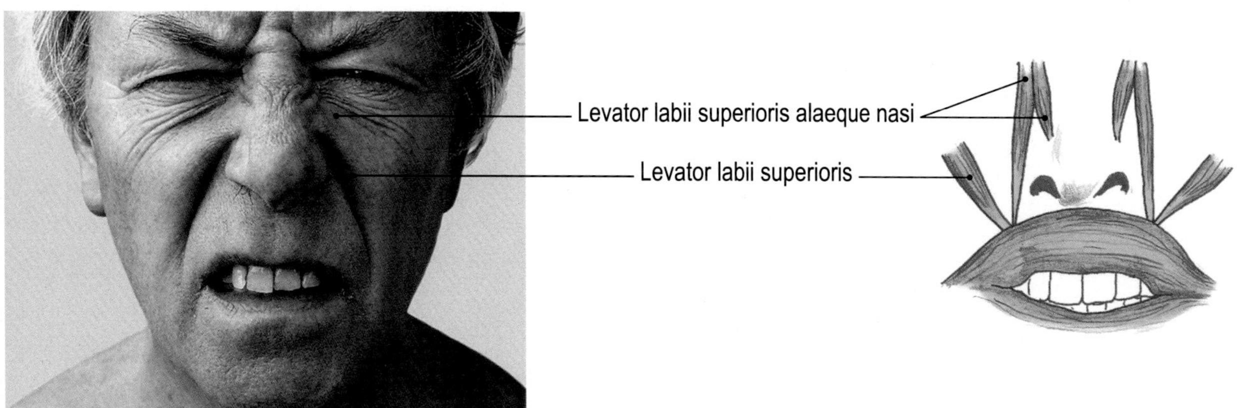

Fig. 4.10 (g, h) Muscles raising the upper lip and opening the nasal cavity (sneering). Levator labii superioris alaeque nasi attaches above to the maxillary bone and below to the greater alar cartilage and skin covering it. Levator labii superioris attaches above to the maxilla and zygomatic bone and below to the upper lip halfway between the angle of the mouth and the mid point

- **Orbicularis oculi** (Fig. 4.10e, f). This muscle closes the eye. The muscle can be palpated easily. Ask the model to close the eye. With your fingers gently resting on the eyelids, ask the model to squeeze the eyes shut tightly. A hard muscular covering can be felt.
- **Levator labii superioris alaeque nasi** (Fig. 4.10g, h). Ask the model to attempt a sneer. Place your fingers over the corner of the nose and the upper lip where you will feel the muscle contracting. The alae of the nose will also be raised and move apart while the upper lip is raised at its centre.

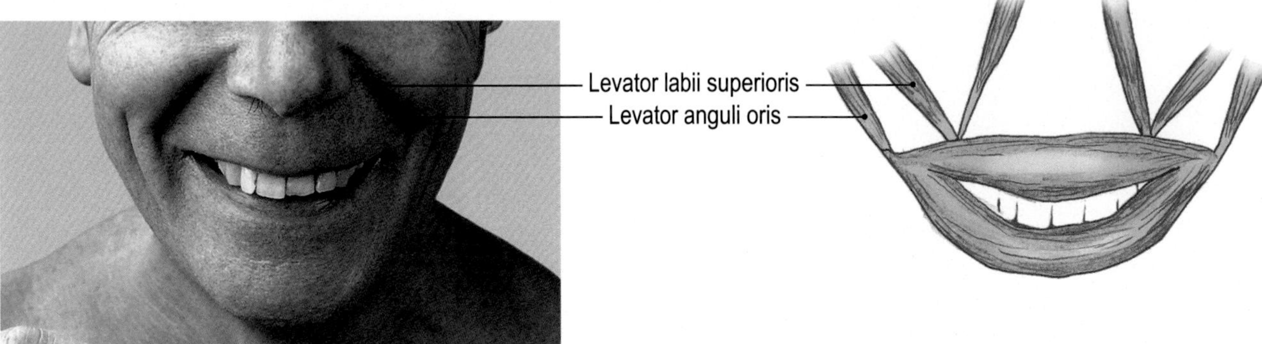

Fig. 4.11 (a, b) Muscles raising the corners of the mouth (smiling). The levator anguli oris attaches above to canine fossa just below the infraorbital foramen of maxilla and attaches below to the corner of the mouth

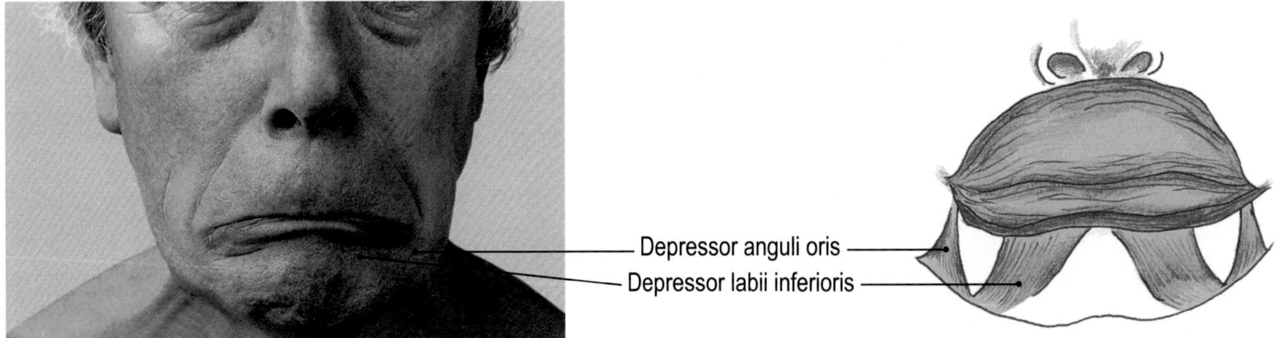

Fig. 4.11 (c, d) Muscles pulling the corners of the mouth and lower lip downwards (indicating sadness). Depressor anguli oris attaches to the mental tubercle of the mandible below and to the angle of the mouth above. Depressor labii inferioris attaches below to the oblique line close to the mental foramen and above to the centre of the lower lip

- **Levator anguli oris, zygomaticus major** and **minor** (Figs 4.9 and 4.11a, b). Ask the model to smile and note that the corners of the mouth are drawn upwards and laterally. This movement is produced by contraction of levator anguli oris and zygomaticus major and minor. These muscles are all palpable between the angle of the mouth and the zygomatic bone (the point of the cheek).
- **Depressor anguli oris** (Fig. 4.11c, d). This muscle can be palpated just below the angle of the mouth.
- **Depressor labii inferioris** (Fig. 4.11c, d). Ask the model to draw the mouth downwards, as in the expression of sadness. The muscle is palpable between the lower lip and the chin. It curls the whole lower lip downwards, thereby exposing the lower teeth.

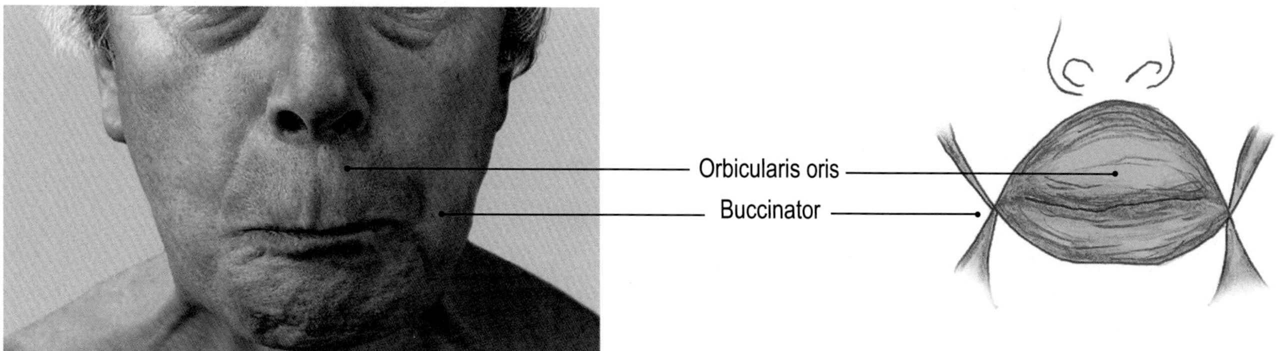

Fig. 4.11 (e, f) Muscles closing or pursing the lips. Orbicularis oris is a highly complex raphe of fibres surrounding the mouth composed of eight blending sections and functionally acting in four quadrants. In addition it receives fibres from all the surrounding muscles. Buccinator basically attaches to the molar area of the maxilla and mandible. Its fibres pass forwards, blending with the orbicularis oris, its upper fibres into the upper lip, its lower fibres into the lower lip, but its middle fibres crossing at the corners of the mouth

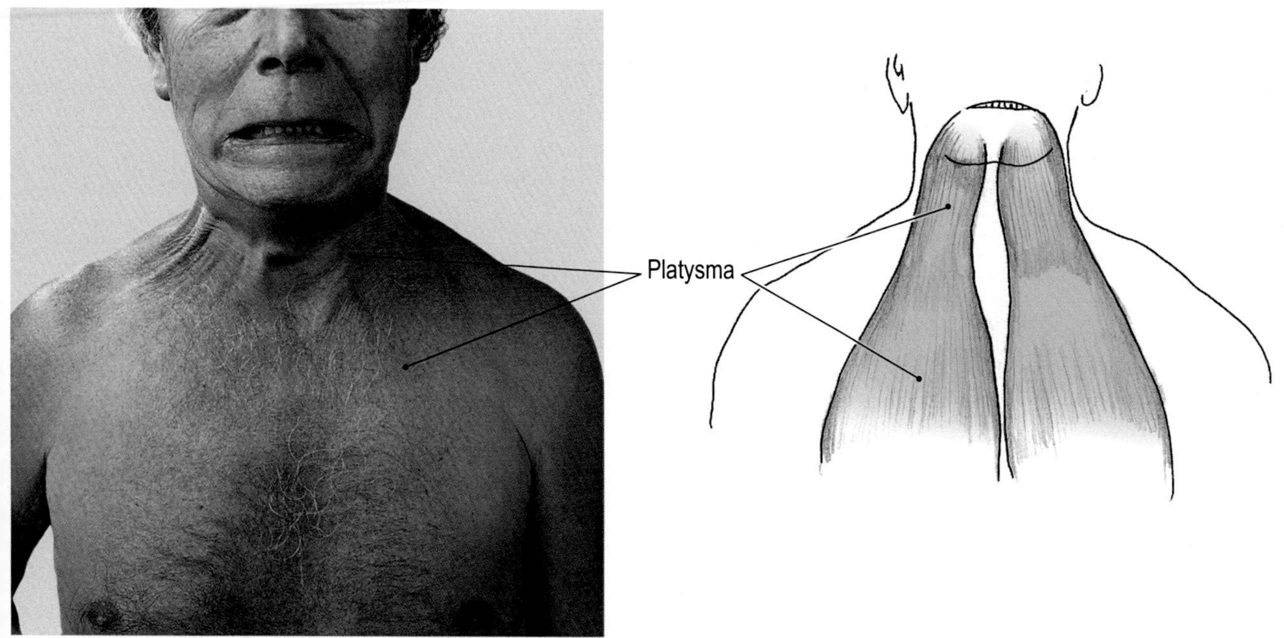

Fig. 4.11 (g, h) Muscles drawing fascia around the mouth downwards (protecting the structures in the neck and producing a snarling expression). Below it attaches to the fascia covering the upper part of pectoralis major and deltoid. Above it attaches to the inferior border of the mandible with some of its lateral fibres passing over to the lower lip and its medial fibres crossing over to the opposite side

- **Orbicularis oris** (Fig. 4.11e, f). Ask the model to close the lips tightly. The hard ring of muscle surrounding the mouth can be palpated.
- **Buccinator** (Fig. 4.11e, f). Ask the model to attempt to blow through the closed mouth and palpate the muscle contraction in the cheeks.
- **Platysma** (Fig. 4.11g, h). Ask the model to clench the teeth together as in a 'snarling' expression. The muscle can be palpated anywhere between the mandible and the superior part of the chest. This muscle appears to expand the neck volume. It will also be brought into action if you apply resistance to hands being tightened around the neck.

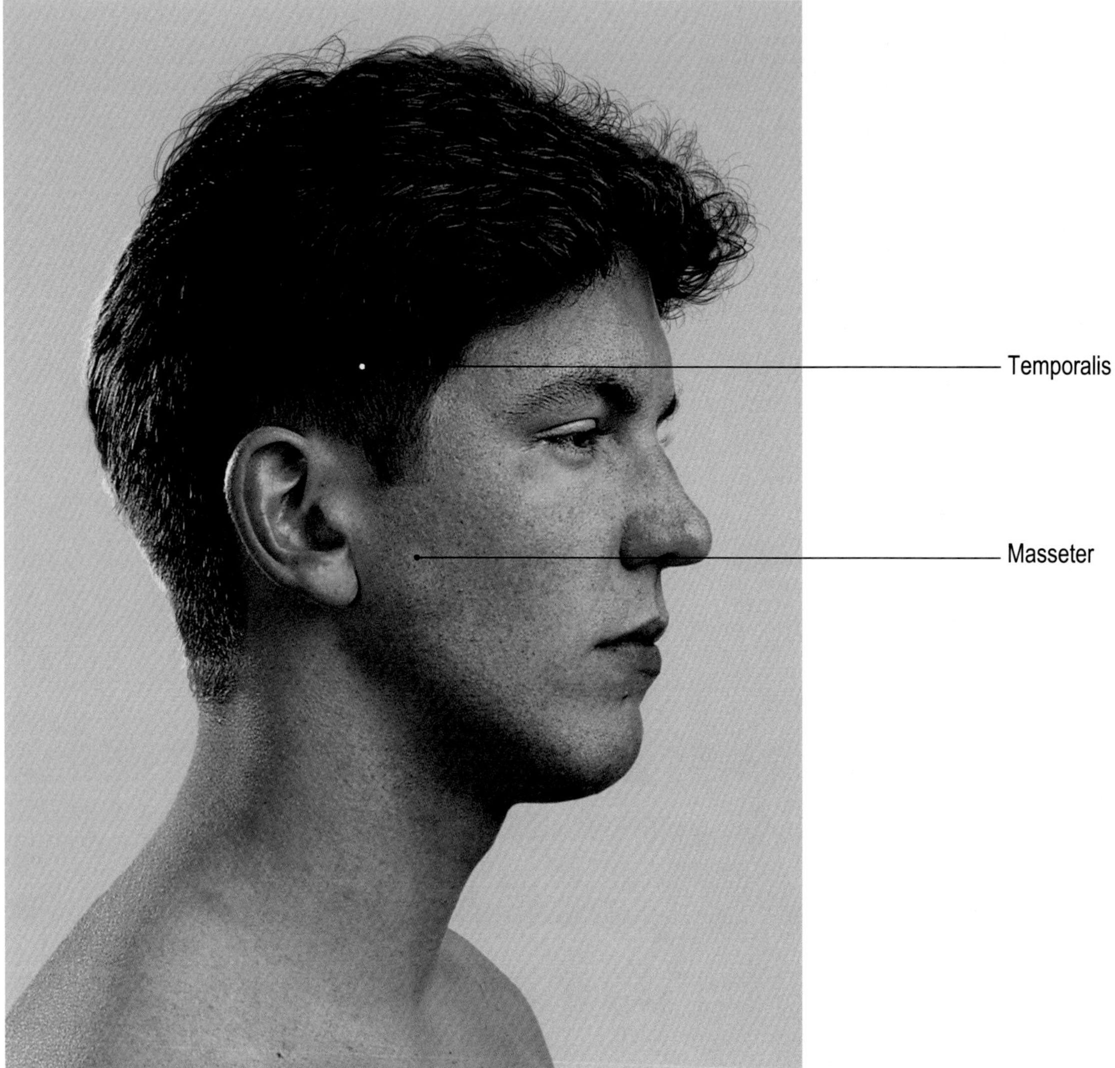

Fig. 4.12 (a) Two of the more superficial muscles of mastication (lateral aspect)

Muscles of mastication (Fig. 4.12)

These are powerful muscles situated more deeply on the lateral side of the face. Temporalis is a fan-shaped muscle attaching above to the lateral side of the temporal bone, reaching as high as the suture between it and the parietal bone. The muscle passes down under the zygomatic arch to the coronoid process of the mandible. Masseter attaches above to the zygomatic arch, its fibres passing downwards and backwards to attach to the lateral surface of the mandible close to its angle.

The medial and lateral pterygoid muscles lie deep to the upper part of the ramus and coronoid process of the mandible. The medial pterygoid attaches above to the medial side of the lateral pterygoid plate and palatine bone to pass downwards and backwards to the medial side of the ramus and angle of the mandible. The lateral pterygoid attaches above to the lateral side of the lateral pterygoid plate and the temporal bone and passes backwards to attach to the neck of the mandible and the capsule and disc of the temporomandibular joint.

Palpation

- Temporalis. Ask the model to alternatively clench and relax the teeth. Place your fingers just above the zygomatic arch. Although hidden to a certain extent by the thick fascia which covers it, the contraction of the fan-shaped belly of temporalis can be palpated. Passing almost vertically deep to the zygomatic arch of the mandible, its fibres become too deep to be palpated.

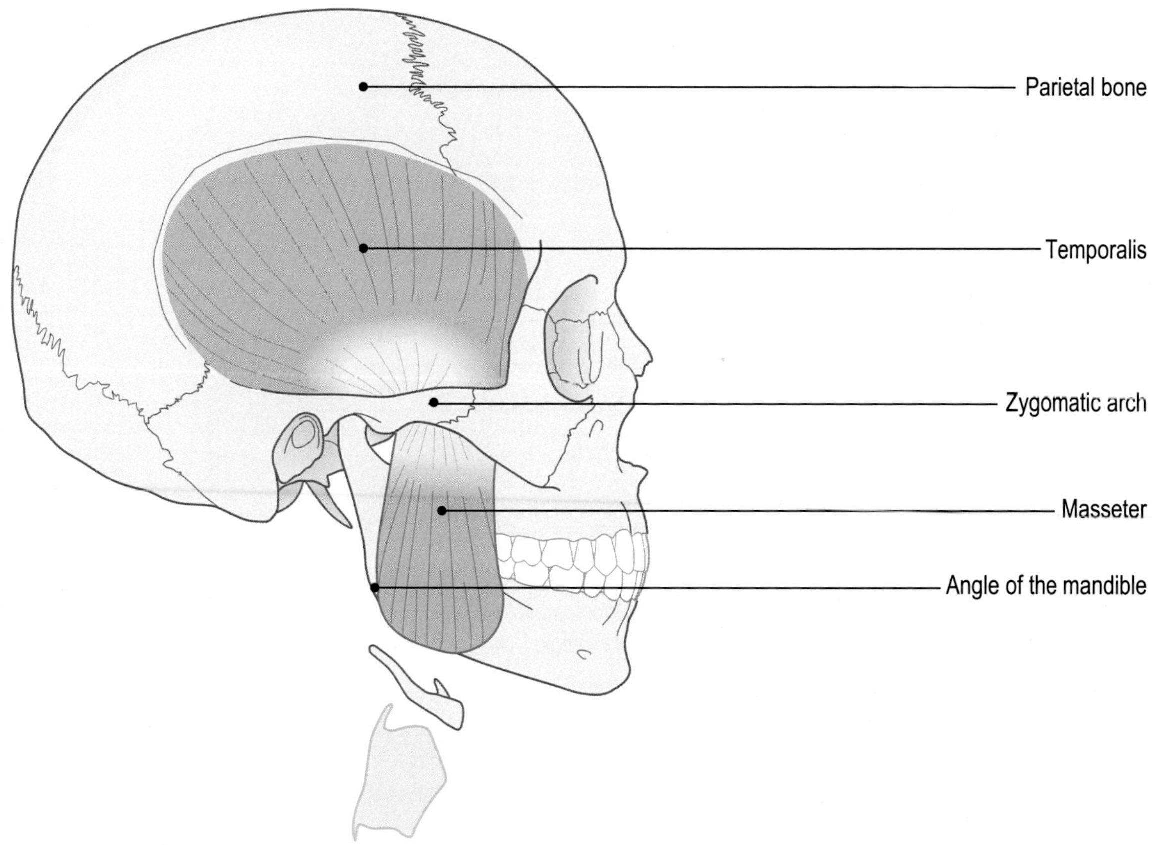

Fig. 4.12 (b) Two of the more superficial muscles of mastication (lateral aspect)

- Masseter. Again, ask the model to clench and relax the teeth. Place your fingers over the side of the mandible just above and in front of the angle. The powerful masseter muscle can be felt contracting and relaxing. A series of ridges can be palpated, indicating the direction and power of its fibres. In some subjects, particularly lean males, the coarse muscle fibres can be seen crossing the side of the jaw obliquely. The lower fibres can be traced as far as the lower border of the mandible inferiorly, and the anterior end of the zygomatic arch superiorly.
- Note 1. Palpation of the medial and lateral pterygoid muscles is impossible, as they are too deeply situated. It will be noted that the temporalis and the masseter muscles are concerned with closing the mouth and with powerful biting. Although the mandible acts as a third-order lever in the initial bite, as the food moves backwards between the molars it changes so that the food is first in line with the muscle pull and then nearer to the temporomandibular joint than the muscles. The mandible then becomes a second-order lever, with its decrease in range but increase in power. It is at this point that the act of chewing takes place.
- Note 2. During the act of chewing, place your fingers over the posterior part of the cheeks. As the food makes its way backwards, the muscles contract harder and the jaw moves from side to side in a grinding action, utilizing the pterygoid muscles. If the food is tough, these muscles will ache.

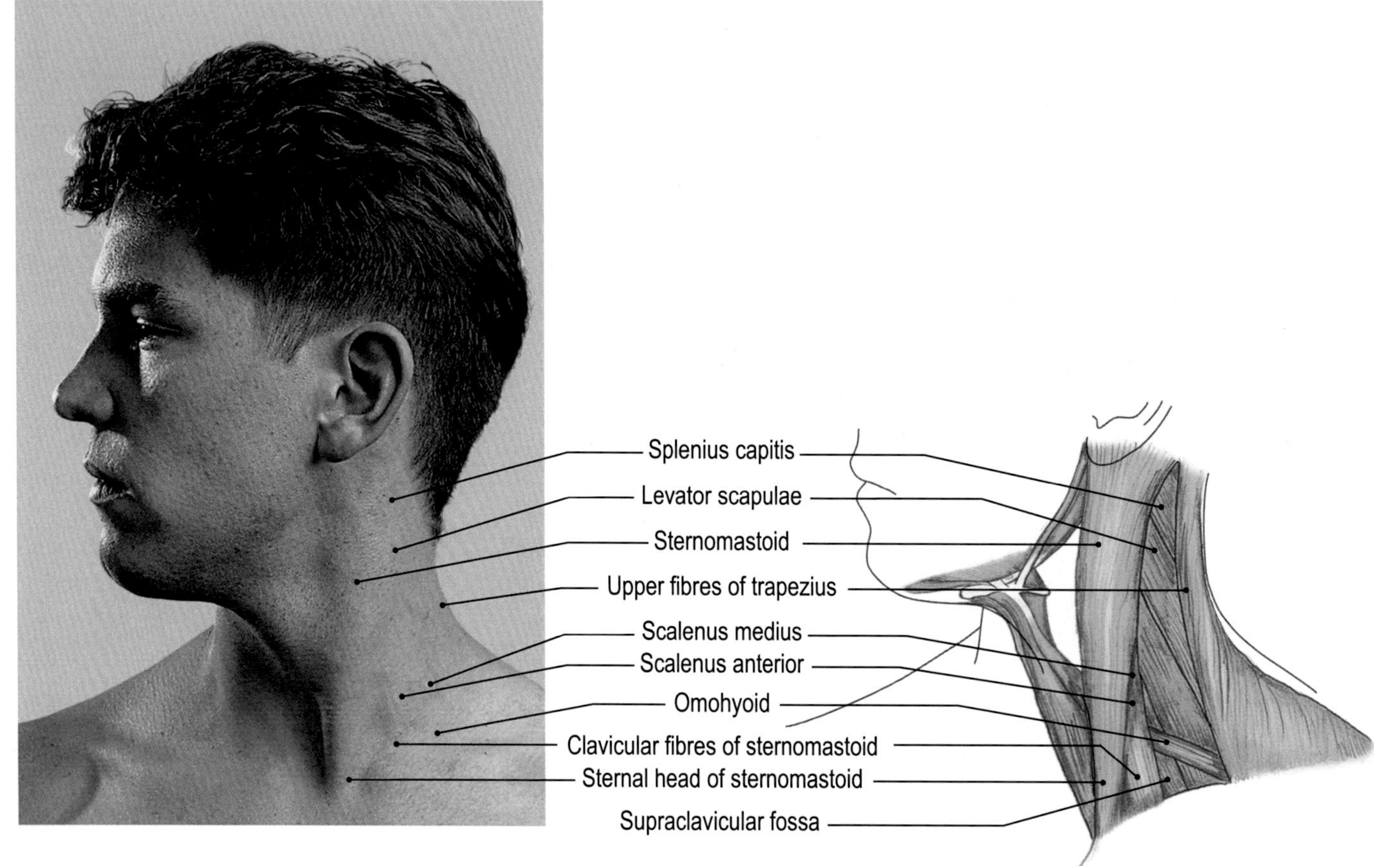

Fig. 4.13 (a, b) Muscles of the neck (lateral aspect, posterior group)

Muscles of the neck (Fig. 4.13)

The neck is surrounded by layers of muscle. These vary in their function, which may include moving the neck itself, moving the head, mastication, swallowing and moving the shoulder girdle. Some are involved in a combination of several of these functions.

The more superficial muscles tend to be the more powerful and are therefore easier to find and palpate. Because of their size, however, they do tend to cover the smaller, deeper muscles.

Some of the muscles are only attached to different parts of the vertebral column: some attach the column to the head and thoracic cage. Others, usually the longer, attach to the head and the thoracic cage. All the attachments are complex, but have a direct bearing on the resultant movement and function. Thorough knowledge of this region is essential and further study must be undertaken. (See Palastanga et al 2002, Standring 2004).

Palpation on movement

For palpation in this region, the model is in the sitting position.

- The **upper fibres of trapezius** (Fig. 4.13a, b). Place your hands over the posterosuperior area of the neck, halfway between the occiput and the acromion process. Ask the model to raise the pectoral girdle, as in a shrugging movement. The powerful upper fibres of trapezius can now be felt contracting. Trace the muscle superiorly to its aponeurotic attachment to the medial third of the superior nuchal line of the occipital bone, external occipital protuberance and the sides of the ligamentum nuchae. Trace the muscle inferiorly to its attachments to the posterior border of the lateral third of the clavicle, medial border of the acromion and lateral part of the upper lip of the spine of the scapula.
- The central muscular fibres of trapezius. These sometimes appear to be stringy and are often quite tender, particularly after a period of sustained activity.
- **Sternomastoid (sternocleidomastoid)** (Fig. 4.13a, b). This muscle attaches to the mastoid process above, and the upper surface of the medial end of the clavicle and upper border of the sternum below. Place your fingers over the lower attachment. Ask the model to turn the head to the opposite side. Two distinct attachments can be felt, one more cord-like from the sternum and the other more aponeurotic from the clavicle. These appear to twist on each other as they are traced upwards.

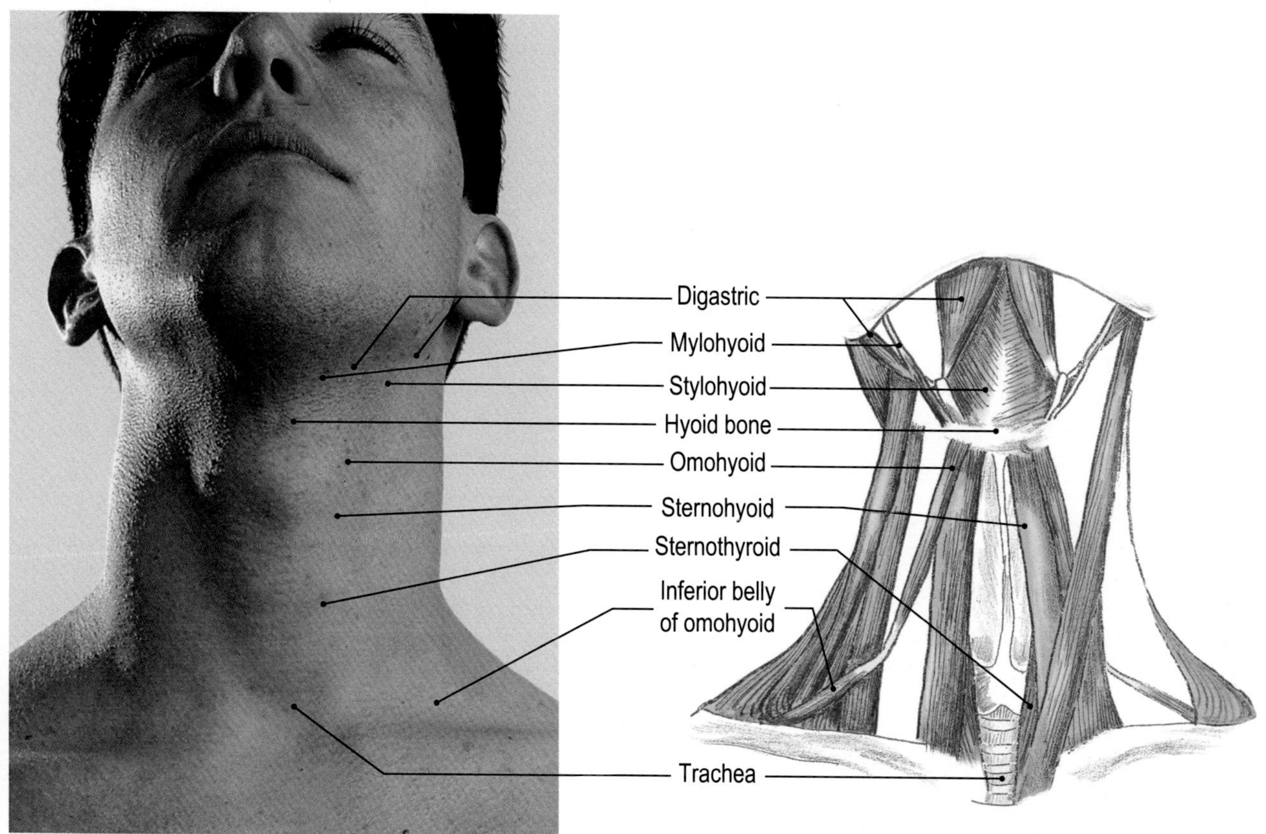

Fig. 4.13 (c, d) Muscles of the neck (anterior aspect, anterior group)

The thick strap-like sternomastoid stands away from the neck when contracted. It becomes cord-like again as it approaches and attaches to the mastoid process, spreading as a sheet to the lateral part of the superior nuchal line.

- Both sternomastoid muscles. When both muscles contract strongly they are easily palpable. The model is in the supine lying position. Ask the model to raise the head.
- Contraction of sternomastoid and trapezius. This can be produced by asking the model to move the head and neck to the same side (lateral flexion). Now resist this movement. Ask the model to rotate the head to the opposite side and, again, resist this movement. Palpate the contracting muscle.
- The scalene muscles (Fig. 4.13a, b). These lie just behind and deep to sternomastoid. The model is in the sitting position. These muscles can be palpated deep in the hollow between sternomastoid and the upper fibres of trapezius in the posterior triangle of the neck. These cord-like muscles, running down to attach to the first and second ribs, appear to be continuously contracted while the head is in the upright position.
- The inferior belly of the omohyoid muscle (Fig. 4.13a, b). During coughing, it is often possible to palpate the inferior belly of the omohyoid muscle as it crosses the lower anterior part of the posterior triangle of the neck.
- Note. Posterosuperior to this is scalenus anterior, and a little higher, scalenus medius.
- Levator scapulae (Fig. 4.13a, b). Ask the model to elevate the pectoral girdle. The fibres of levator scapulae can be palpated nearer the top of the posterior triangle.
- Mylohyoid (Fig. 4.13c, d). During swallowing, the muscles between the mandible, hyoid, thyroid cartilage and sternum contract and relax. Place your fingers on either side of the throat between the mandible and the hyoid during swallowing. Myohyoid can be observed, contracting and lifting the hyoid bone.
- Sternohyoid. This is difficult to palpate during swallowing, but in yawning its fibres can be observed on either side of the thyroid cartilage passing downwards towards the sternum.

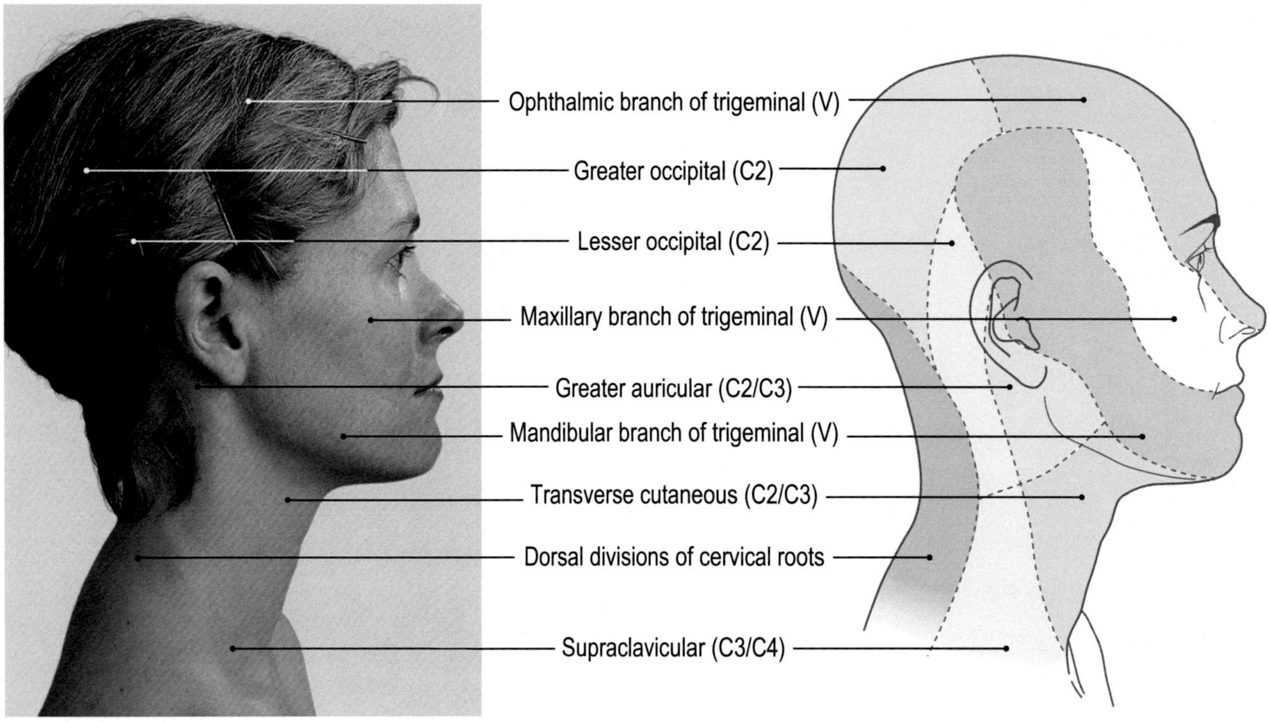

Fig. 4.14 (a, b) Cutaneous supply of the head and neck, lateral aspect

NERVES (FIG. 4.14)

The cutaneous innervation of the face, including forehead, is by the cranial nerves. These are mainly the **ophthalmic**, **maxillary** and **mandibular branches of the trigeminal nerve**. The occipital, temporal and posterior parts of the parietal regions are supplied by the **greater auricular**, and greater and **lesser occipital**, branches of the cervical plexus. The neck is supplied almost entirely through the anterior and posterior rami of the cervical nerve roots, via the **transverse cutaneous** and **supraclavicular** branches of the cervical plexus (Fig. 4.14a, b). The muscles of facial expression are supplied by the facial nerve (cranial VII), the muscles of mastication via the mandibular branch of the trigeminal (cranial V). All the muscles of the neck are supplied by the cervical nerve roots via the cervical or brachial plexuses. Some of these roots receive communication from other cranial nerves: for example, the glossopharyngeal (cranial IV), accessory (cranial XI) and hypoglossal (cranial XII).

Palpation on movement

Very few nerves are palpable in the head and neck region. Usually only the terminal branches reach the surface and even these are difficult to find.

- The greater occipital nerve (Fig. 4.14a, b). The model is in the prone lying position. Posteriorly it is possible to palpate the greater occipital nerve (root value C2) as it passes vertically to supply the skin over the back of the skull as far forwards as the vertex. This cord-like structure can be palpated over the lower part of the occipital bone approximately 3 cm from the midline. Pressure on the nerve, produced either by your fingers

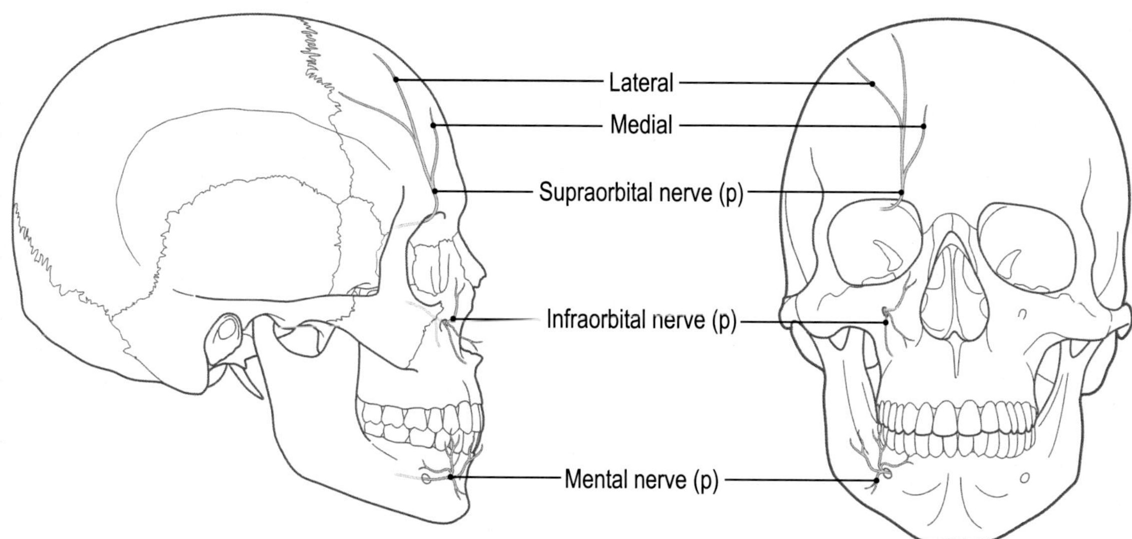

Fig. 4.14 (c, d) Cutaneous branches emerging onto the face, lateral and anterior aspect (p, palpable)

or muscle tension due to poor posture, or long periods of continuous contraction, can lead to unpleasant sensations and headaches. Care should be taken, therefore, when palpating in this area.

- Note. Massage to relieve the tension of the muscles surrounding the nerve can produce almost immediate relief from the resulting headache.
- The orbital nerves. Pressure on the **supraorbital nerve** as it crosses the superomedial rim of the eye orbit and on the **infraorbital nerve** as it emerges from the maxilla just below the centre of the eye orbit (Fig. 4.14c, d) causes discomfort over these areas and the area supplied by the nerves. They are, however, quite difficult to palpate.
- The mental nerve (Fig. 4.14c, d). On the anterior surface of the mandible, approximately 1 cm lateral to the midline and approximately 1 cm above the inferior border, the **mental nerve** (a continuation of the inferior dental nerve) emerges on to the surface. The nerve is often palpable in this region. If you apply pressure to the area, the model will experience an unpleasant sensation.
- Note. This is the area which appears to become numb first when the dentist gives an anaesthetic injection for drilling the lower teeth.
- The trunks of the brachial plexus. Just above the central part of the clavicle in the supraclavicular fossa, you will be able to palpate a series of 'cord-like' structures running downwards and laterally. These are the trunks of the brachial plexus emerging from between scalenus anterior and scalenus medius before passing deep to the clavicle to enter the axilla. Pressure in this area will cause discomfort locally and possibly also result in a 'tingling', pain or numbness over the distribution of these nerves in the upper limb.

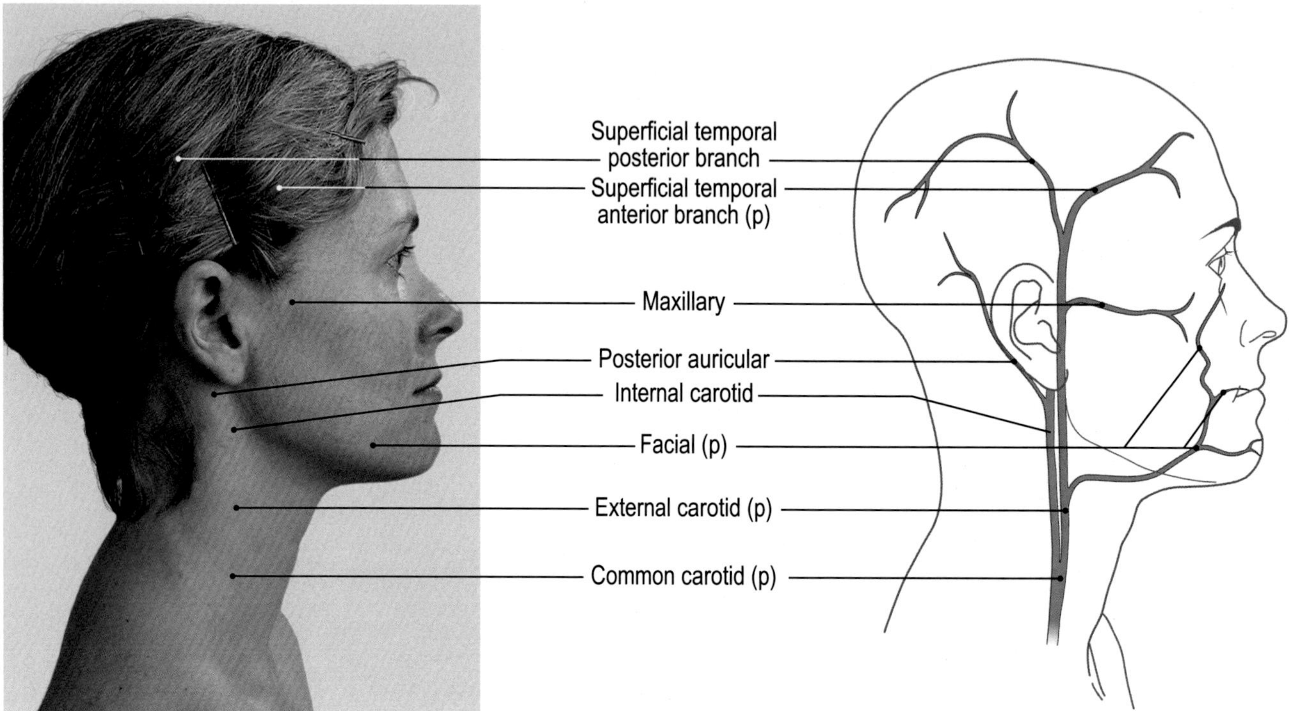

Fig. 4.15 (a, b) Main arteries of the head and neck, lateral aspect (p, palpable)

ARTERIES (FIG. 4.15)

The left common carotid artery arises from the arch of the aorta, while the right is a division of the brachiocephalic artery. They pass up on either side of the neck deep to sternomastoid to the level of the upper border of the thyroid cartilage, where each divides into the internal and external carotid arteries.

The former passes superiorly, anterior to the upper three transverse processes, to enter the skull through the carotid canal. Each supplies the cerebral hemisphere, orbit and nose of its own side.

The external carotid artery passes vertically from the upper border of the thyroid cartilage, deep to the parotid gland behind the ramus of the mandible, where it divides into the superficial temporal and maxillary arteries (Fig. 4.15a, b).

Palpation on movement

- The common carotid artery. This artery can be palpated on either side of the thyroid cartilage deep to sternomastoid. The muscle has to be moved laterally so that your fingers can be slipped from the anterior aspect into the cleft between the cartilage and the muscle. The pulsations of the artery can be felt on the lateral side of the upper part of the thyroid cartilage, close to the greater cornua of the hyoid bone as the artery divides.
- Note. This point is important for checking the pulsations of the carotid arteries and it is worth spending some time practising the technique.
- The superficial temporal artery. Between the tragus of the ear and the neck of the mandible the pulsations of the superficial temporal artery can be felt. It can also be palpated above the upper limit of temporalis.
- The maxillary artery. Just below the zygomatic bone, this artery is not quite so obvious as it is covered by muscle and fascia, although, with practice, it is palpable running anteriorly.
- The facial artery (Fig. 4.15a, b). This artery can be palpated as it crosses the lower border of the body of the mandible, halfway between the angle of the mandible and the mental tubercle. With care, it can be traced upwards to the corner of the mouth and cheek.
- The supraorbital artery. Finally, above the eye the pulsations of the supraorbital artery can be palpated as it crosses the medial superior margin of the orbit.
- Note. It is at this point that injuries, particularly in the sport of boxing, occur. The artery is often ruptured and large quantities of blood pulse out on to the eye and face. It is worth remembering that if pressure were applied to this point for just a few minutes, this loss of blood would cease and the area could be cleaned up, exposing the injury which is usually just a minor trauma.

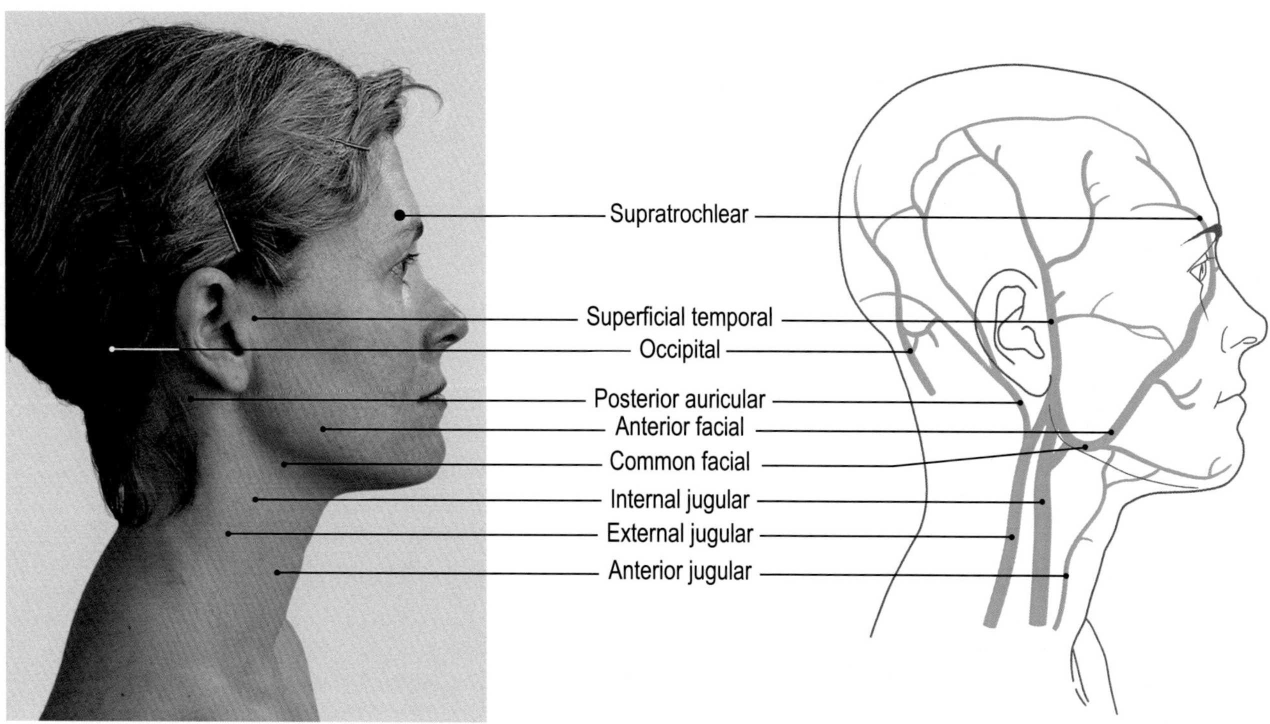

Fig. 4.16 (a, b) Veins of the head and neck, lateral aspect

VEINS (FIG. 4.16)

The veins of the head, neck and face are divided into two main groups: (a) those that drain the exterior of the cranium and deep tissues of the face, and (b) those that drain the brain, the neck and the superficial areas of the face. The former mainly drain into the **external jugular** vein, while the latter mainly drain into the **internal jugular vein**.

Palpation

None of these veins are easy to palpate but is important to be able to locate their general outline. The lower part of the external jugular vein contains two valves: one, as it joins the subclavian vein and the other, 4 cm above. The valves do not prevent regurgitation of blood. The area between them often bulges and is termed 'the sinus'.

For identification of the veins, the model is in the sitting position.

- The external jugular vein. The surface marking of the external jugular vein is from the angle of the mandible to the middle of the clavicle.
- The internal jugular vein. The surface marking of the internal jugular vein is by a broad line drawn from the lobe of the ear to the medial end of the clavicle.
- **Note.** This vein also contains a valve at its junction with the subclavian vein and is often distended just above. This vein lies deep to sternocleidomastoid muscle and cannot be palpated.

5 The thorax

Contents

At the end of this chapter you should be able to:

1. Find, recognize and name the constituent bony components of the thorax, including the clavicle, scapula, ribs and vertebrae, noting their size and position.
2. Palpate many of the bony features, being able to relate one to another.
3. Locate, name or number the spines and transverse processes of all the thoracic vertebrae.
4. Recognize and palpate all 12 of the ribs, noting their extent.
5. Name all the joints in which the clavicle, scapula, ribs, sternum and vertebrae are involved and palpate the joint lines where possible.
6. Give the class and type of all the joints named.
7. Demonstrate any accessory movements which may be possible in the joints of the thorax.
8. Locate and name the muscles which cover the thorax.
9. Draw the shape of the muscle on the surface and give its attachments.
10. Demonstrate the actions of all of the muscles covering the thorax.
11. Describe the position and attachments of the diaphragm.
12. Give an account of its actions and functional significance.
13. Demonstrate the cutaneous distribution of the thoracic nerves, giving an outline of the course each takes.
14. Describe the arrangement of chambers in the heart.
15. Give the surface markings of the main boundaries of the heart.
16. Describe the arrangement of the main arteries in the thorax, giving their surface markings.
17. Describe the arrangement of the main veins in the thorax, giving their surface markings.

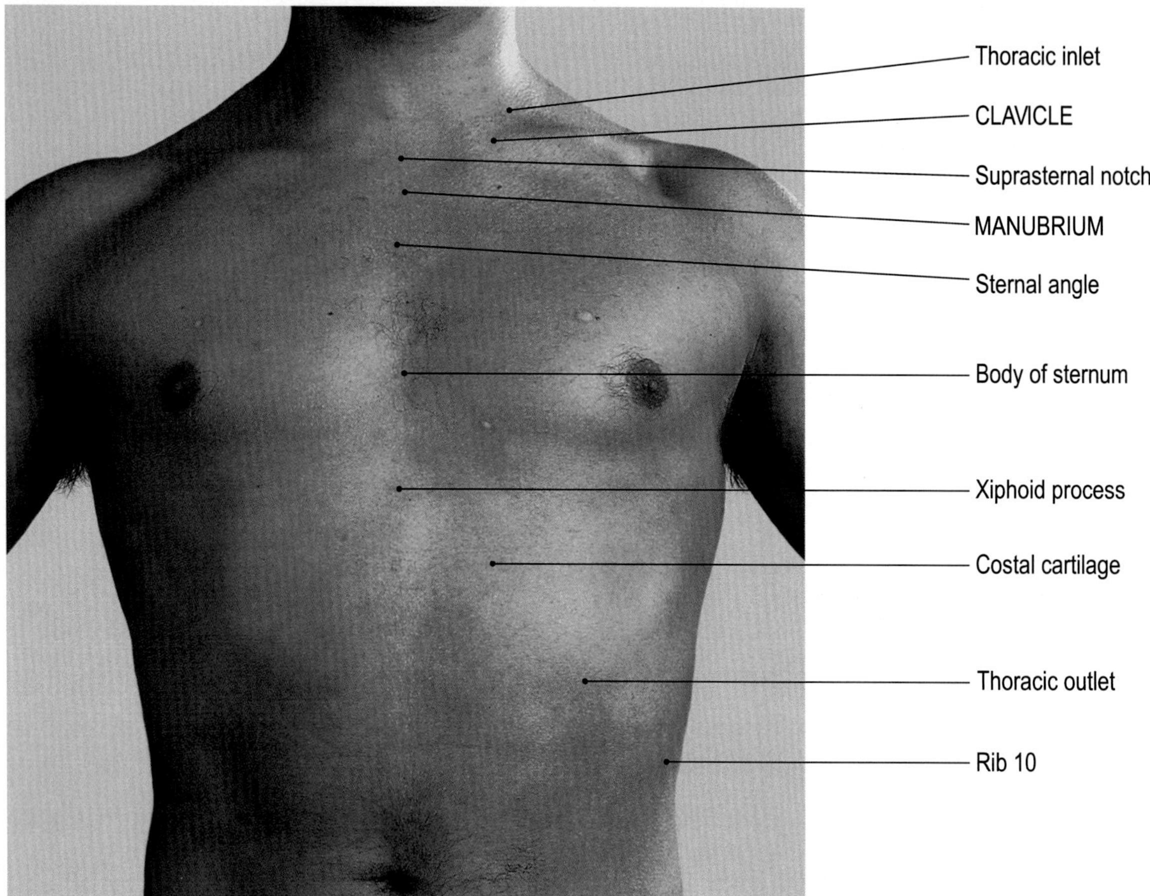

Fig. 5.1 (a) The thorax (anterior aspect)

BONES

The thoracic cage

The bony structure of the thoracic cage consists of:

- the **sternum** [*stereos* (Gk) = solid, hard] anteriorly
- the twelve thoracic vertebrae [*vertebra* (L) = joint; from verto – I turn] posteriorly, the first thoracic vertebra being the smallest and the twelfth the largest (see Figs 5.2–5.4), and
- the twelve ribs on either side linking the vertebrae with the sternum.

The sternum is angled forward at the manubriosternal joint and angled backwards at the xiphisternal joint, forming a concavity backwards. The ribs are concave inwards and the vertebral column is concave forwards in this region. This forms a large cavity for the protection of vital organs such as the heart and lungs.

The rib spaces are filled with a musculofibrous sheet made up of the intercostal muscles and membrane. This forms a sealed unit in front, to the sides and behind. There are, however, openings at the top and bottom. The former is smaller and consists of the first thoracic vertebra posteriorly, the **first rib** on either side and the **manubrium** sterni anteriorly. This is termed the '**thoracic inlet**'. Below there is a much larger opening: the '**thoracic outlet**'. This comprises the twelfth thoracic vertebra posteriorly, the **xiphoid** anteriorly and the **costal cartilages** of **ribs** 7, 8, 9 and **10**, the tip of rib **11** and the full length of rib **12**.

The sternum

The sternum lies centrally at the front of the chest. It comprises three flat plates of bone: the **manubrium** [*manubrium* (L) = a handle; the sternum, as a whole, resembles a sword] superiorly, the body centrally and the pointed **xiphoid** [*xiphos* (Gk) = a sword] **process** inferiorly. The xiphoid usually remains cartilaginous until approximately 40 years of age.

The clavicle and scapula

The **clavicle** lies almost horizontal, articulating with the superolateral part of the manubrium. Posterolaterally the scapula rests on the second to eighth ribs, with the acromion at the lateral end of the spine articulating with the lateral end of the clavicle at the acromioclavicular joint (see Fig. 2.7).

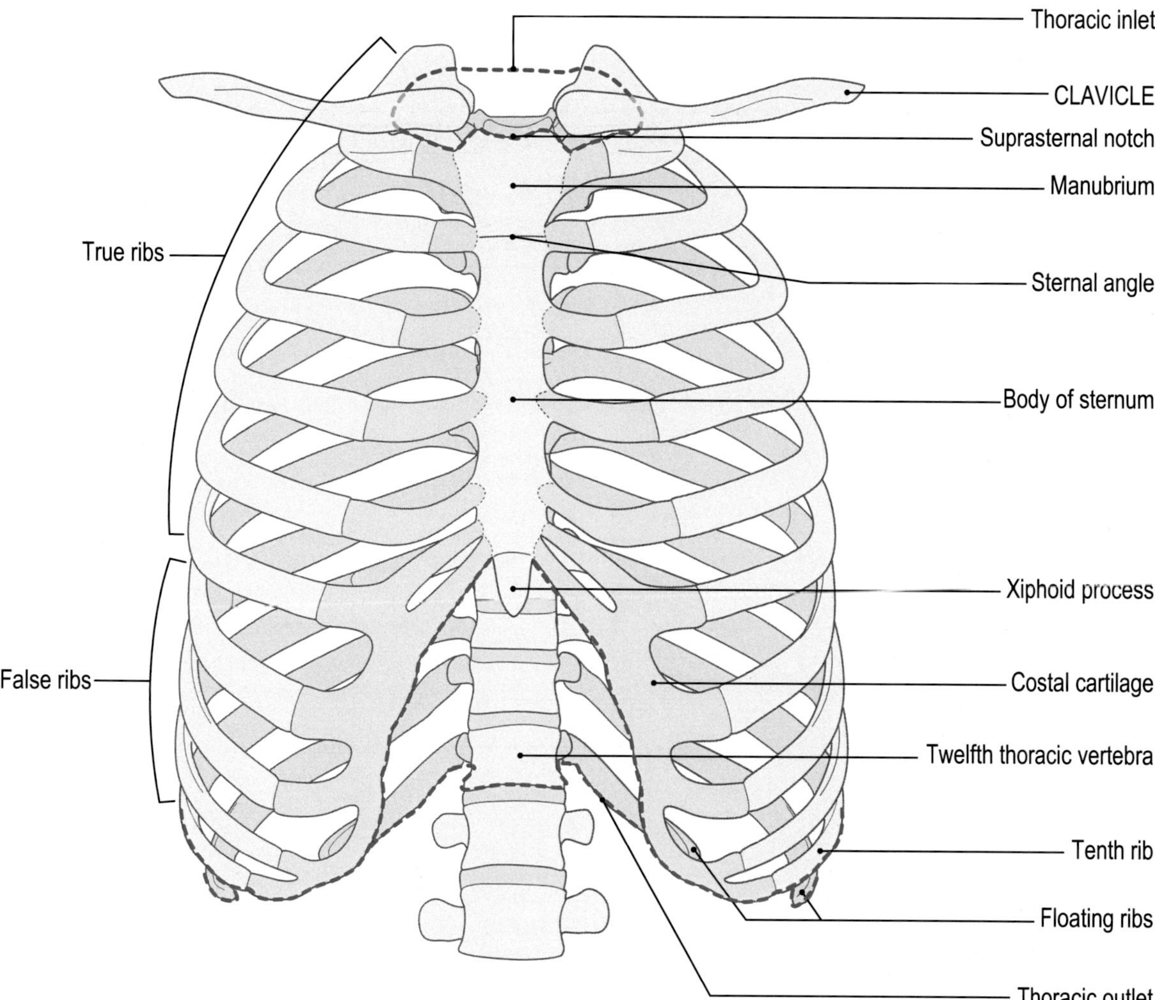

Fig. 5.1 (b) Bones of the thorax (anterior aspect)

Palpation

For palpation in this region, the model can be in either the sitting or standing position.

- The suprasternal notch. Identify the suprasternal notch which can be located at the upper border of the manubrium (Fig. 5.1a, b).
- The medial ends of the clavicle. On either side of the suprasternal notch, palpate the medial ends of the clavicle which project above the line of the manubrium sterni.
- The first rib. Just below the medial end of the clavicle, find the enlargement at the lateral end of the manubrium sterni. This is actually the anterior end of the first rib.
- The sternocostal joint. With careful palpation, you will be able to locate the joint between the first rib and the manubrium sterni running vertically, concave laterally 1 cm below and 1 cm lateral to the medial end of the clavicle.
- The manubriosternal joint (sternal angle). Trace down the anterior surface of the manubrium until you find a raised horizontal line. This is where it joins the body of the sternum at the manubriosternal (sternal angle) joint (Fig. 5.1a, b). The reflex angle between the manubrium and body of the sternum is of the order of 200°, changing some 5–7° between full inspiration and full expiration.
- The costal cartilages of the second ribs. On either side of the manubriosternal junction the costal cartilages of the second ribs can be palpated, with the lateral border of the manubrium just above.
- Ribs 3–6. Continue to trace down either side of the sternum and identify the third to sixth ribs and their costal cartilages with the lateral border of the sternum lying between their medial ends.
- The xyphoid process of the sternum. The sternum narrows inferiorly and usually dips inwards to join the cartilaginous xiphoid process. The costal cartilage of the seventh rib usually articulates with the sternum at the xiphisternal junction.
- Note 1. The whole of the sternum is subcutaneous and is commonly used to take samples of bone marrow.
- Note 2. The xiphoid process varies in its formation: it may appear to be pointed, double pointed or even rounded. Normally it projects forwards and can therefore easily be palpated. Occasionally it projects downwards and backwards and is then difficult to palpate.

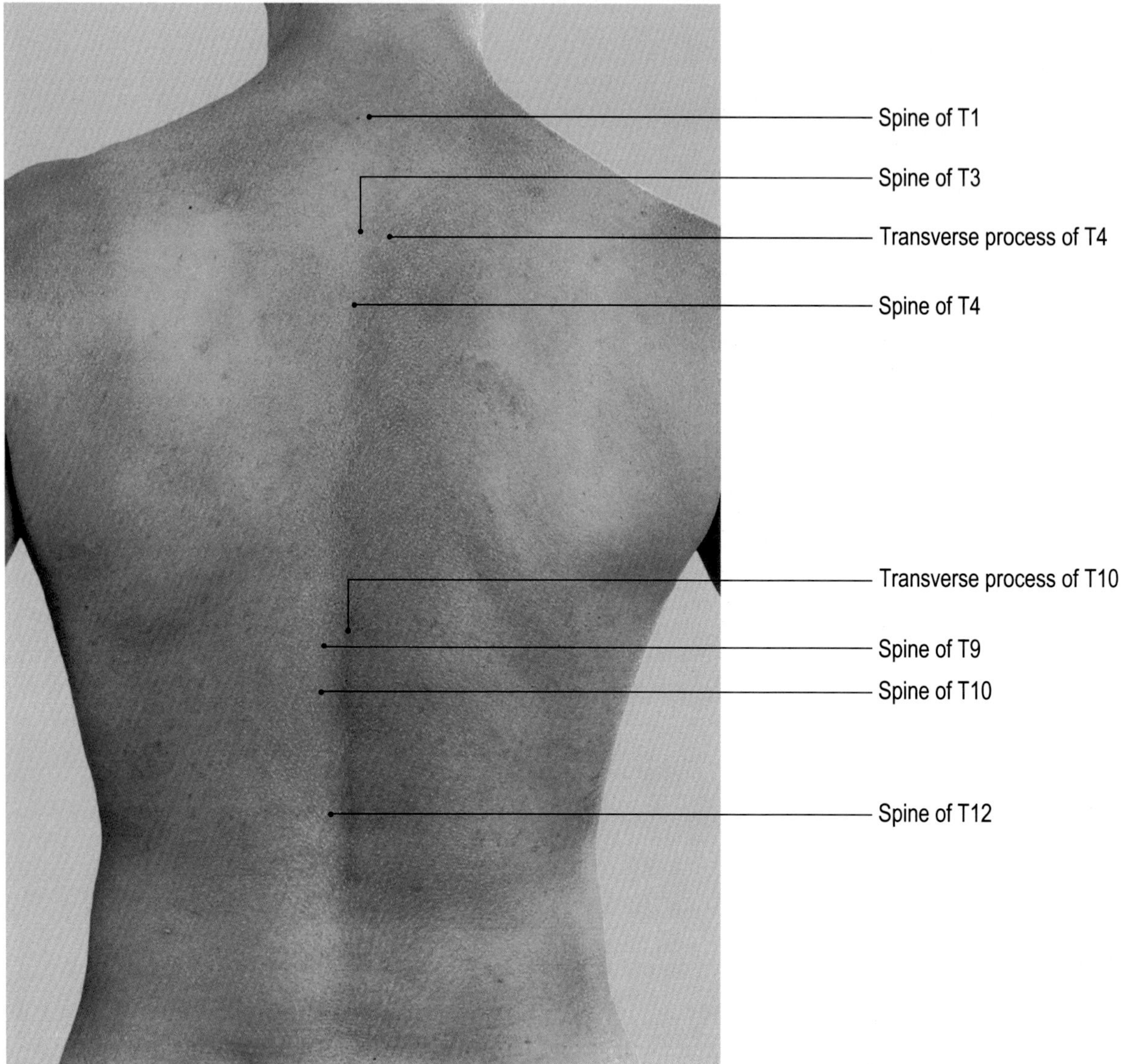

Fig. 5.2 (a) The thoracic vertebrae

The vertebrae

The thoracic part of the vertebral column can only be palpated posteriorly where it presents spines and transverse processes. These either overlap each other or are covered with strong, thick muscles and fascia, and so prove difficult to identify, even by an experienced practitioner.

The spines form a line of tubercles down the midline of the thorax. They are not uniform in length but pass downwards and backwards with a tendency to overlap the spine below. The tips of those near the upper part of the thorax are level with the upper surface of the vertebral body below. The lower vertebrae have longer spines which reach to the lower border of the vertebra below. The tip of the spine of T3 is roughly level with the root of the spine of the scapula; that of T7 is level with the inferior angle of the scapula. The spine of T12 is atypical as it is squared posteriorly and resembles that of a lumbar vertebra. It is level with the disc between T12 and L1. Accurate location of these spines must therefore be carried out by palpation. The usual method is to count down from an identifiable point above or below.

The transverse processes are much more difficult to palpate as they are covered by strong, thick muscles even in the leaner subject. The tips of the transverse processes are level with the upper border of their own vertebral body (Fig. 5.2).

Palpation

For palpation in this region, the model is in the slump sitting position.

- The thoracic spines. The back is rounded by asking the model to place the chin on the chest. In this position, the tips of the spines become more identifiable.
- The spines of C7 and T1. First, identify the spines of C7 and T1, these are the two most prominent spines at the base of the neck.

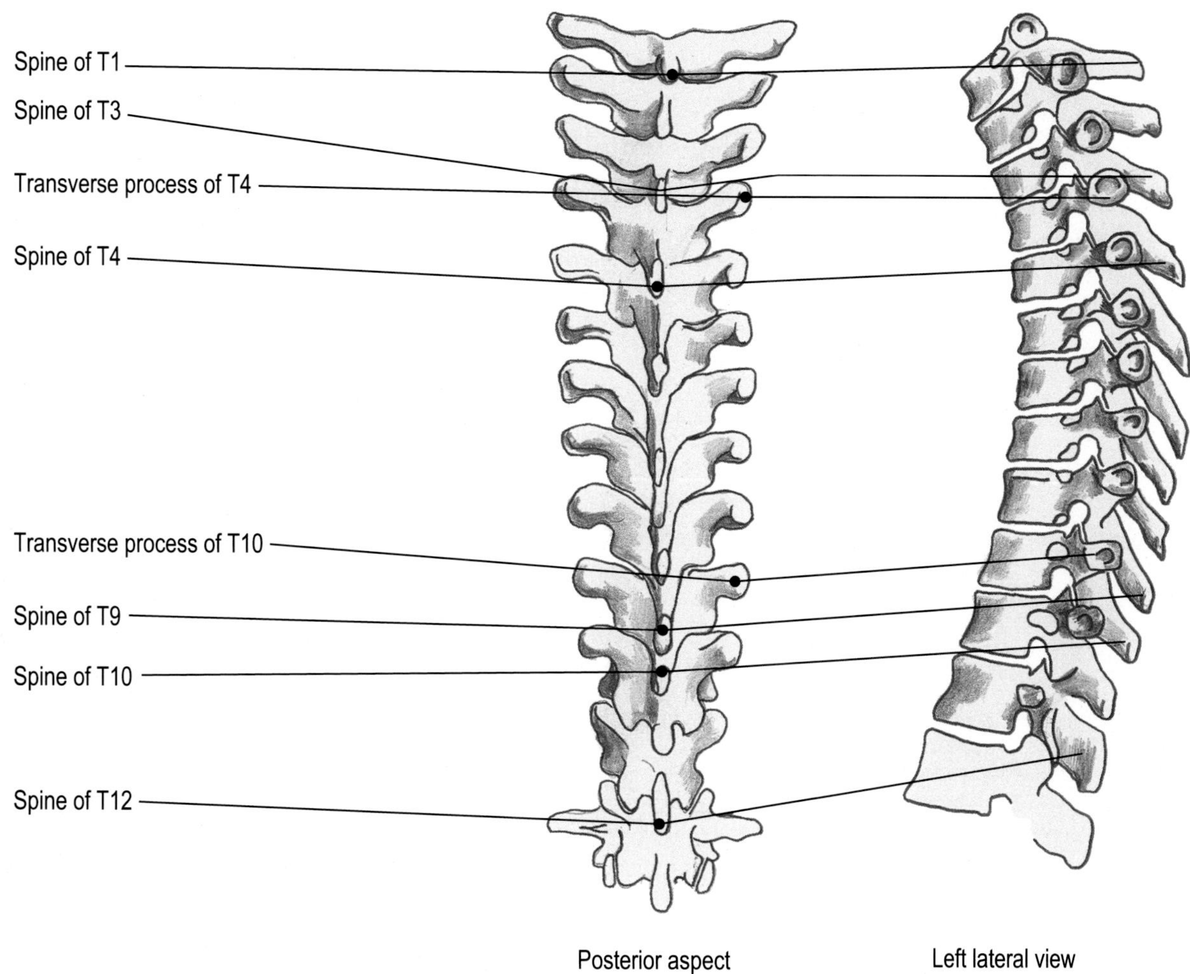

Fig. 5.2 (b) The thoracic vertebrae

- The thoracic spines. Carefully count down the tips of the spines, being sure to mark the upper spine with the fingers of one hand while seeking the spine below with the other. Each spine will feel quite pointed until the level of T12 where the spine becomes flattened. This is because the spine has features similar to those of a lumbar vertebra.
- **Note.** If you find that palpation is difficult, use the technique suggested on p. 6 where the fingertips are moved rapidly up and down the spine, in a scanning manner. This method of palpation is useful for locating and mapping structures which lie below the surface. It is, however, rarely used, as it gives the impression of merely moving the skin on the underlying structures. It amounts to the building up of a total picture by adding together many disparate pieces of information. Use the pads of all fingers of one hand (the most sensitive) if possible, to sweep across an area, allowing your fingers to move the skin and superficial fascia on the deeper structures. By using this technique, you will be building up a picture similar to that which would be achieved by the scanning beam of a video camera. Use the other hand to mark certain points and mark from where the previous information was obtained. More refined palpatory techniques can then be used on selected areas.
- The lateral tips of the thoracic transverse processes. These lie 3 cm lateral and parallel to the spines.
- **Note.** The tip of the spine lies 1 cm below the level of the transverse process of the vertebra below. This measurement remains constant because the shorter spines in the upper thorax are compensated for by the transverse processes being slightly raised.
- The costotransverse joints. Lateral to the tips of the transverse processes is a groove marking the line of the costotransverse joints.

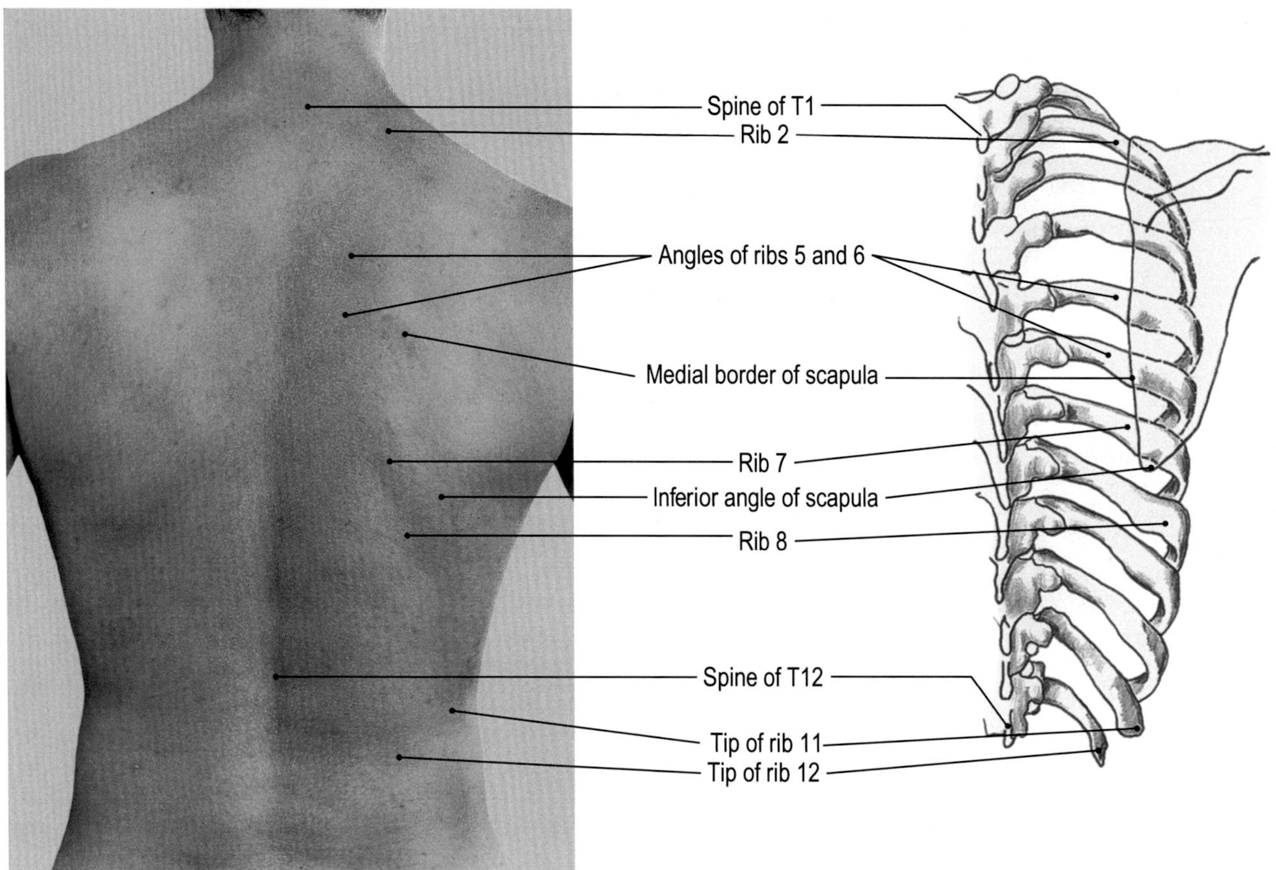

Fig. 5.3 (a, b) The ribs of the right side (posterior aspect)

The ribs (Fig. 5.3)

There are 12 ribs on either side. They are convex outwards, the eighth being the longest and the twelfth the shortest. The upper seven ribs articulate with the vertebral bodies and transverse processes posteriorly by the facets on their heads and tubercles. The first, tenth, **eleventh** and **twelfth** ribs have only one facet; the rest have two. The eleventh and twelfth ribs have no tubercles. Ribs 1–7 articulate with the sternum anteriorly via a varying length of costal cartilage. These are termed **'true' ribs**. Ribs 8–10 articulate anteriorly via their costal cartilage, with the costal cartilage above, and are termed **'false' ribs**. Ribs 11 and 12 do not articulate with their transverse process posteriorly and are free anteriorly. They are therefore termed **'floating' ribs** (see Fig. 5.1).

Palpation

To facilitate the palpation of the ribs, the back muscles need to be relaxed. This is best achieved if the model is in the prone lying position.

- The posterior section of the ribs. Just lateral to the tip of each transverse process the posterior section of each rib can be palpated, being separated from the transverse process by a depression.
- Ribs 1–10. Ask the model to hang the arm over the side of the plinth (i.e. the pectoral girdle is in protraction). Now find and trace the first to tenth ribs laterally. The rib angle lies approximately 3–4 cm lateral to the tips of the transverse processes. It can readily be palpated in the mid-thoracic region, becoming less clear above and below. The first rib does not possess an angle and those of the eleventh and twelfth ribs are slight if present.

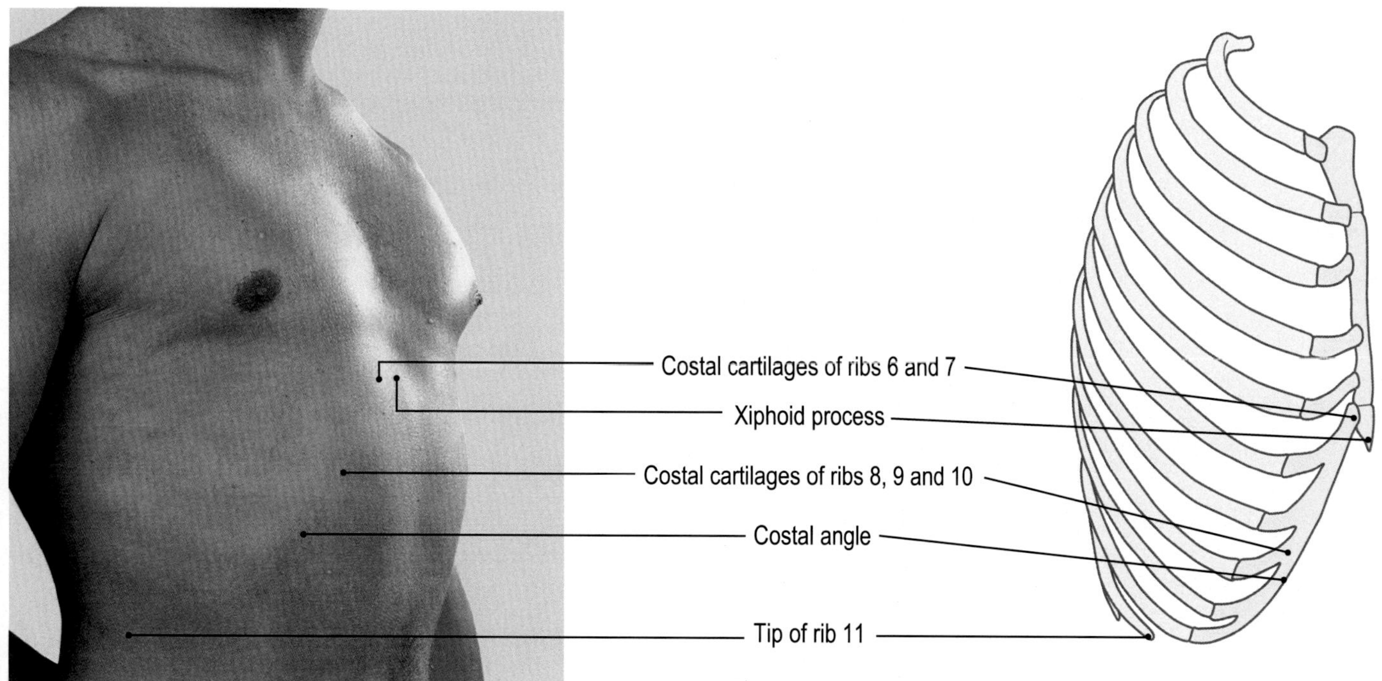

Fig. 5.3 (c, d) The ribs of the right side (lateral aspect)

- Ribs 1–12 and the intercostal spaces. Each rib, together with the intercostal spaces above and below, can be traced anteriorly to where it joins the sternum. The second to seventh or eighth ribs are usually hidden posterolaterally by the scapula, while the eleventh and twelfth ribs only exist posterolaterally.
- The first rib. This rib is the most difficult to palpate. It lies deep to the clavicle anteriorly and deep to the trapezius and levator scapulae muscles posteriorly. If you apply deep pressure immediately below the clavicle, 1 cm lateral to its medial end, you will be able to palpate the junction of the rib with the manubrium. By applying deep pressure above the middle of the clavicle in the supraclavicular fossa, it is possible to feel the lateral border of the first rib.
- **Note.** This area is particularly tender and may produce unpleasant reactions in the upper limb due to pressure on the trunks of the brachial plexus and subclavian artery.
- The neck and tubercle of the first rib. Posteriorly, the neck and tubercle of the first rib can be palpated running downwards and laterally approximately 2 cm lateral to the tip of the spine of C7. This, however, is dependent on the thickness of the upper fibres of trapezius.
- Ribs 8–10 and the costal angle. The **costal cartilages** at the anterior end of the **eighth to tenth ribs** form the anterior part of the costal margin, running superomedially to join the **xiphoid process**. At the level of the ninth costal cartilage an angle and projection are formed: the '**costal angle**'. This lies on a level with the transpyloric plane, in common with the spine of L1 and the tip of the twelfth rib.
- Ribs 11 and 12. Just above the twelfth, the eleventh rib can easily be identified, ending in a point just anterior to the mid-axillary line.

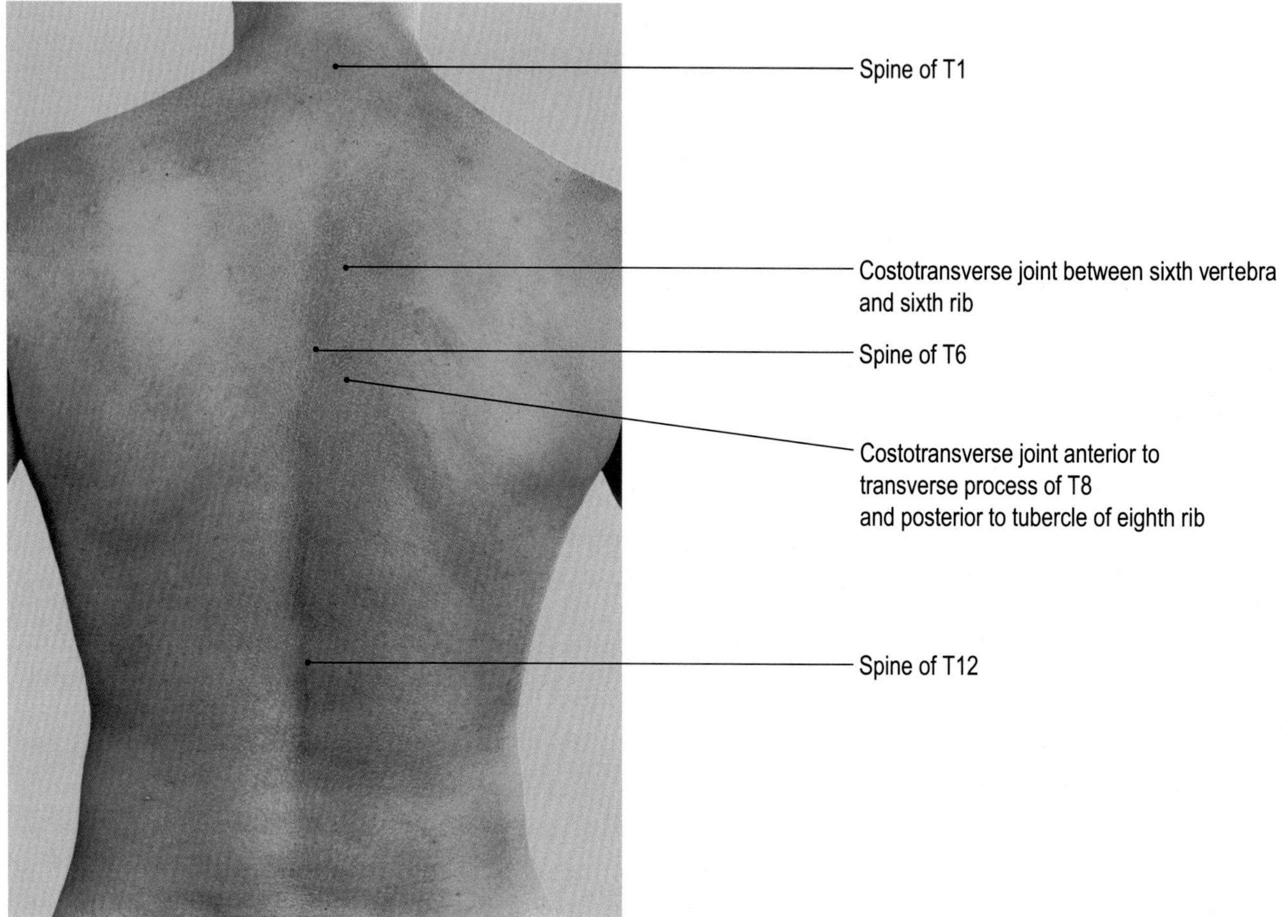

Fig. 5.4 (a) The costotransverse joints of the right side (posterior aspect)

JOINTS

The thoracic vertebral column (Fig. 5.4)

The joints of the thoracic vertebral column are similar to those in the cervical region. They do not, however, possess uncovertebral joints. They do have facets on the side of all of the bodies and the upper 10 transverse processes for the articulation of the ribs. The vertebral bodies articulate centrally by a series of intervertebral discs. These joints are complex cartilaginous symphyses. The intervertebral discs are made up of an outer ring of fibrous bands passing obliquely from one body to the other (the annulus fibrosus) and a central nucleus (the nucleus pulposus) composed of a soft highly hydrophilic substance. These discs are supported by many ligaments, including the very strong anterior and posterior longitudinal ligaments.

On either side are the **zygapophyseal joints** (Fig. 5.4d, e) between the articular facets, two above and two below. In addition there are **costovertebral joints** (Fig. 5.4c) between the heads of the ribs and the side(s) of the body of the vertebrae and costotransverse joints between the tubercle of the rib and the transverse process (Fig. 5.4 a–c). The zygapophyseal, costovertebral and costotransverse joints are all synovial, surrounded by a capsule which is lined with synovial membrane and supported by ligaments. (For detailed study refer to Palastanga et al 2002.)

Palpation

All but the costotransverse and possibly the zygapophyseal joints are impossible to palpate.

For palpation in this region, the model is in the prone lying position with the forehead resting on the backs of the hands.

- The costotransverse joints. These joints lie in the furrow between the transverse processes and the ribs. They can be located either by following backwards along the line of a known rib to the point where it is obscured by the transverse process or finding the tip of the spinous process of a known vertebra and tracing out laterally to the furrow mentioned above.

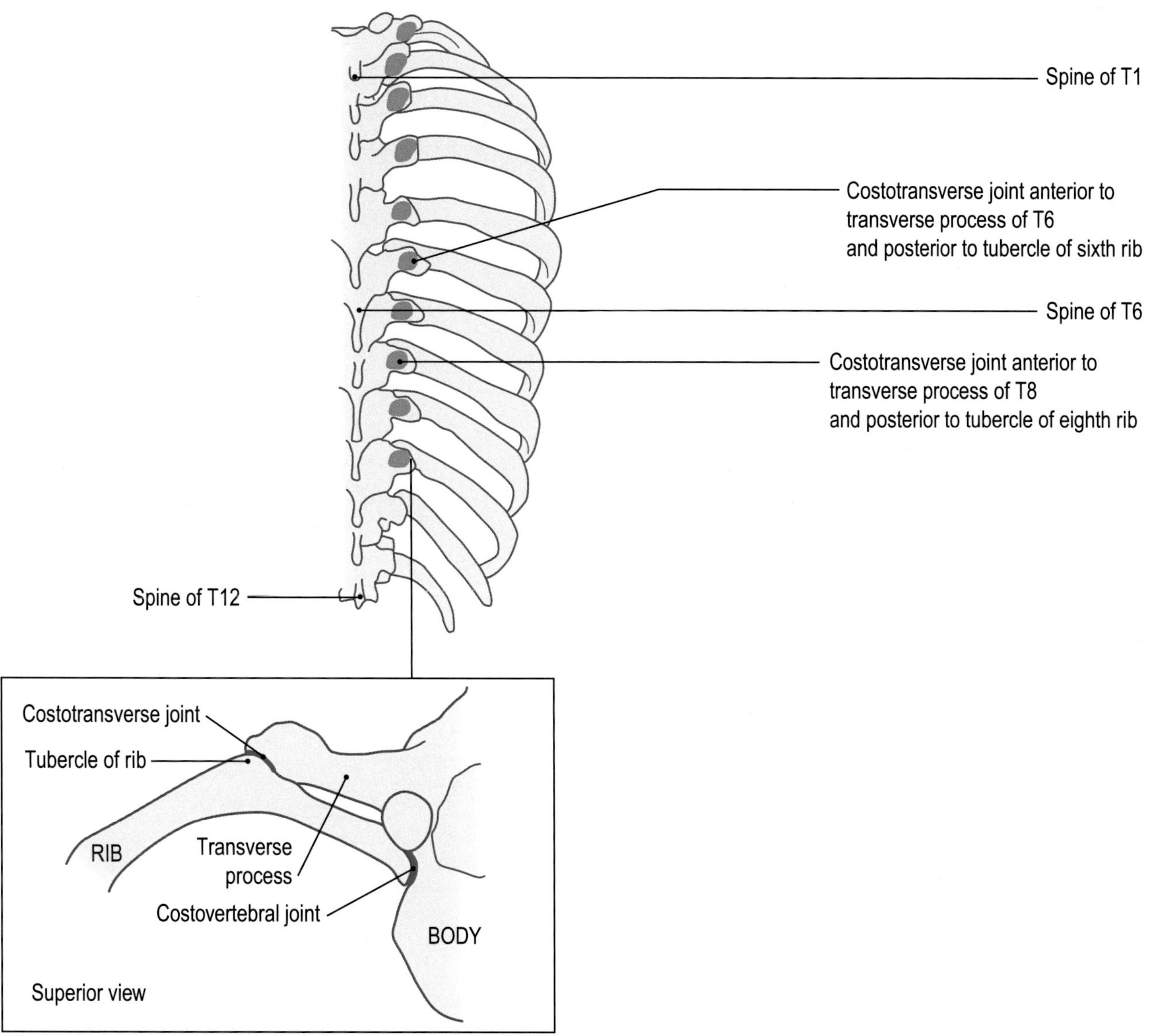

Fig. 5.4 (b, c) The costotransverse joints of the right side (posterior aspect)

- **Note.** Due to the length of the spines in the thoracic area, the transverse process you can feel is that of the vertebra below.
- The laminae of the thoracic spines. The joints between the articular facets of the thoracic vertebrae lie at the upper edge of the lamina as it meets the lamina above. The joint is virtually impossible to palpate but the lamina can be traced a little laterally from the spines. Slip your fingers down the side of the spinous process. Note that the lamina you feel is that of the vertebra below.

Accessory movements

As stated above, pressure on the lamina of one vertebra can part the zygapophyseal joint surfaces above and compress those below on the ipsilateral side (Fig. 5.4c).

- Posterior-to-anterior pressure to a thoracic spine. Applying this technique to the tip of a thoracic spine causes it to act as a lever, parting the upper zygapophyseal joint and compressing the lower (Fig. 5.4f, g).
- Lateral pressure. Pressure applied to the lateral side of the spinous process causes rotation of the body of the vertebra to the opposite side. This results in gapping of the upper zygapophyseal joint on the side to which the spine is moved, but compressing the lower joint. It has the opposite effect on the joints of the ipsilateral side.
- Traction. Traction on the thoracic intervertebral joints is difficult to produce, resulting in virtually no movement. To a limited extent, movement certainly does occur during lumbar or cervical traction.
- Pressure on the rib angles. Laterally, the heads of the ribs articulate with the bodies of the vertebrae; the tubercles of the ribs articulate with the transverse processes of the vertebrae (Fig. 5.4). Pressure on the angle of the rib will part the costotransverse joint. If you move your thumbs slightly medially to an area just lateral to the joint, the gapping is increased.
- **Note.** If you apply pressure even more medially, it will encroach upon the back of the transverse process, producing exactly the opposite effect and resulting in compression of the costotransverse joint (Fig. 5.4c).

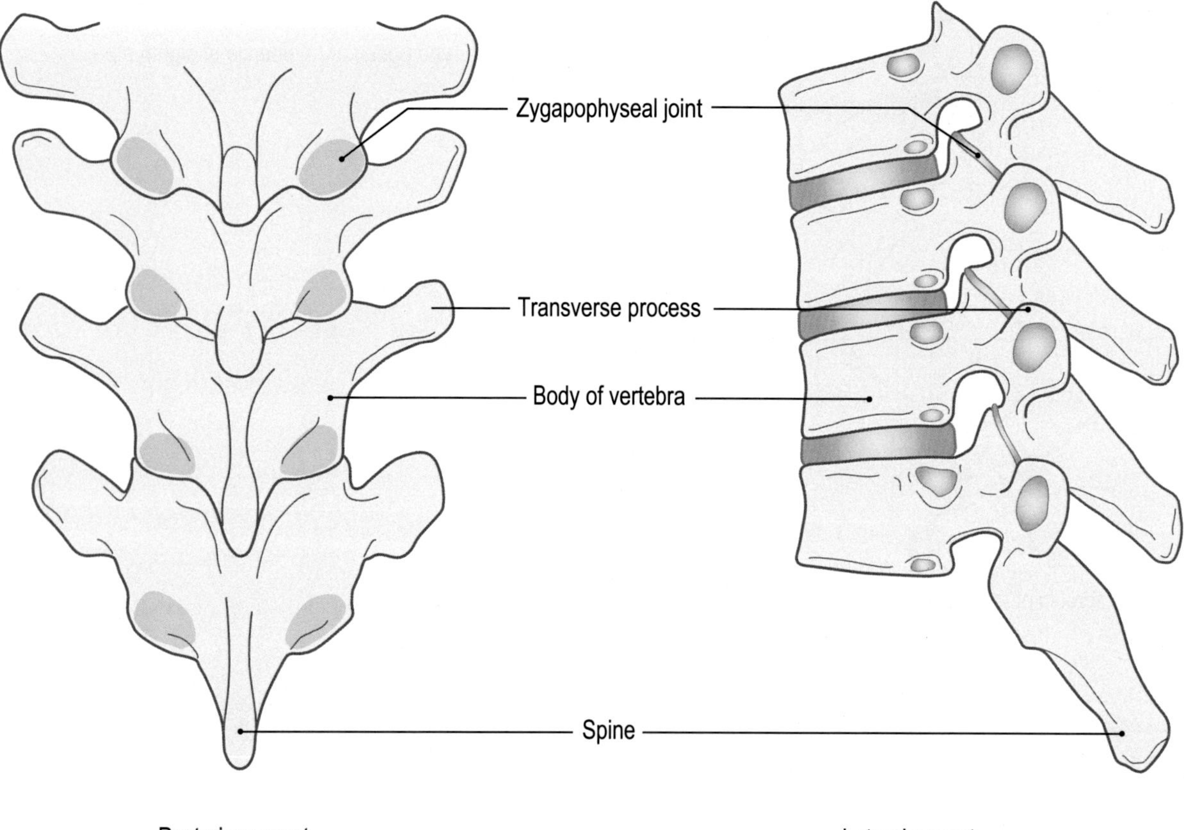

Fig. 5.4 (d, e) Zygapophyseal joints of thoracic spine. Shaded areas show joint surface deep to inferior articular processes

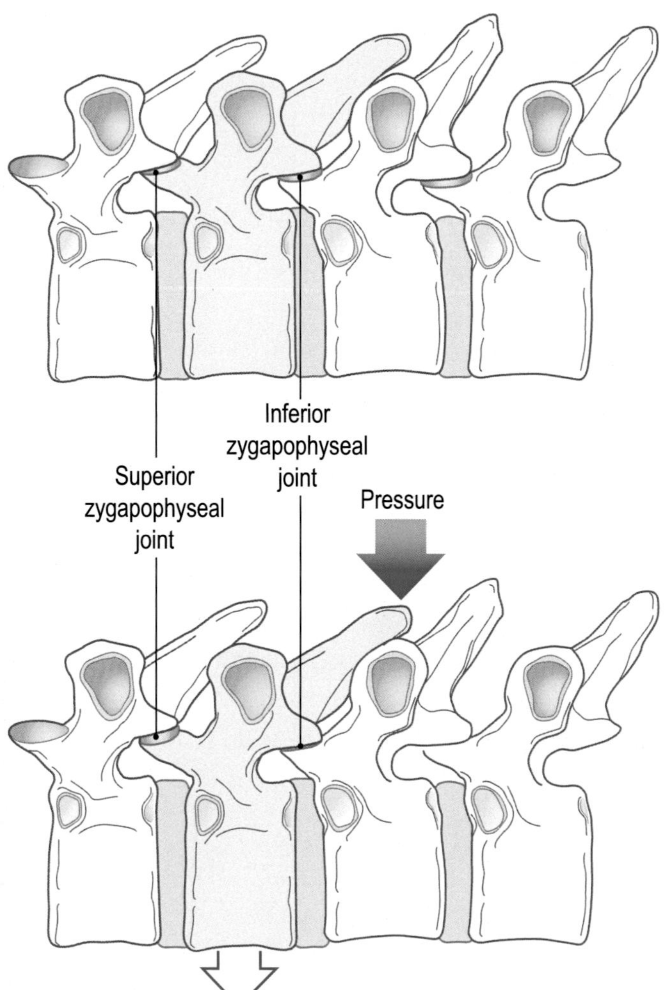

Fig. 5.4 (f, g) Vertebrae in horizontal position showing effect of pressure on spine in direction of arrow

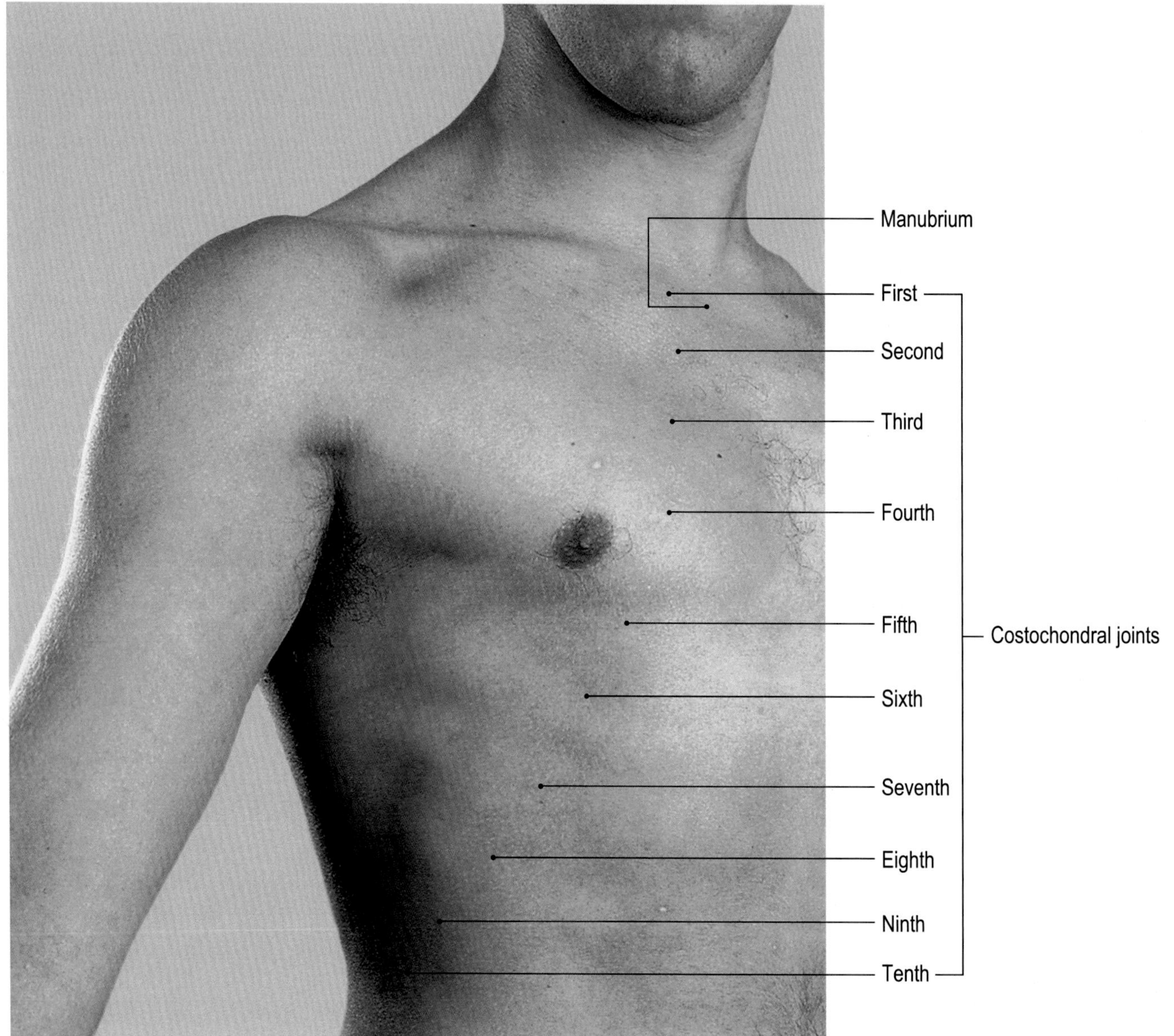

Fig. 5.5 (a) Costochondral joints of the right side (anterior aspect)

The joints of the anterior end of the ribs

Anteriorly, the upper seven ribs articulate with the sternum via their costal cartilages. These are termed true ribs. The costal cartilages of ribs eight to ten articulate with the costal cartilage above and are termed false ribs. The two lower ribs are only capped with costal cartilage and do not link up with the sternum and are termed floating ribs.

There are three sets of joints in this area: the costochondral, the interchondral and the sternocostal joints.

The costochondral joints

These joints are really the junction between the rib and its cartilage. The rounded end of the cartilage fits into the depressed roughened end of the rib. Its periosteum is continuous with its perichondrium.

Palpation

- The costochondral joints (Fig. 5.5a, b). These joints can be identified in some subjects. They lie approximately 3 cm lateral to the sternum at the second rib, progressing to some 12 cm from the xiphoid at the seventh rib and approximately 18 cm from the xiphoid process at the tenth rib.

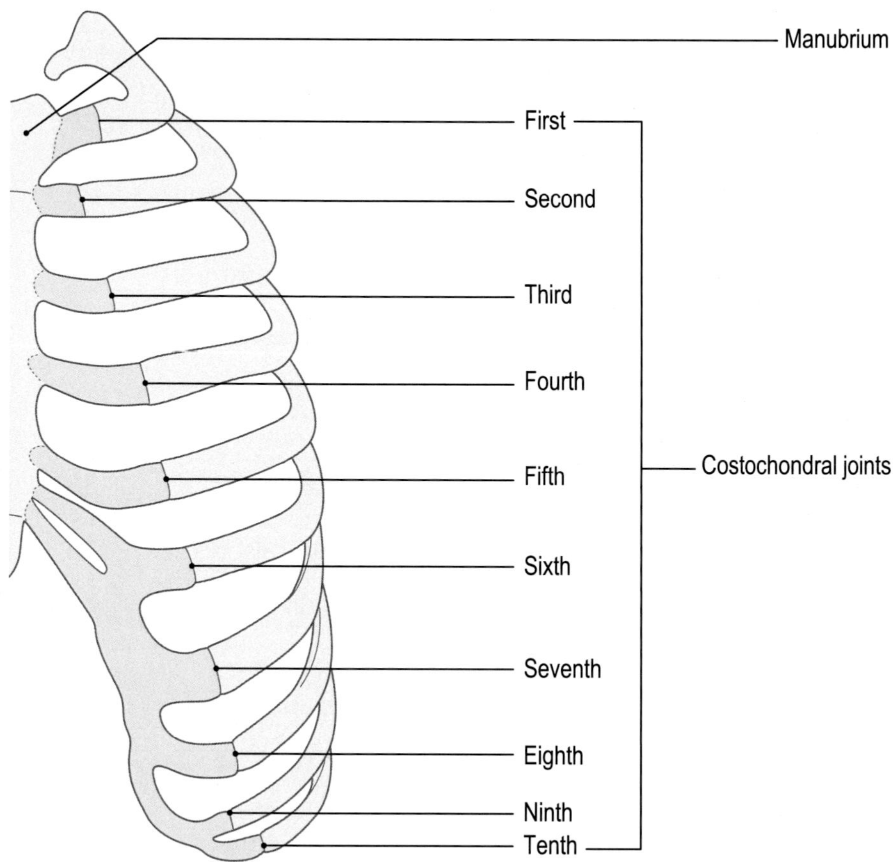

Fig. 5.5 (b) Costochondral joints of the right side (anterior aspect)

- Note. Pressure on the anterior surface of these joints can often be unpleasant and too much palpation may lead to the area becoming very tender, the symptoms lasting for some time.

Accessory movements

The model is in the supine lying position.

- Compression of the joints. Applying pressure to the sternal area of the chest achieves quite marked compression of the joints. This is due in part to the flexibility of the ribs and costal cartilage and in part to the slight gliding and bending movements occurring between the costochondral, interchondral, sternocostal and intersternal joints.
- Movement of individual joints. It is possible to produce movement of each individual joint. Using two thumbs, apply pressure to the rib or to the costal cartilage close to either side of the joint. The movement is minimal in some joints, such as that of the first and second ribs with the sternum. It is quite considerable lower down the thorax, particularly at the interchondral joints.
- Note. Some of these joints can be traumatized and become inflamed. This is usually following a blow on the chest or stress on the rib cage due to resting heavily against a beam or bar. This produces acute pain over that area of the chest. If the pain is over the area of the heart, it may erroneously be associated with a heart attack.

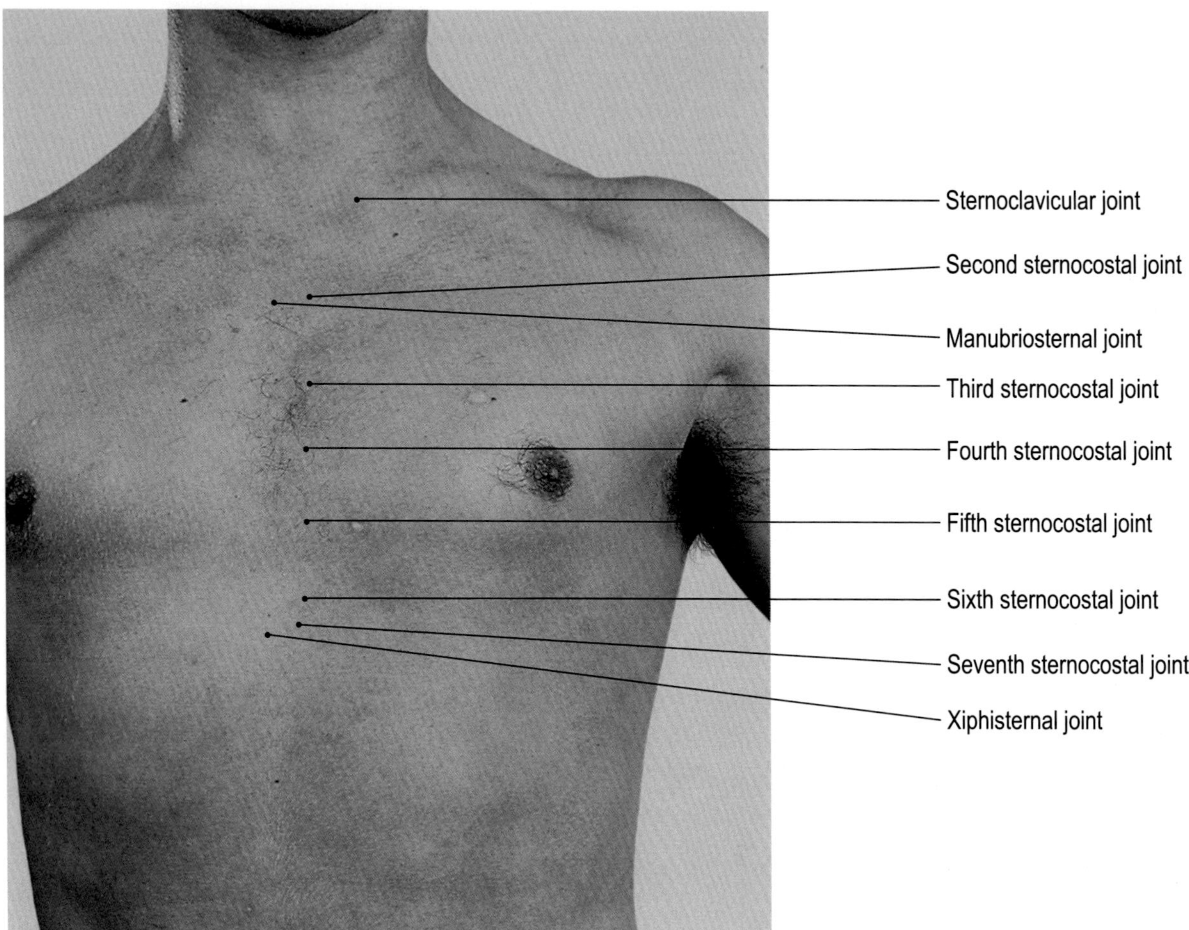

Fig. 5.5 (c) Joints of the sternum (anterior aspect)

The sternocostal (chondrosternal) joints (Fig. 5.5c, d)

These are the joints between the anterior rounded end of the costal cartilages of the upper seven ribs and the small hollow cavities on the side of the sternum.

The first articulates with the side of the manubrium just below the clavicular notch. It is a synarthrosis and has a similar structure to a symphysis, so forming a fairly rigid union. It is close to the midline of the body, a location where most symphyses are found.

The second to the seventh are all synovial joints. They are surrounded by a capsule which is lined with synovial membrane and supported by ligaments that radiate from the front of the cartilage on to the anterior aspect of the sternum (the sternocostal radiate ligaments). The second costal cartilage joins the sternum at the side of the manubriosternal joint. It has the extra support of an interosseous ligament which attaches to the disc of the manubriosternal joint. The seventh costal cartilage joins a small shallow facet formed by the lower part of the sternum and the xiphoid process. It is supported in front and behind by costoxiphoid ligaments. This synovial joint is often replaced by a symphysis.

Palpation

- The costomanubriosternal joint. At the side of the manubriosternal joint, approximately 7 cm below the sternal notch, you can palpate the articulation of the second costal cartilage, the manubrium (Fig. 5.5b) and body of the sternum. It is identified as a small V-shaped notch, with the concavity facing laterally.
- Ribs 3–7 and costal cartilages. Below this, on either side, the third to seventh ribs and their costal cartilages can be palpated as they articulate with the lateral border of the sternum at the costosternal or chondrosternal joints. The section of the sternum between each costal cartilage is concave laterally, being the anterior limit of the intercostal spaces.

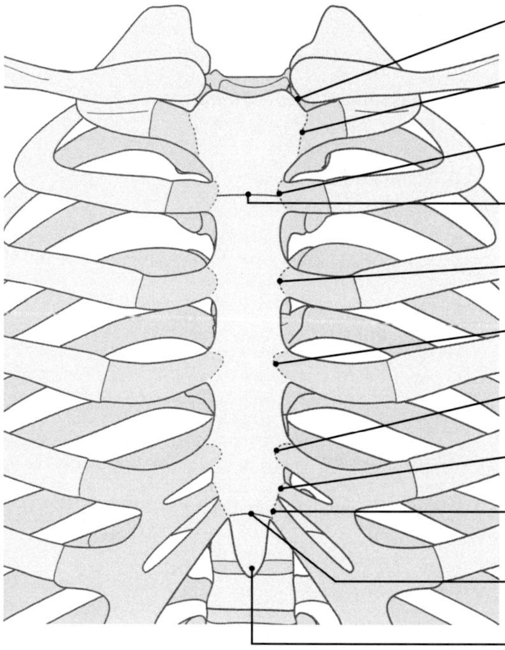

Fig. 5.5 (d) Joints of the sternum (anterior aspect)

- The manubriocostal joint. The joint between the first rib and the manubrium lies 1 cm below, and 1 cm lateral to, the medial end of the clavicle and is more difficult to identify. You can, however, palpate the anterior limit of the rib.
- Ribs 8–10 and their costal cartilages. The costal cartilage of the eighth to tenth ribs can be identified. They articulate medially, with the costal cartilage above, at the interchondral joints and form the costal margin.

Joints of the sternum

The sternum is composed of three segments: the manubrium superiorly, the body centrally, and the small, pointed xiphoid process inferiorly. The joints between these sections are secondary cartilaginous symphyses.

Palpation

- The manubriosternal joint (Fig. 5.5c, d). This joint is easy to identify. It is approximately 7 cm below the upper border of the sternum at the sternal angle. It is level with the articulation of the second costal cartilage with the sternum.
- The xiphisternal joint (Fig. 5.5c, d). The joint between the body and the xiphoid process is more difficult to palpate, although the body and the xiphoid are both easily identifiable.

Accessory movements

- Bilateral pressure. There is very little accessory movement of the manubriosternal joint, although pressure on either the body or the manubrium, close to the joint, will produce slight angling of the two sections.
- Anterior-posterior pressure. At the xiphisternal joint, however, the xiphoid process can normally be moved backwards some considerable distance by pressure applied to its anterior surface. This produces an angling at the joint.

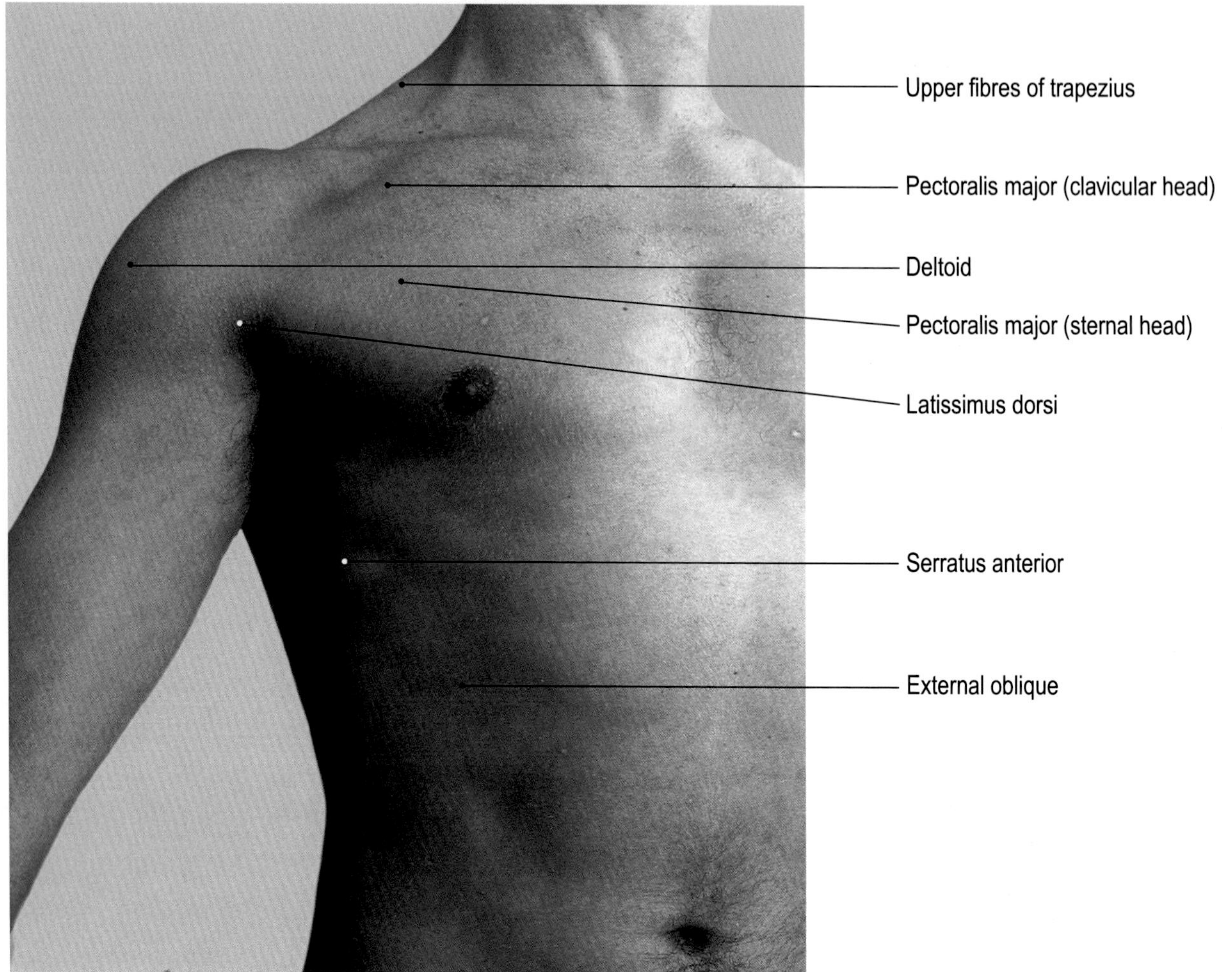

Fig. 5.6 (a) Muscles of the right shoulder region (anterior aspect)

MUSCLES

The anterior aspect of the chest

The muscle that dominates the upper part of the chest is pectoralis major. Lying deep to it are pectoralis minor and the upper intercostal muscles. In the lower part of the chest, rectus abdominis and the external oblique muscle of the abdomen have their upper attachment (see Fig. 6.5).

Pectoralis minor is a triangular muscle. Its base attaches to the third, fourth and fifth ribs at approximately the mid-clavicular line; its apex attaches to the coracoid process of the scapula. It is very difficult to palpate. The intercostal muscles attach to the lower border of the rib above and to the upper border of the rib below. They are easier to palpate in the lower region of the chest (see p. 199).

The external oblique muscle attaches above to the external surface of the lower border of the lower eight ribs.

Palpation

For palpation in this region, the model is in the supine lying position.

- External oblique. Place your fingers under the lower border of the rib cage, on the right, just lateral to the costal angle. Now ask the model to turn to the left. You will be able to feel the contraction of the muscle.

The rectus abdominis attaches above to the fifth, sixth and seventh costal cartilages just lateral to the sternum.

Palpation

- Rectus abdominis. Place your fingers just below the rib cage just lateral to the xiphoid process. Now ask the model to raise the head. Immediately the powerful contraction of the muscle will be palpated. (See also p. 229.)

Pectoralis major

Pectoralis major (Figs 5.6 and 5.7) is a large, thick triangular muscle situated on the upper anterior area of the chest wall. It is composed of two main groups of fibres: clavicular and sternal. The clavicular fibres attach medially to the anterior surface of the medial half of the clavicle. The sternal fibres attach the anterior

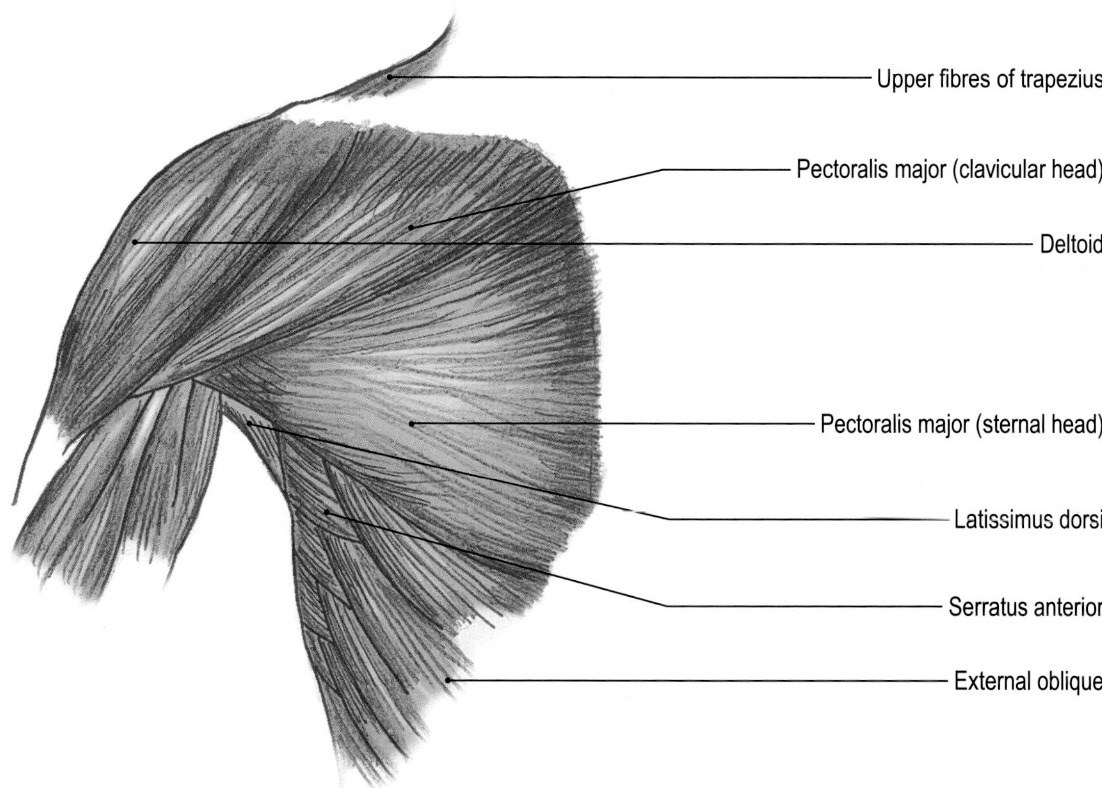

Fig. 5.6 (b) Muscles of the right shoulder region (anterior aspect)

surface of sternum on the same side, the anterior surface of the upper seven costal cartilages and the upper part of the aponeurosis covering the abdominal muscles. Both sets of fibres pass laterally, leaving a small space between them, and join together laterally to form a bilaminar tendon which attaches to the lateral lip of the intertubercular groove of the humerus. The lower sternal fibres tend to fold up behind the upper fibres to form the double bilaminated tendon. The muscle forms a lower border which becomes the anterior border of the axilla laterally.

Palpation

For palpation in this region, the model is in the sitting position.

- Pectoralis major. This muscle is easily recognizable and palpable in even the less muscular subject. Ask the model to press the hands against the iliac crest and feel the contraction of the whole muscle.
- The sternal fibres. Identify the lower border of the anterior wall of the axilla. This is rounded due to the lower sternal fibres of pectoralis major twisting upwards posterior to its upper fibres. The muscle can be traced medially and inferiorly on to the anterior aspect of the chest as far down as the costal cartilage of the seventh rib and xiphoid process. Now ask the model to extend the arm from the flexed position against resistance. Palpate the lower sternal fibres. These are identifiable as a thick triangular shape forming the lower boundary of the muscle which can be traced out laterally to the intertubercular groove of the humerus (Fig. 5.7c, d).
- Note. The bulk of the muscle forms a rounded shape on the upper anterior chest wall. It is the muscle that men try to develop to produce a characteristic shape to the upper part of the chest. It is almost entirely covered by the breast in the female, particularly in its lower section.
- The clavicular fibres. Now ask the model to flex the arms against resistance. Palpate the clavicular fibres which are easily identified, just below the medial half of the clavicle, as a column of muscle standing clear of the chest wall (Fig. 5.7a, b) passing downwards and laterally.
- The sternal and clavicular fibres together. To observe the two sets of fibres working in concert, ask the model to press the two hands together in front of the chest. Palpate both sets of fibres which will now stand clear of the chest wall.

Functional anatomy

It is interesting to note that pectoralis major has two functionally distinct sets of fibres, a bilaminal tendon, and is supplied through

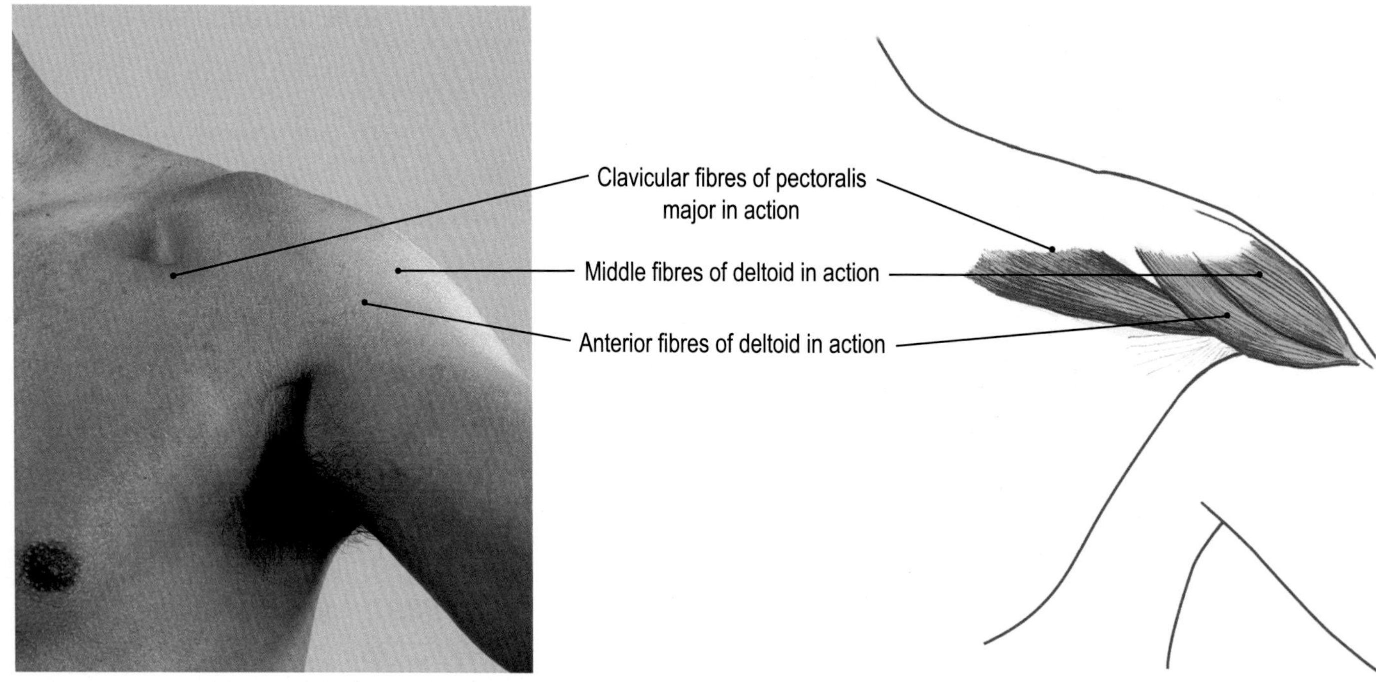

Fig. 5.7 (a, b) Sternal fibres of pectoralis major and deltoid of left shoulder (anterior aspect)

two nerves (lateral and medial pectoral). In addition, it is involved in two actions which appear to oppose each other. The clavicular fibres will flex and the sternal fibres will extend the shoulder joint. In prone kneeling, both sets of fibres act to stabilize the upper trunk posture, preventing sway either forwards, backwards or from side to side. In crawling, the limb is taken forwards by the clavicular fibres and backwards by the sternal fibres. This important muscle must have had a greater significance in our evolution and recognition of its residual function may help in its re-education.

In patients suffering from respiratory embarrassment, pectoralis major may be used as an accessory muscle of inspiration. In this case the arms have to be fixed, as in gripping a post or beam, thus fixing the lateral attachment of the muscle to the humerus. The medial attachment of the muscle may then be used to expand the chest a little more.

Comparative anatomy

The pectoralis muscle(s) also play an important role in the animal, bird, fish, reptile and insect worlds. In the quadruped this muscle acts as a stabilizing muscle for the forelimb in the standing position, similar to that in the human prone kneeling position, and because of its shape takes part in both the propulsive and recovery phase of the forelimb in locomotion. It also acts as a sling for the thorax, holding it up between the two limbs. In the bird and insect it creates the enormous thrust for take-off and flight, while at the same time controlling the intricate movements of the wings. In

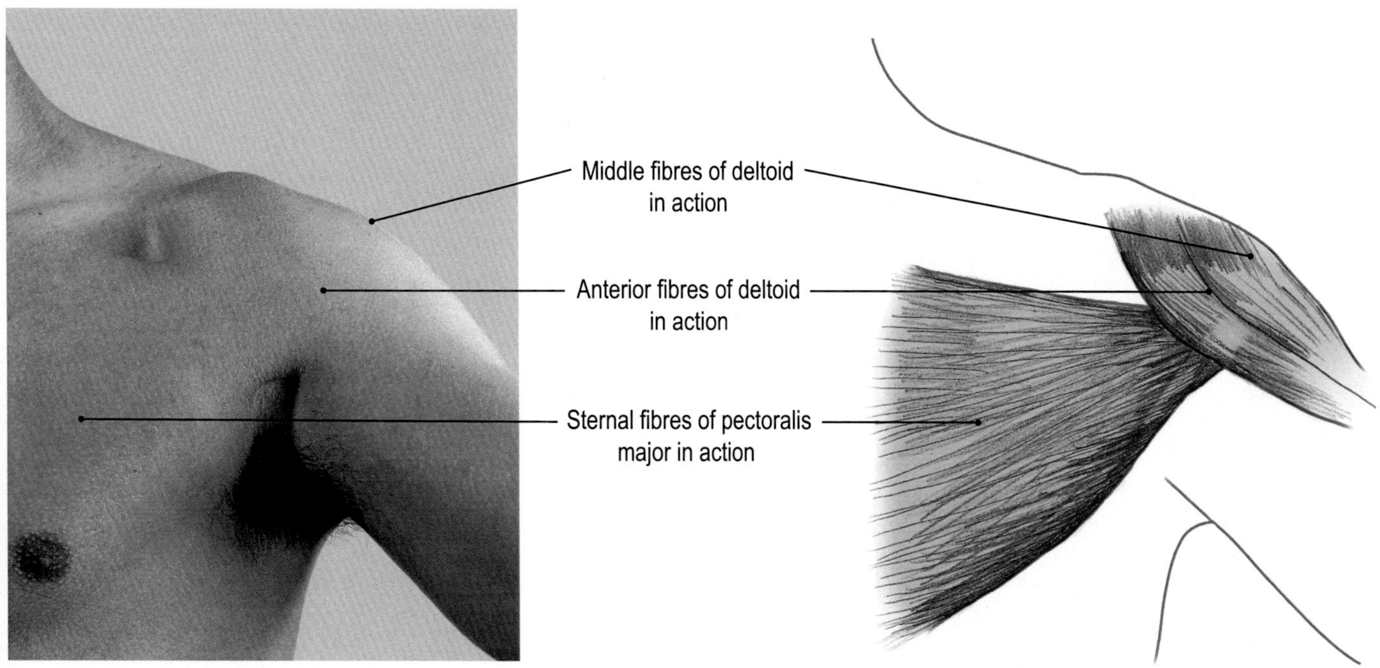

Fig. 5.7 (c, d) Sternal fibres of pectoralis major and deltoid of left shoulder (anterior aspect)

the fish it controls the fine movements of the pectoral fin in a comparatively simple up-and-down motion, but occasionally may have fibres which are extended into the neck region. The pectorals in the forelimb of a reptile normally have the adaptability of being functional in water and on land.

Biceps brachii and coracobrachialis (see Ch. 2)

Palpation

For palpation in this region the model is in the sitting position.

- Biceps brachii and coracobrachialis tendons. Running vertically from the coracoid process the combined tendon of the biceps brachii and coracobrachialis can be palpated just below the coracoid process but is soon hidden by the broad tendon of pectoralis major. It emerges below and can be identified passing down into the anteromedial aspect of the arm and splitting into its anterior (bicipital) and posterior (coracobrachialis) section.
- The intercostal muscles. Place your fingers between the ribs and identify a tight membranous sheet. This consists of the external and internal intercostal muscles and their covering fascia. These are most easily palpated just below pectoralis major and slightly lateral to the line of the nipple. On muscular subjects they are possibly hidden by larger, more superficial muscles.

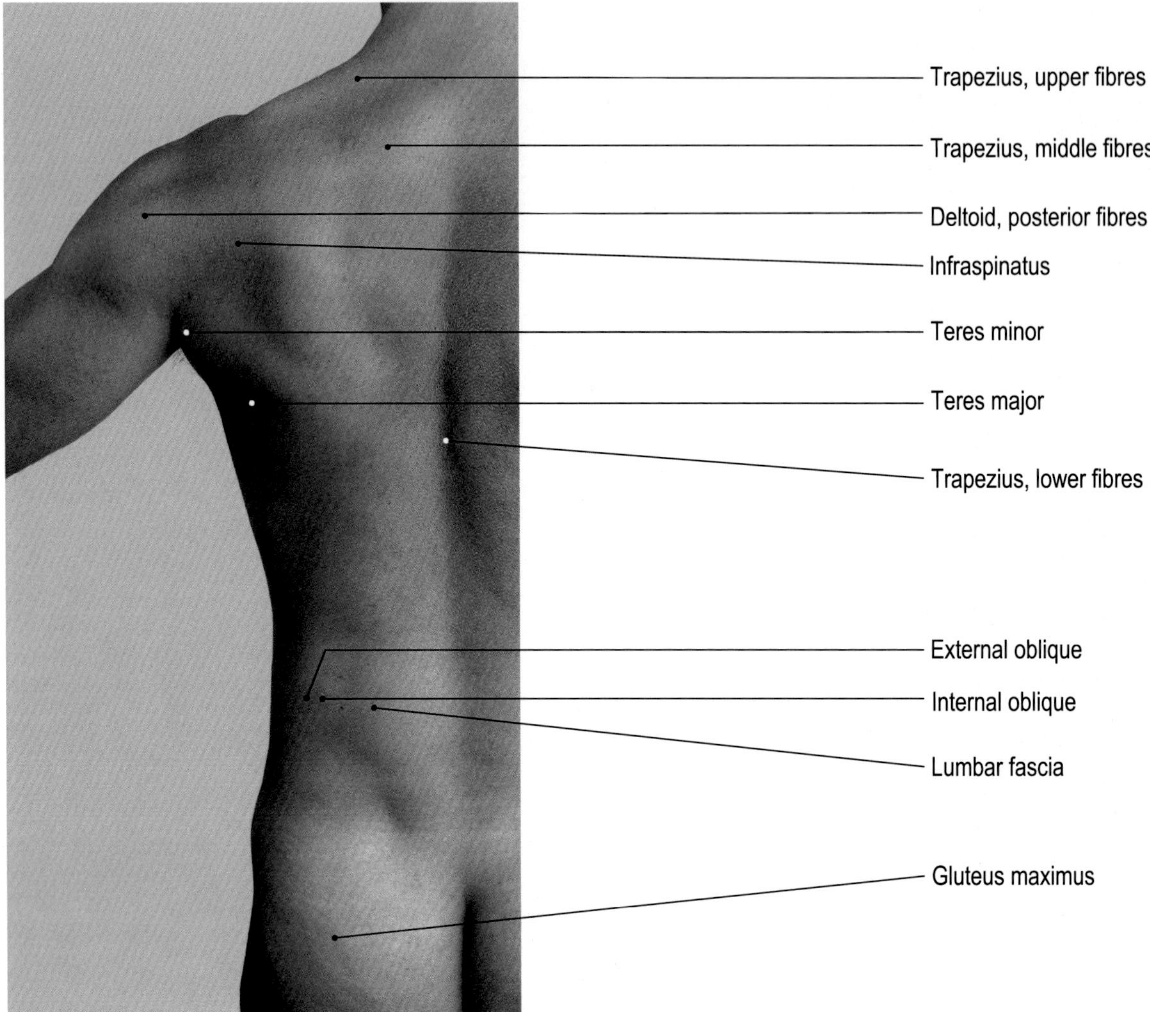

Fig. 5.8 (a) Muscles of the neck, thorax, lumbar and gluteal region (posterior aspect)

The posterior aspect of the chest

Trapezius (Fig. 5.8a, b)

The two trapezius muscles cover most of the posterior aspect of the neck and upper thorax, connecting the skull, ligamentum nuchae, seventh cervical and all the thoracic spines to the lateral end of the clavicle, acromion and superior border of the spine of the scapula.

Palpation

For palpation in this region, the model is in the sitting position.

- The upper fibres of trapezius. These are easier to identify if the model is asked to shrug the shoulders: raising the shoulder girdle. They can be palpated halfway between the external occipital protuberance and the acromion process, forming the contour of the upper lateral aspect of the shoulder.
- The middle fibres of trapezius. These are easier to identify if the model is asked to retract the shoulder girdle. They can be palpated between the upper border of the spine of the scapula and the lower cervical and upper thoracic regions.
- The lower fibres of trapezius. These are more difficult to identify as they pass from the lower thoracic spines to the medial end of the spine of the scapula. Palpation is, however, facilitated if you ask the model to depress the shoulder girdle.

Levator scapulae, rhomboid major and rhomboid minor

These muscles lie deep to the trapezius. Levator scapulae attaches above to the transverse processes of the upper four cervical vertebrae and below to the upper part of the medial border of the scapula. The rhomboid muscles attach above to the lower part of the ligamentum nuchae, the spine of the seventh cervical vertebra and the spines of the upper five thoracic vertebrae. They pass downwards and laterally to attach to the lower two-thirds of the medial border of the scapula.

Palpation

- Levator scapulae and the rhomboid muscles. These muscles add bulk to the area between the scapula and lower neck and can be palpated in this region when the shoulders are raised and braced back.

Supraspinatus and infraspinatus

Supraspinatus arises from the supraspinous fossa of the scapula passing laterally to the top of the greater tuberosity of the humerus

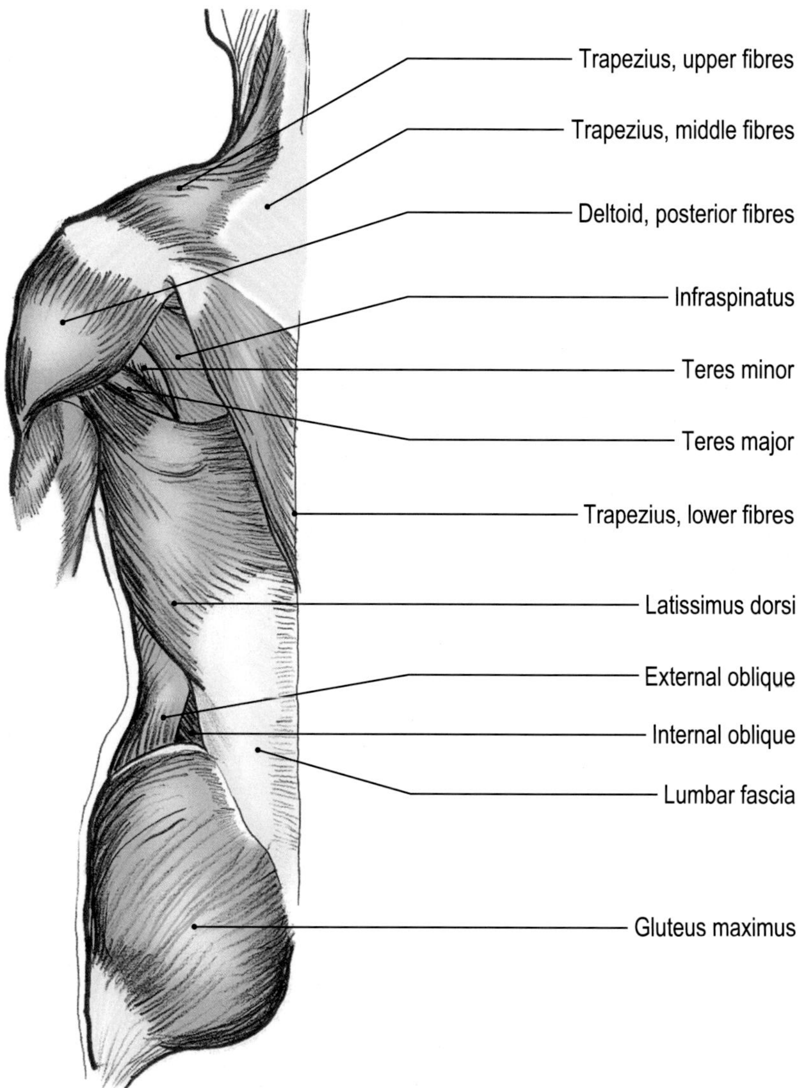

Fig. 5.8 (b) Muscles of the neck, thorax, lumbar and gluteal region (posterior aspect)

Infraspinatus arises from the infraspinous fossa, passing laterally to the posterior aspect of the same tuberosity.

Palpation

- Supraspinatus. Ask the model to begin to raise the arm from the side. Supraspinatus can be identified just above the spine of the scapula in the supraspinous fossa.
- Infraspinatus. Ask the model to rotate the arm laterally. Below the spine, infraspinatus can be felt contracting.

Teres major and latissimus dorsi

These two muscles are triangular in shape and cover the lateral border of the scapula, **teres major** actually arising from the border. **Latissimus dorsi** comes from an extensive attachment to the spines of the lower six thoracic vertebrae, the thoracolumbar fascia and the posterior section of the iliac crest. It passes over the inferior angle of the scapula, taking a few fibres of origin, and then twists under the axilla with teres major to attach to the floor of the intertubercular groove of the humerus. Teres major attaches to its medial lip.

Palpation

- Teres major. Ask the model to extend the arm from a flexed position against resistance. The triangular bulk of teres major lies over the lateral border of the scapula.
- Latissimus dorsi. Again, ask the model to extend the arm from a flexed position against resistance. The tendon of latissimus dorsi can be traced, laterally and forwards, forming the posterior wall of the axilla. This tendon can be traced to its muscle fibres medially over the dorsum of the chest and lumbar area. Ask the model to cough and palpate the muscle.

Serratus anterior (see Fig. 5.6a, b)

Serratus anterior is a flat but powerful muscle attaching to the whole of the medial border of the scapula. Passing deep to the scapula, it attaches anteriorly to the lateral aspect of the first to eighth ribs at the mid-axillary line. Most of the muscle is concealed beneath the scapula, but palpation of its anterior attachment to the ribs is possible.

Palpation

- Serratus anterior. Ask the model to protract the shoulder girdle. Now place your fingers behind the mid-axillary line but in front of the scapula. The anterior attachment of serratus anterior to the ribs can be identified.
- **Note.** Care must be taken to observe the contraction when the pectoral girdle is retracted and begins to move forwards. Once the lateral border of the scapula has passed beyond the mid-axillary line, the muscle is hidden.

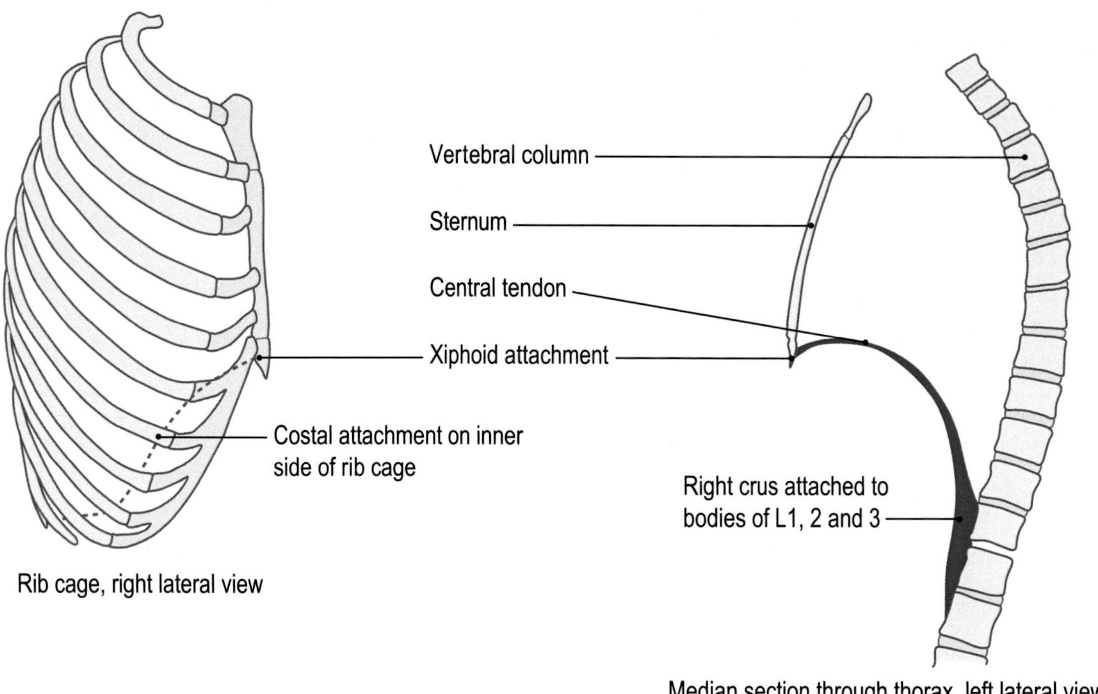

Fig. 5.9 (a, b) Attachments of the diaphragm

The diaphragm (Figs 5.9 and 5.10)

The **diaphragm** is a musculotendinous sheet separating the thoracic and abdominal cavities. It forms a double **cupola** within the thorax, with the heart resting upon its **central tendinous part**. Anteriorly it attaches to the xiphisternum, laterally to the inner aspect of the lower six ribs on a line with the inner surface of the **costochondral** joints, and posteriorly to the vertebral column. It is the main muscle of inspiration and moves downwards on inspiration and upwards on expiration. It is therefore more useful to indicate its surface markings after full expiration and then after a deep inspiration. The attachments to the xiphisternum, ribs and vertebral column remain constant, but the two cupolae and central tendon vary in height. It must also be remembered that the position of the diaphragm is influenced by other factors: it lies at a higher level with respect to the rib cage when lying supine than when standing; its downward movement is restricted by food and gas in the stomach, and by increased pressure in the abdominal cavity, for example during pregnancy; in side lying it is pushed up into the thoracic cavity on the lower side by the contents of the abdomen; and in prone lying the liver tends to restrict its downward movement on the right side.

On full expiration, **the right cupola** rises to the level of the fourth rib, **the left** to the fourth intercostal space and the central tendon to the level of the fifth costal cartilage. On full inspiration – which may produce a 6 cm descent of the cupolae – the diaphragm may reach the level of the sixth or seventh ribs. In quiet respiration, the diaphragm normally only moves up and down 1–2 cm.

Palpation: surface marking

It is impossible to palpate the diaphragm. On full inspiration there is a bulging of the abdomen between the two costal margins. Although this is produced by the diaphragm, it is actually the upper section of the abdominals.

- The diaphragm: surface marking. The attachment of the diaphragm to the inside of the chest wall can be marked by an oblique line drawn from the xiphoid process, anteriorly, downwards and laterally slightly concave downwards. It follows the line of the sixth costal cartilage, attaching to the inner surface and anterior end of the sixth to tenth ribs (Fig. 5.9a). It then attaches to the inner surface of the eleventh and **twelfth ribs**. Its vertebral attachment is marked by a line running down the lateral side of the bodies of the **first and second lumbar vertebrae** on the left and the **first to third lumbar vertebrae** on the right (Fig. 5.10b). These can be represented by two vertical lines, 2 cm lateral to the first and second lumbar spines on the left and the first to third lumbar spines on the right.

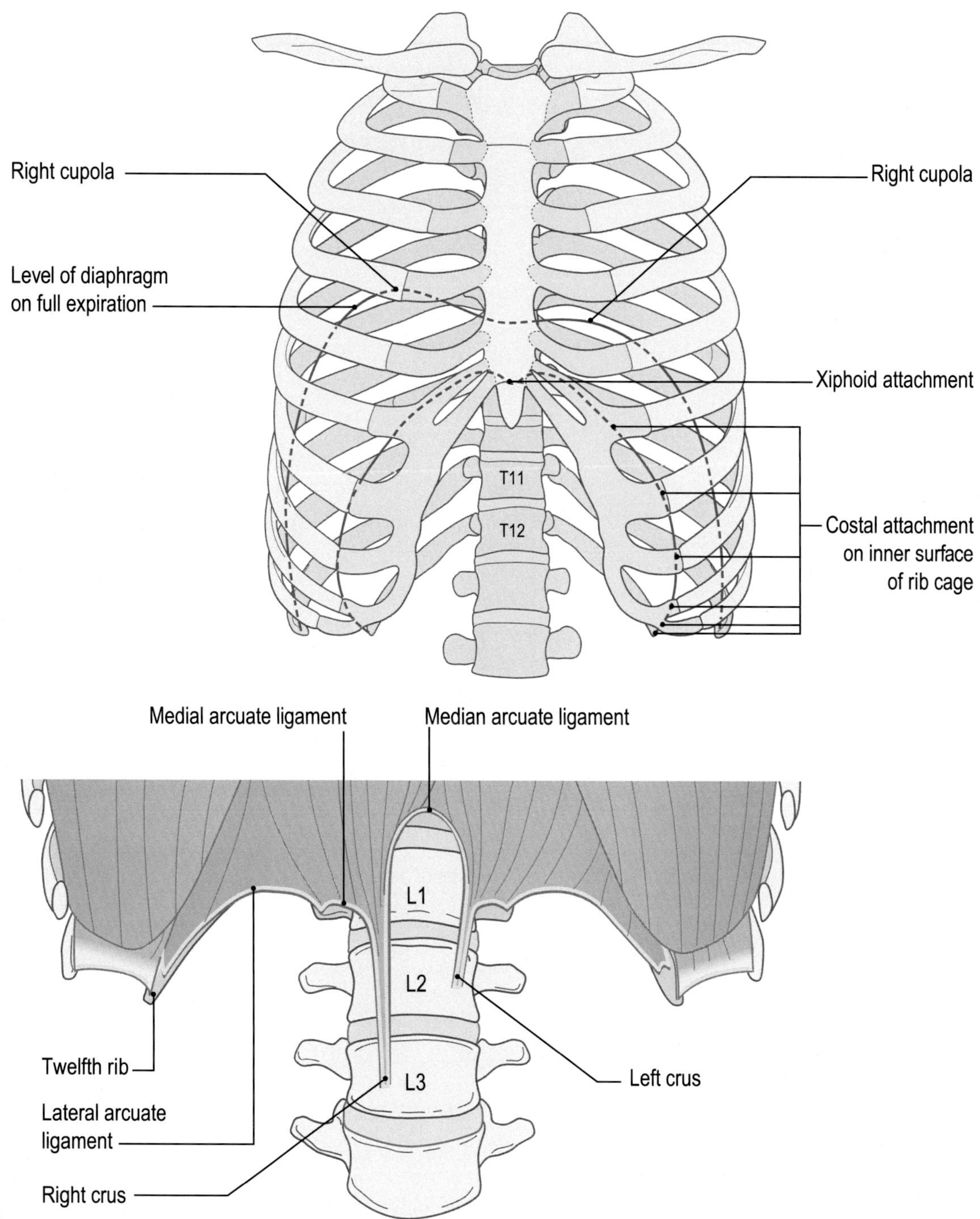

Fig. 5.10 The diaphragm. **(a)** The rib cage (anterior aspect). **(b)** Attachments of diaphragm to the vertebrae and twelfth rib (anterior aspect viewed from inside rib cage)

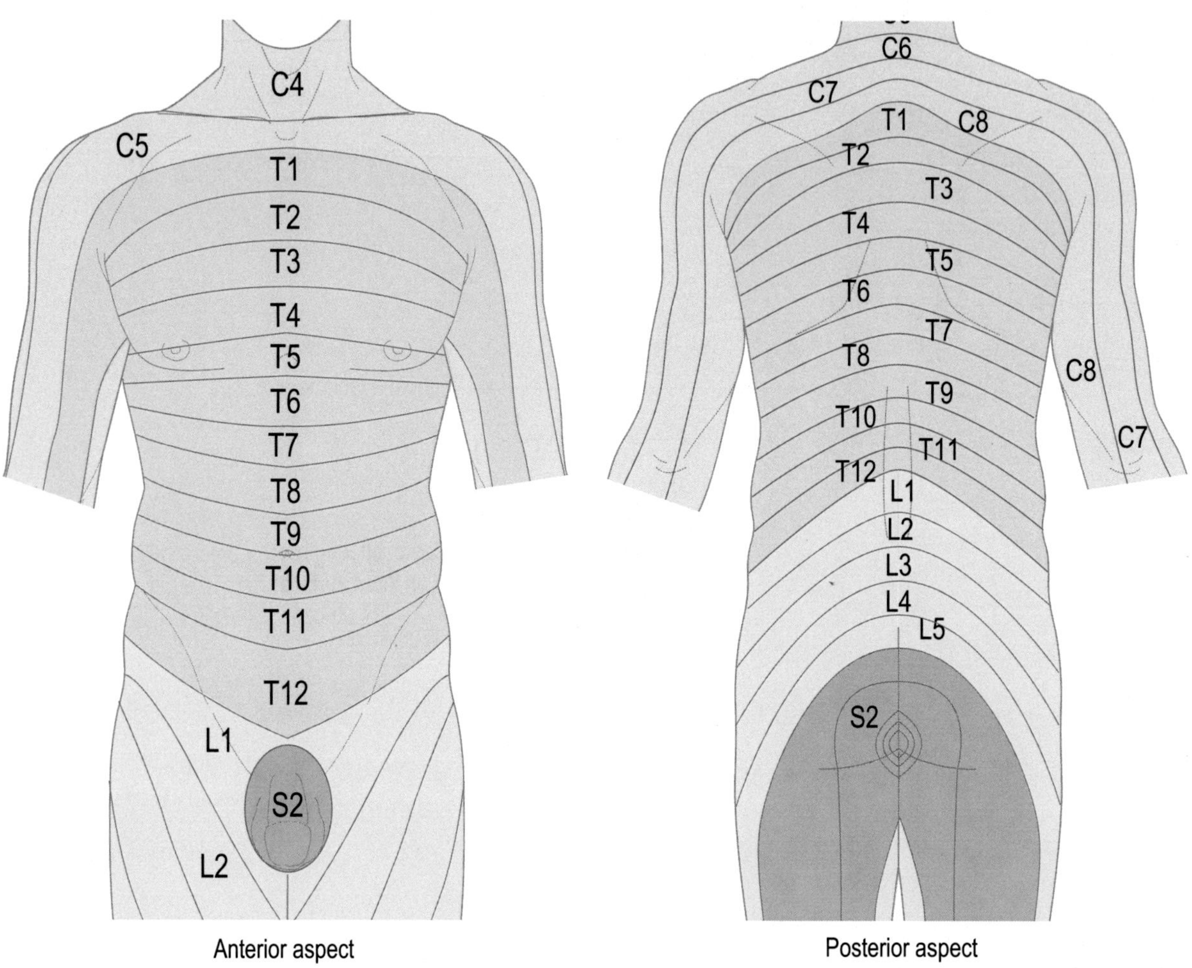

Fig. 5.11 (a, b) Cutaneous nerve supply to the thorax

NERVES (FIGS 5.11 AND 5.12)

The only nerves that become superficial in the thoracic region are those that supply the skin covering the ribs and intercostal spaces. By the time they reach the surface they are fine filaments and impossible to palpate.

Each **intercostal nerve** passes around the inside of the rib cage deep to the **internal intercostal muscle**, normally giving off a **lateral branch** at approximately the mid-axillary line. The area of skin supplied by each nerve usually includes that covering the rib above and below, including the **external intercostal muscle** passing between. Therefore there is an area of overlap of the cutaneous nerves, so that the loss of sensation from one nerve only leaves an area of paraesthesia not anaesthesia.

Below the sixth rib the nerves continue obliquely around the abdominal wall in the same direction as the ribs between which they commenced.

- **Note.** In the condition herpes zoster (shingles), the sensory component of an individual thoracic nerve is often affected by the virus and this leads to small pustules appearing over the area supplied by this particular nerve. The patient presents with a strip around the chest or abdomen following the line of its distribution (Fig. 5.11). Although this condition commonly appears to affect a single thoracic nerve it may affect any nerve in the body.

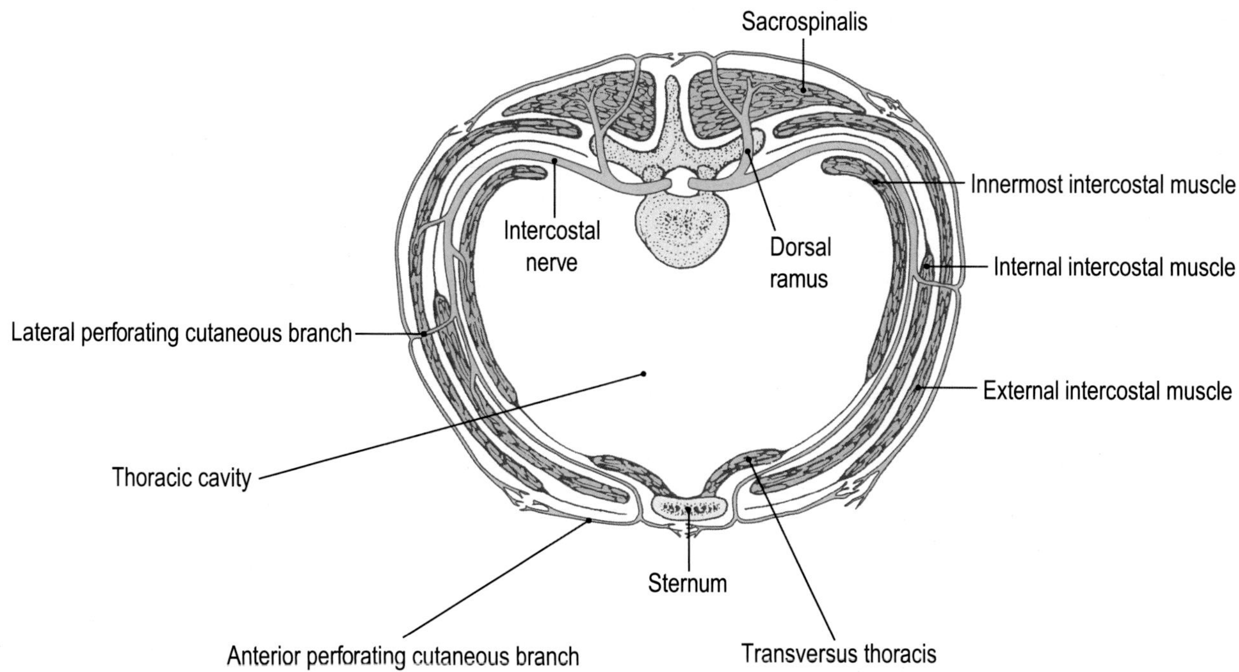

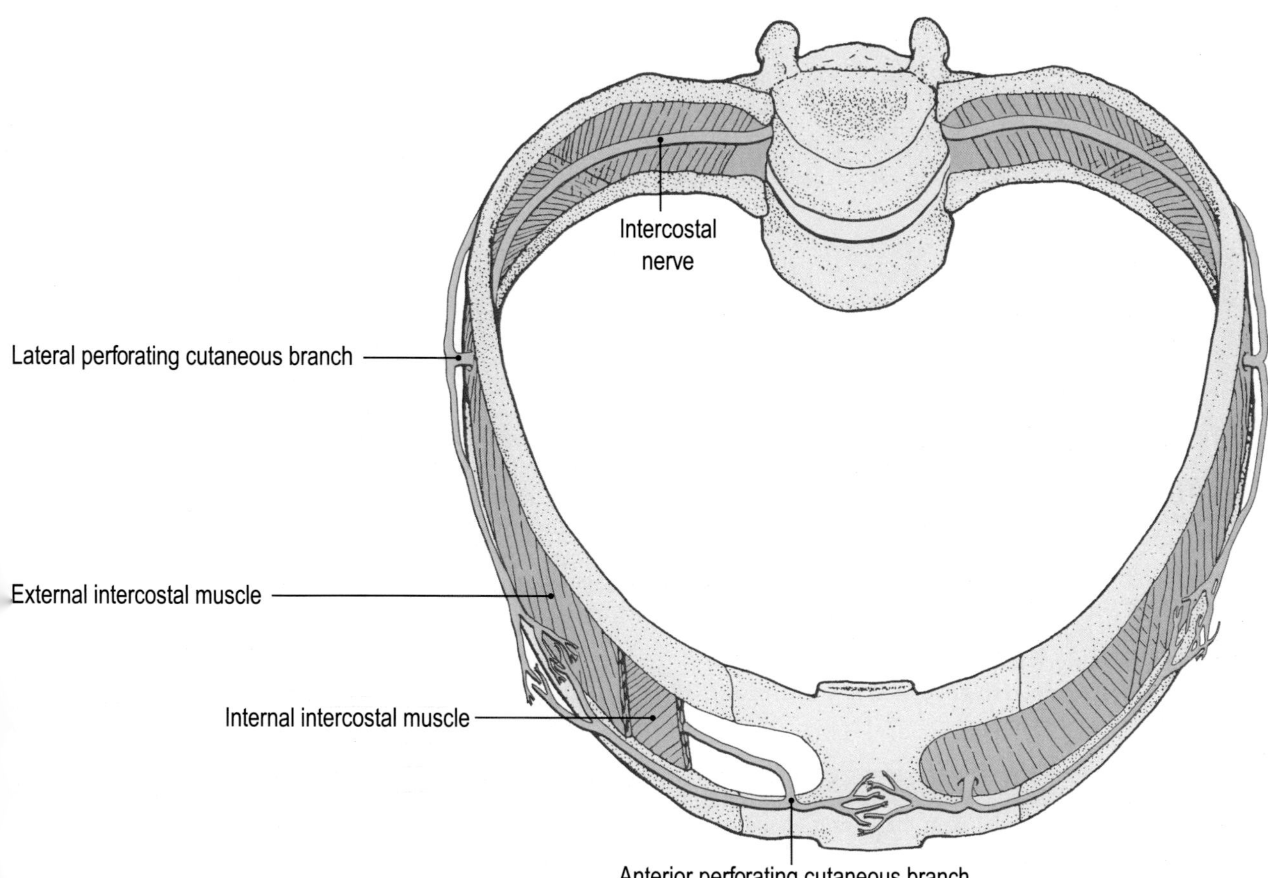

Fig. 5.12 (a, b) The course and distribution of a typical intercostal nerve

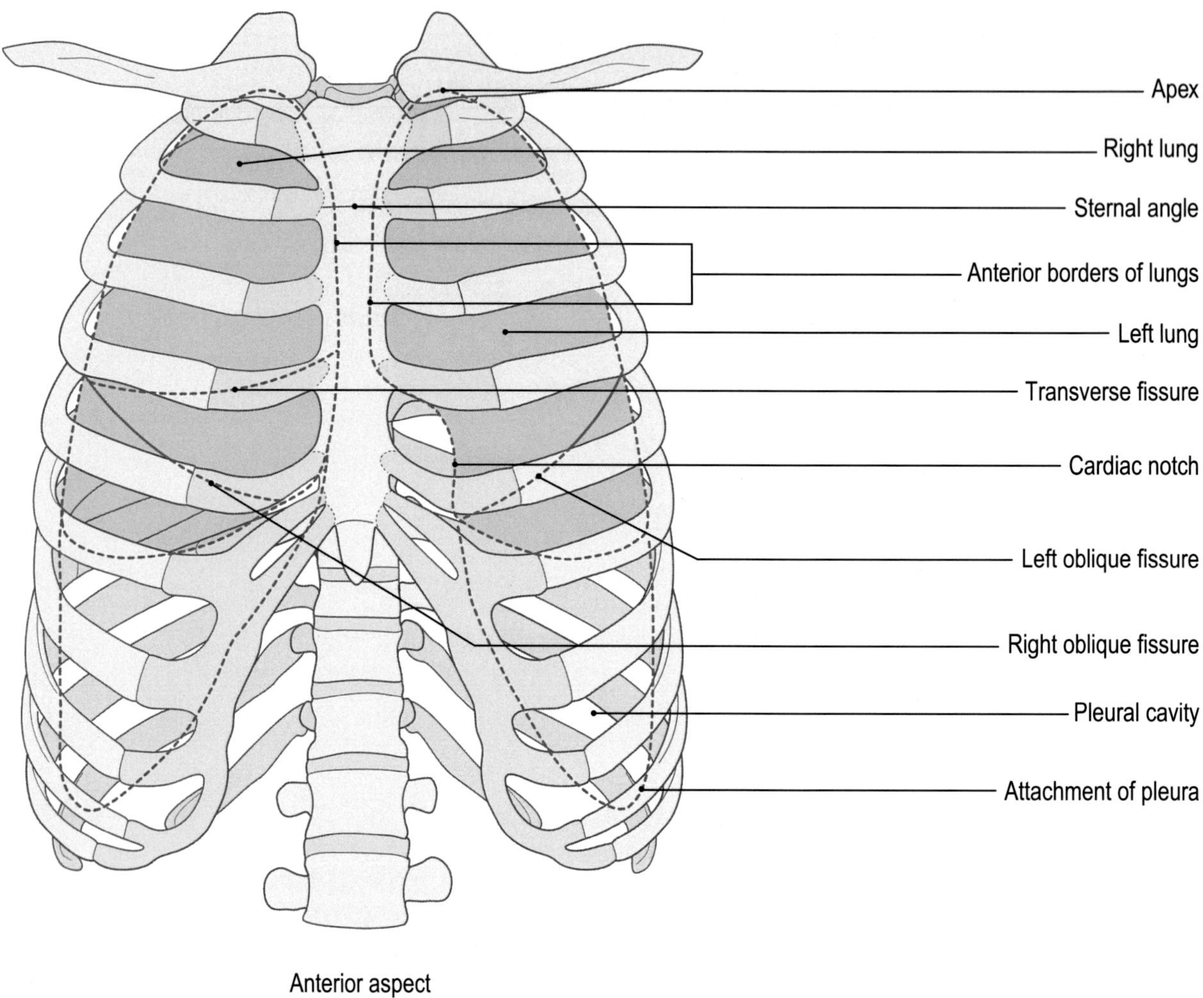

Fig. 5.13 (a) The lungs

STRUCTURES WITHIN THE THORACIC CAGE

Although the structures contained within the thoracic cage are almost totally hidden by the ribs, sternum and vertebral column, it is of some importance to be able to indicate the surface markings of the major organs and vessels. Owing to considerable movement during life, no surface marking can be constant; nevertheless, each organ stays within certain boundaries. These will be indicated by the locations given.

Palpation: surface marking

For palpation in this region, the model is in the sitting, standing or supine lying position.

The lungs (Fig. 5.13)

The **lungs** almost totally fill the thorax on either side of the heart.

The apices of the lungs. The **apex** of each lung can be palpated, on deep inspiration, as it rises behind the middle third of the clavicle. These are the only areas of the lungs which are palpable and may prove to be elusive in some individuals.

Each lung takes on the shape of the deep surface of the rib cage and intercostal muscles, being convex laterally and concave medially and inferiorly. Each lung presents **anterior**, **posterior** and **inferior borders** medially. The borders divide the lung into lateral, medial and inferior surfaces.

Palpation: surface marking

- Both lungs. The surface markings of the anterior borders of the two lungs differ slightly. Both descend from the apex of the lung, behind the sternoclavicular joint of the appropriate side, to come together behind the **sternal angle**. They then pass downwards close to the midline until the level of the fourth costal cartilage.
- The left lung. At the level of the fourth costal cartilage the left anterior border passes laterally in a C-shaped curve concave medially (the **cardiac notch**) to reach the inferior border behind the sixth costal cartilage in the mid-clavicular line.

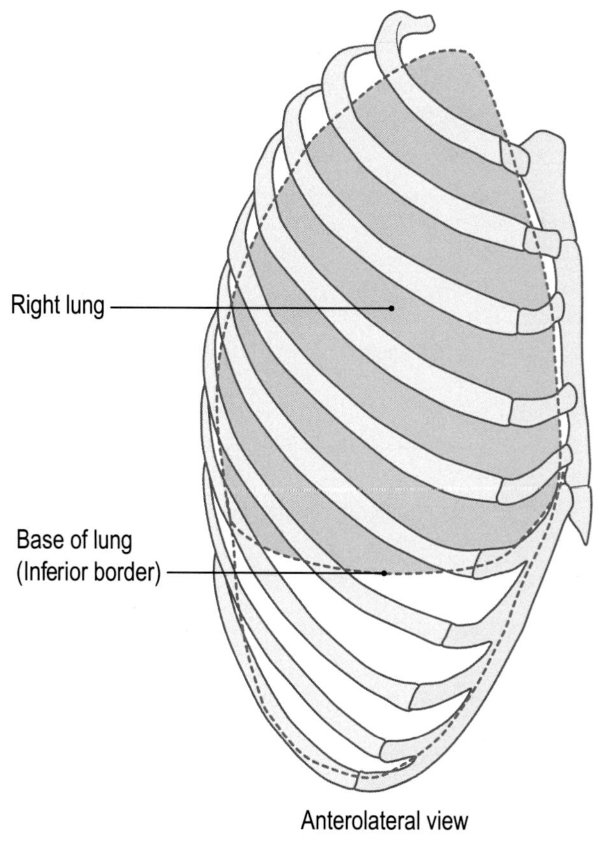

Fig. 5.13 (b) The lungs

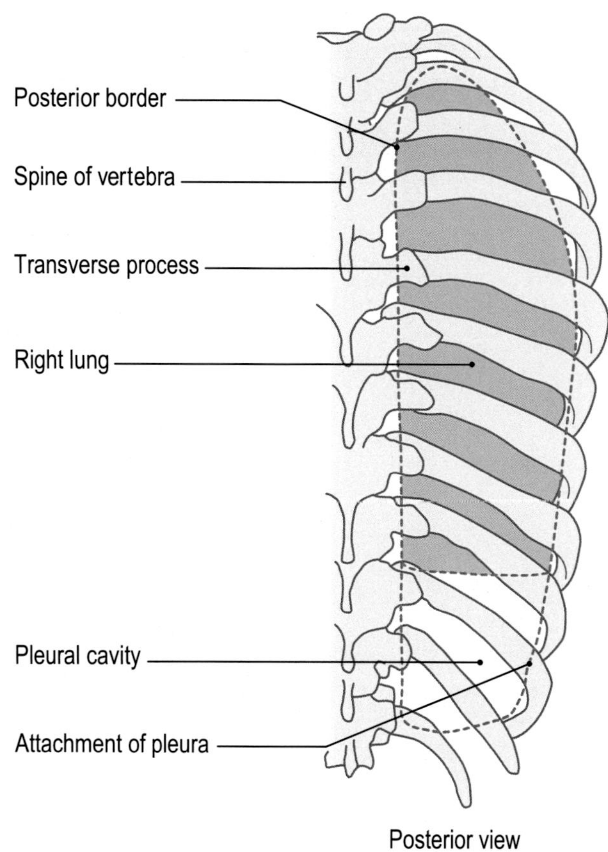

Fig. 5.13 (c) The lungs

- The right lung. The right medial border passes straight downwards, reaching the inferior border at the sixth chondrosternal joint (Fig. 5.13a).
- Both lungs. The posterior borders of both lungs pass vertically downwards in front of the necks of the ribs, approximately 2 cm either side of the **spines of the vertebrae**, from the apex of the lung to the level of the tenth rib (Fig. 5.13c).
- Both lungs. The inferior border of each lung passes almost horizontally around the chest wall, being level with the sixth costal cartilage anteriorly, crossing the eighth rib in the mid-axillary line and the tenth rib posteriorly.
- The right lung. The base of the right lung is usually slightly higher than the left owing to the presence of the liver below it (Fig. 5.13a–c).
- The pleura. Parietal pleura lines the thoracic cage of each side and covers each lung in parts. The lower part of this pleura, however, is prolonged downwards for some 5 cm below the lower border of the lung to the twelfth rib posteriorly, the tenth rib at the mid-axillary line and the sixth costal cartilage anteriorly (Fig. 5.13a–c). This is termed the **pleural cavity**.

The fissures of the lungs

Each lung is marked by an **oblique fissure**; the right lung, in addition, has a **transverse fissure**. These mark the junctions between the various lobes of each lung; the left therefore possesses two lobes, upper and lower, while the right possesses three, upper, middle and lower.

- The oblique fissures. Each oblique fissure can be marked on the chest wall by a line drawn obliquely downwards and forwards from a point 2 cm lateral to the spine of T3, crossing the mid-axillary line at the fifth rib, to reach the inferior border of the lung at the costal cartilage of the sixth rib, 7 cm from the midline (Fig. 5.13a). A good guide for the direction of this line is given by the medial border of the scapula when the arm is raised above the head.
- The transverse fissure. Only the right lung has a transverse fissure, which marks the division of the upper and middle lobes. It is indicated by a line from the fifth rib in the mid-axillary line to the fourth costal cartilage 3 cm from the median plane, essentially running along the lower border of the fourth rib.

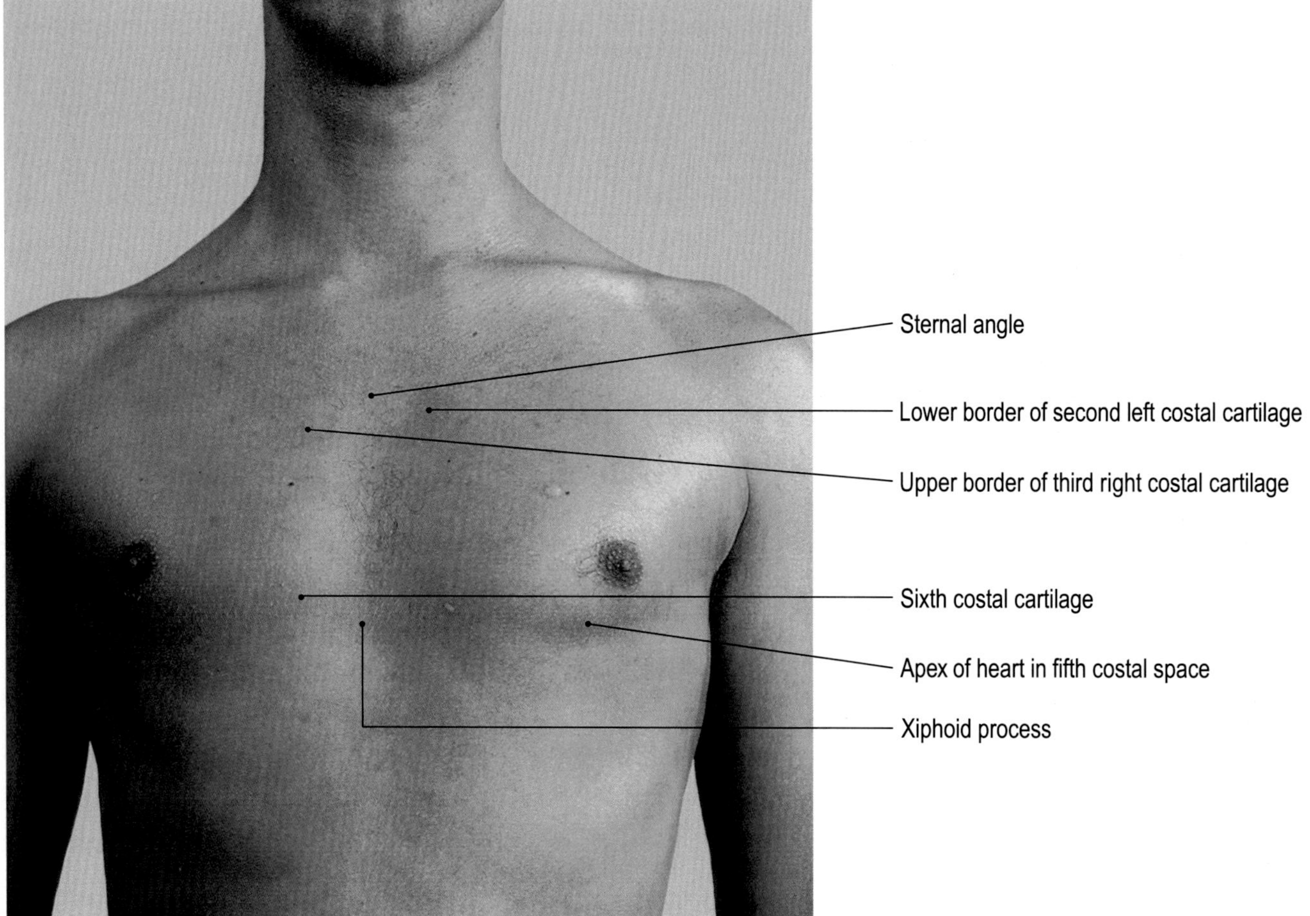

Fig. 5.14 (a) The heart (anterior aspect)

The heart (Fig. 5.14)

The heart is a roughly cone-shaped double muscular pump situated behind the sternum with its apex downward and to the left and its base upward and to the right. It is composed of specialized contractile muscular tissue (myocardium) contained within a double layer of serous pericardium, which is joined around the area where the great vessels enter the heart. The outer layer of the pericardium is attached to the central part of the upper surface of the diaphragm and the inner layer is connected to the heart musculature. The two pumps, although pumping together, are completely separate and are often referred to as the 'left heart' and the 'right heart'. Each pump is composed of an upper receiving chamber, the atrium, and a lower more powerful muscular chamber, the ventricle.

The heart is a rhythmically contractile tissue which is controlled by nerve impulses. The upper chambers or atria are completely separated from the lower ventricles by a fibrous non-conductive layer. The only communication between the two is by a bundle of specialized tissue.

Palpation: surface marking

The position of the heart within the thorax is variable, to some extent, depending on the posture adopted, so that its surface markings are slightly higher when lying compared with standing and sitting.

The projection of the heart on to the anterior surface of the chest is as follows (Figs 5.14 and 5.15).

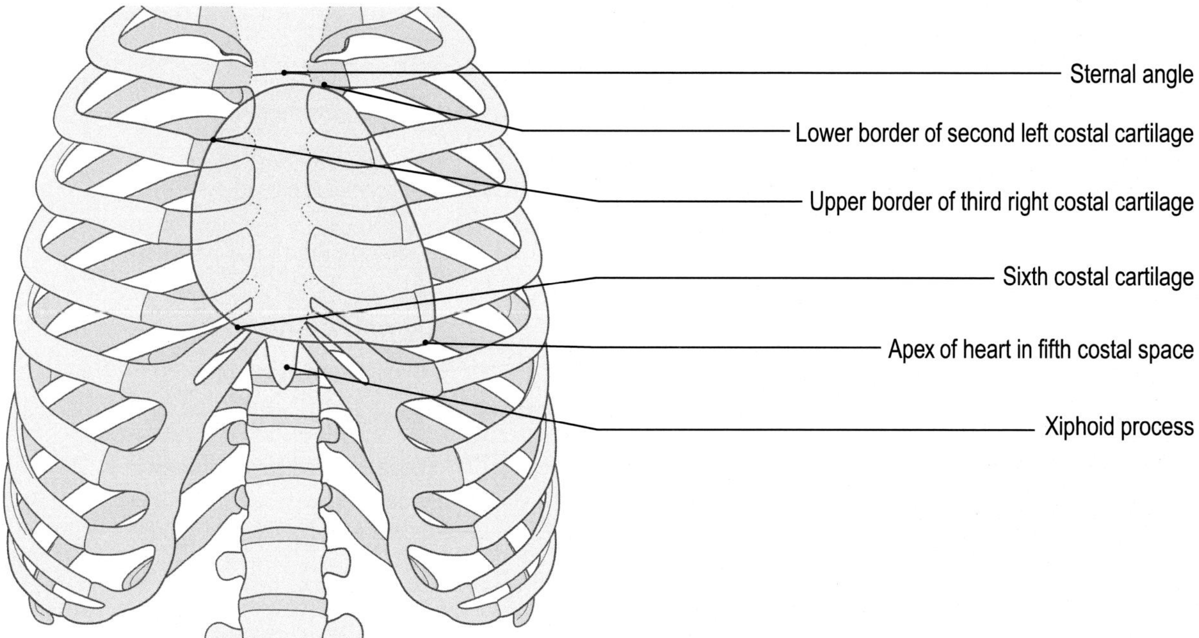

Fig. 5.14 (b) The heart (anterior aspect)

- The **apex**. The apex of the heart points downwards and to the left and can be palpated 9 cm from the midline in the fifth left intercostal space. The model is in the sitting position. Ask the model to lean slightly forward; in this position, the pulsations are enhanced because the apex of the heart is pressed against the chest wall.
- The upper limit of the heart is marked by two points, one at the **lower border of the second left costal cartilage**, 3 cm to the left of the midline, and the other at the **upper border of the third right costal cartilage**, 3 cm to the right of the midline.
- The lower right border of the heart can be indicated on the lower border of the **costal cartilage of the right sixth rib**, 3 cm from the midline. The boundaries are curved, joining the above points and making an area approximately the size of the model's clenched fist.

Function

The heart is responsible for pumping the blood around the body. The deoxygenated blood enters the right atrium from the systemic circulation through the large veins, e.g. the inferior and superior vena cavae. It is then pumped down into the right ventricle through the right atrioventricular (tricuspid) valve, which contracts, sending the blood into the pulmonary circulation and lungs, passing via the pulmonary valve.

Oxygenated blood is received into the left atrium from the lungs and is propelled down into the left ventricle through the left atrioventricular (mitral) valve. When full, the left ventricle contracts, pumping the blood through the aortic valve into the aorta and back into the systemic circulation. Equal volumes of blood must be expelled from the two ventricles at each stroke, the right into the pulmonary circulation and the left into the systemic circulation. This will maintain an equal rate of flow in both systems.

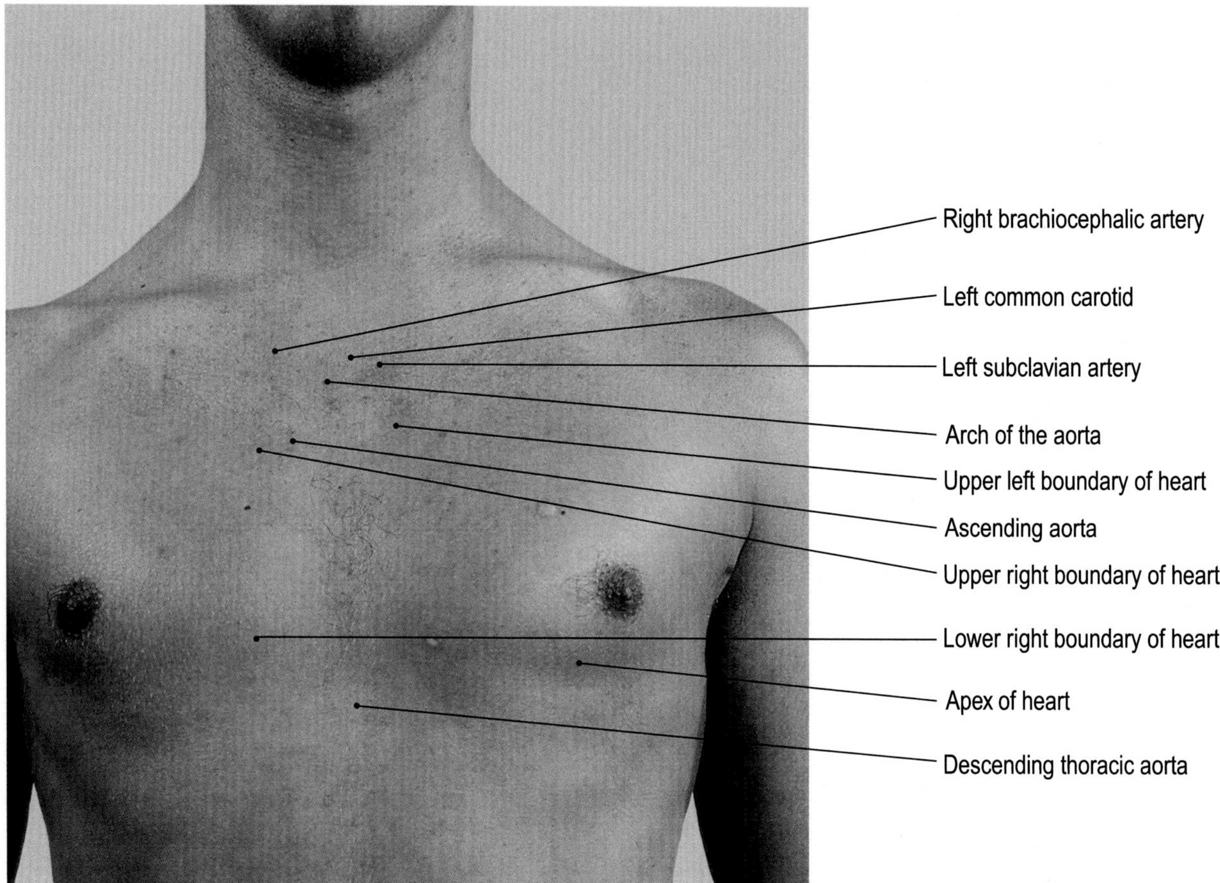

Fig. 5.15 (a) Arteries of the thorax (anterior aspect)

MAJOR ARTERIES (FIG. 5.15)

The aorta

The aorta is the main artery carrying oxygenated blood to the body. It leaves the heart at the base of the left ventricle, immediately giving off the two coronary arteries which supply the heart itself with blood. It passes upwards, slightly forwards and to the right before arching backwards and to the left over the right pulmonary vessels. It then passes inferiorly through the thorax on the left side of the vertebral bodies, behind the heart. As it does so it gradually comes to lie more in the midline, finally leaving the thorax in front, but slightly to the left of the body of T12, passing between the two crura and behind the median arcuate ligament of the diaphragm.

Palpation: surface marking

- The aortic valve. The aortic valve lies deep to the sternum adjacent to the third intercostal space. From here the ascending aorta, a band 2.5 cm wide, passes upwards and to the right as far as the second right chondrosternal joint.
- The aortic arch. The arch of the aorta then passes behind the sternal angle (and the lower part of the manubrium) over the heart, to end behind the second left costal cartilage.
- The descending aorta. This can be represented by a line extending from this point to its exit from the thorax just left of the midline and above the transpyloric plane, which is on a level with the tips of the ninth costal cartilages.

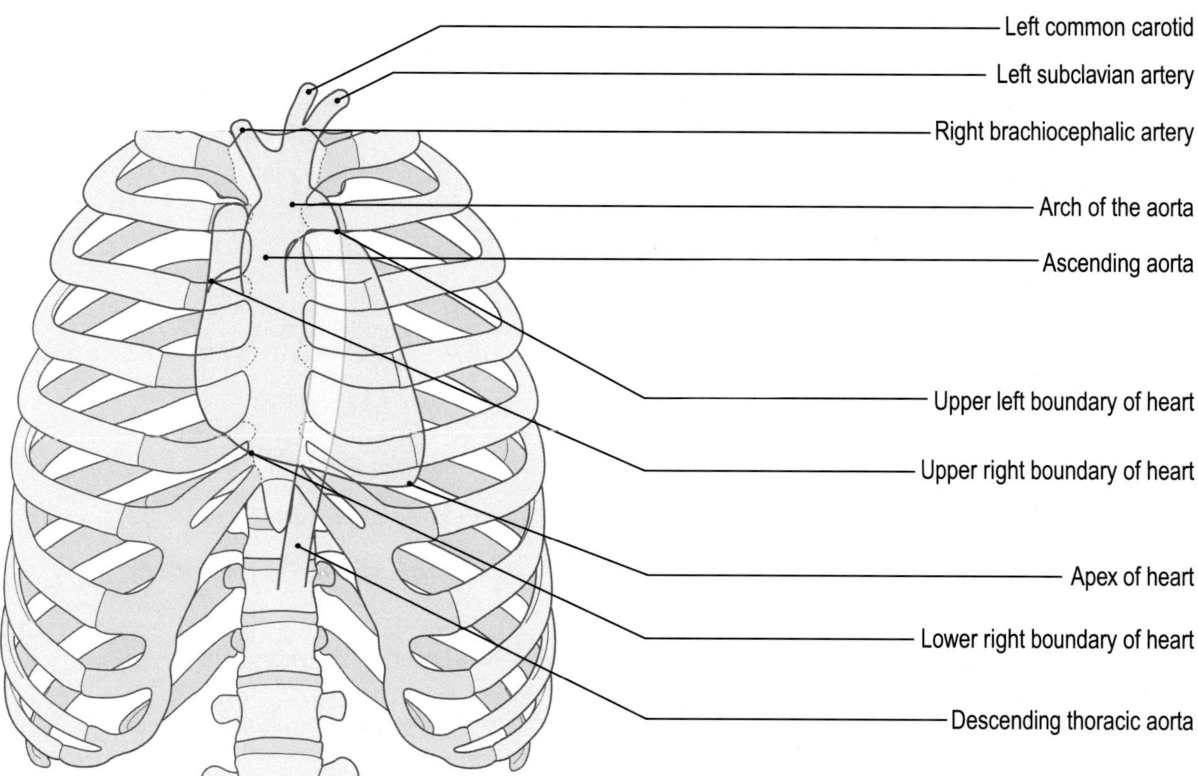

Fig. 5.15 (b) Arteries of the thorax (anterior aspect)

The brachiocephalic, left common carotid and left subclavian arteries

From the upper convexity of the arch of the aorta, three major vessels arise. The **brachiocephalic** (innominate) **artery** is anterior and to the right. Immediately behind and to the left is the **left common carotid**. Behind and to the left of the left common carotid is the left subclavian.

The brachiocephalic artery supplies oxygenated blood to the right side of the head and neck via the right common carotid artery through its internal and external branches. It also supplies blood to the right arm via the right subclavian artery. The left common carotid artery supplies blood to the left side of the head and neck via its internal and external branches. The left subclavian supplies blood to the left arm.

Palpation: surface marking

- The brachiocephalic artery. The brachiocephalic artery arises from the **arch of the aorta** behind the manubrium slightly right of centre and passes upwards, backwards and to the right for approximately 5 cm. It divides behind the right sternoclavicular joint into the right subclavian and right common carotid.
- The left common carotid artery. This artery arises from the aorta just to the left of the mid point of the manubrium and passes upwards, backwards and to the left for approximately 4 cm to enter the neck behind the left sternoclavicular joint.
- The left subclavian artery. This artery arises from the posterior part of the arch of the aorta behind the first intercostal space on the left, just lateral to the manubrium. It passes upwards and to the left for approximately 7 cm behind the first chondrosternal joint on the left to the inner borders of the left first rib. It passes over the rib en route to the left upper limb.

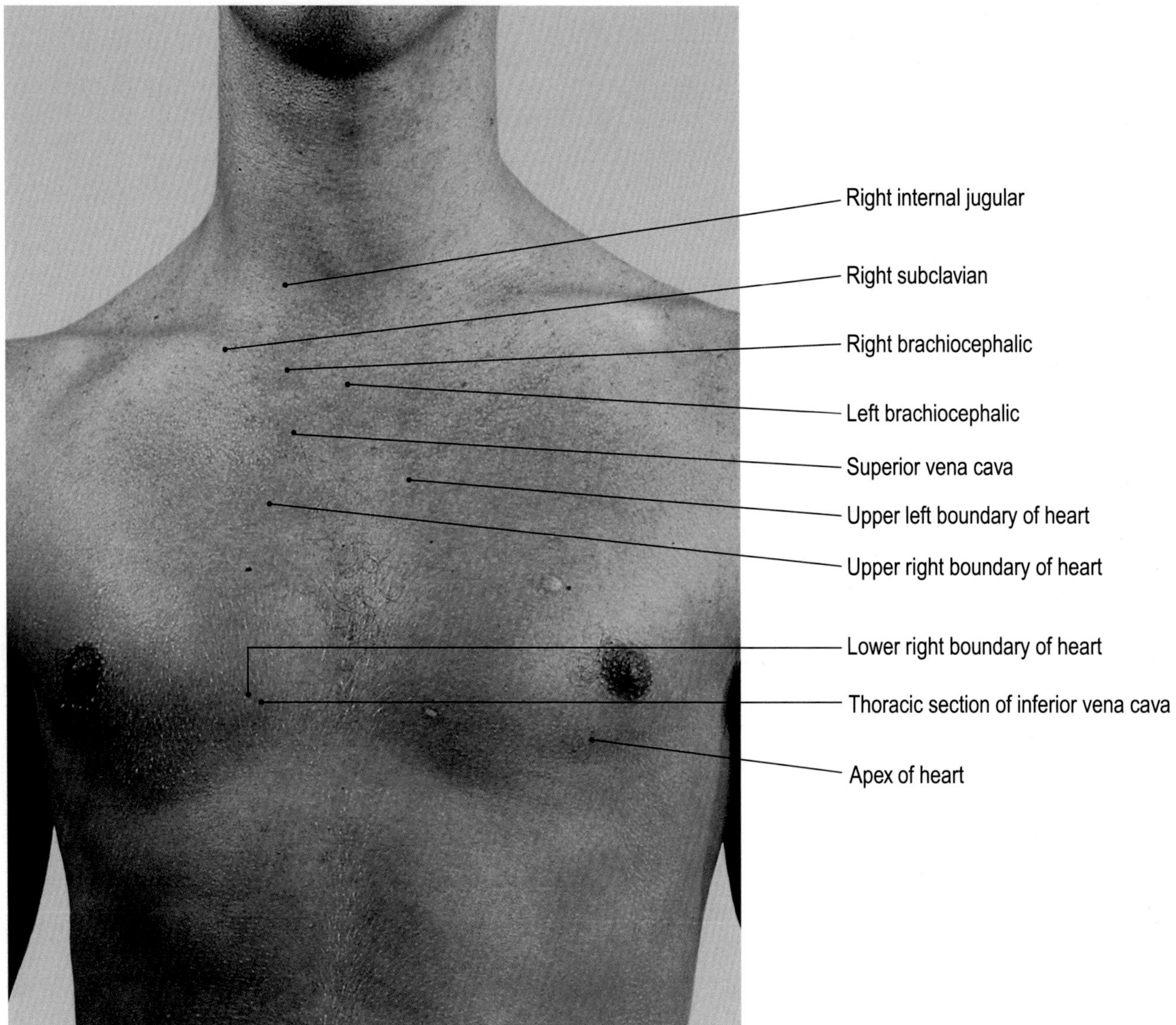

Fig. 5.16 (a) Veins of the thorax (anterior aspect)

VEINS (FIG. 5.16)

The large veins of the thorax are also situated deep within the thoracic cage and are impossible to palpate. Nevertheless, it is of some value to know where they lie in relation to palpable surface markings. It must, however, be remembered that the chest wall, the heart, diaphragm and lungs are all moveable structures and this will lead to small differences in their relationship to one another. Surface markings, therefore, will be as accurate as possible but a little leeway must be expected in this area.

Outline of the venous network

Venous blood from the head, neck, both upper limbs and upper trunk enters the left and right brachiocephalic (innominate) veins. It then passes into the **superior vena cava** and then into the upper part of the right atrium of the heart.

Venous blood from the two lower limbs and lower trunk passes, via the internal and external iliac veins, into the abdominal inferior vena cava, entering the thoracic cavity, for just a short distance, forming its **thoracic section**. This empties into the lower part of the right atrium of the heart.

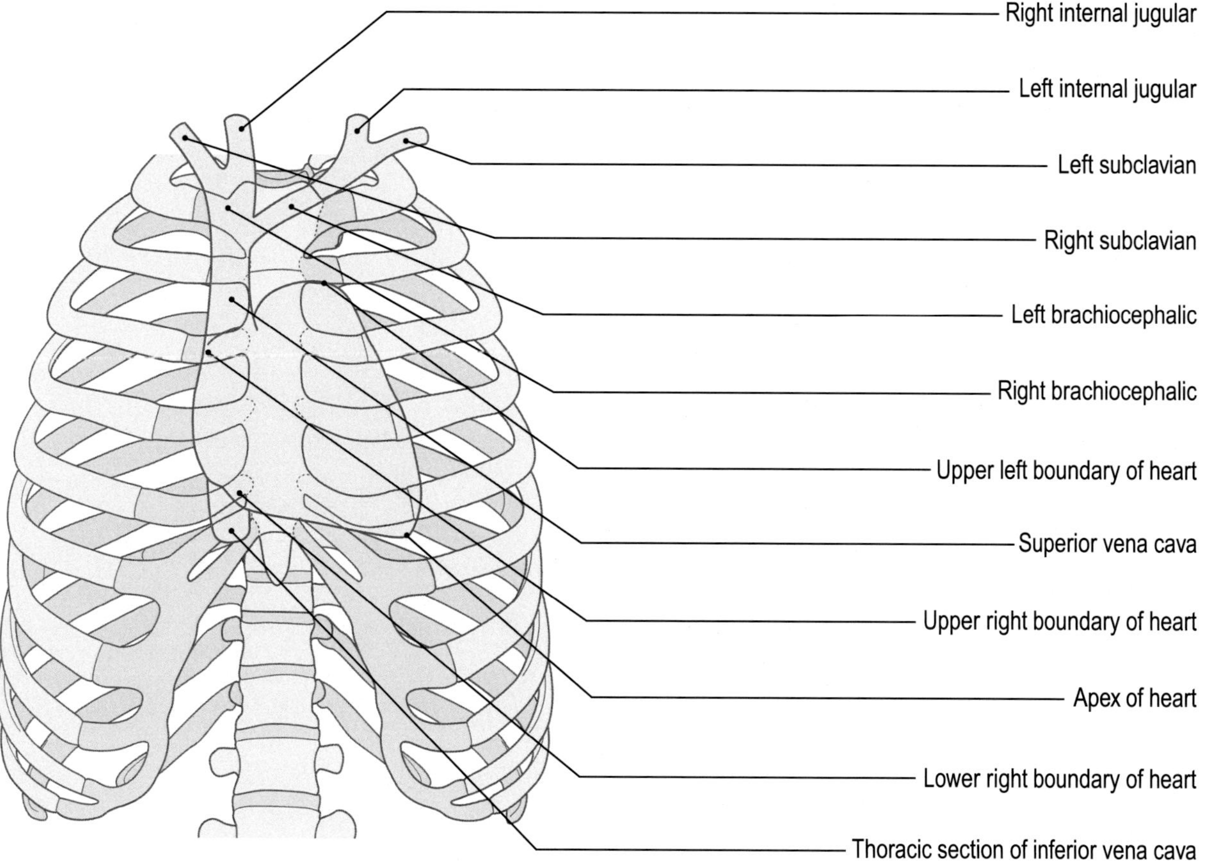

Fig. 5.16 (b) Veins of the thorax (anterior aspect)

Palpation: surface marking

- The innominate veins. In the upper thorax, the left and right brachiocephalic (innominate) veins are formed by the internal jugular and the subclavian veins of their respective sides, just lateral to each sternoclavicular joint.
- The left brachiocephalic vein. This vein passes downwards and to the right for approximately 6 cm to join the right brachiocephalic behind the sternal end of the first right costal cartilage. At this point they form the superior vena cava.
- The superior vena cava. This vein passes vertically downwards for approximately 7 cm from behind the costal cartilage of the first rib on the right to enter the right atrium behind the sternal end of the third costal cartilage.
- The inferior vena cava. In the lower thorax, the inferior vena cava enters the thoracic cavity through the upper fibrous part of the diaphragm, entering the lower part of the right atrium of the heart almost immediately, lying behind the sternal end of the sixth right costal cartilage.

The abdomen 6

Contents

At the end of this chapter you should be able to:

1. Find, recognize and name the constituent bony components of the boundaries of the abdomen, including the lower ribs, cartilages, xiphoid process, lumbar vertebrae and pelvic girdle.
2. Palpate many of the bony features, being able to relate one to another.
3. Locate, name or number the spines and transverse processes of all the lumbar vertebrae.
4. Recognize and palpate the main bony landmarks of the pelvis, sacrum and coccyx.
5. Name all the joints of the lumbar spine and pelvis, noting their active and passive range of movement.
6. Give the class and type of all the joints named.
7. Palpate the joint lines, where possible, and give their surface markings.
8. Demonstrate any accessory movements which may be possible in the joints of the lumbar spine and pelvis.
9. Locate and name the muscles which surround the abdomen.
10. Draw the shape of the muscle on the surface and give its attachments.
11. Demonstrate the actions of all of the muscles covering the abdomen.
12. Give an account of their actions and functional significance.
13. Describe the main anatomical regions of the abdomen.
14. Give the surface markings of the liver, spleen, pancreas, gall bladder, small intestine, large bowel, kidneys and bladder.
15. Demonstrate the cutaneous distribution of the nerves covering the abdomen, giving an outline of the course each takes.
16. Describe the arrangement of the main arteries in the abdomen, giving their surface markings.
17. Describe the arrangement of the main veins in the abdomen, giving their surface markings.

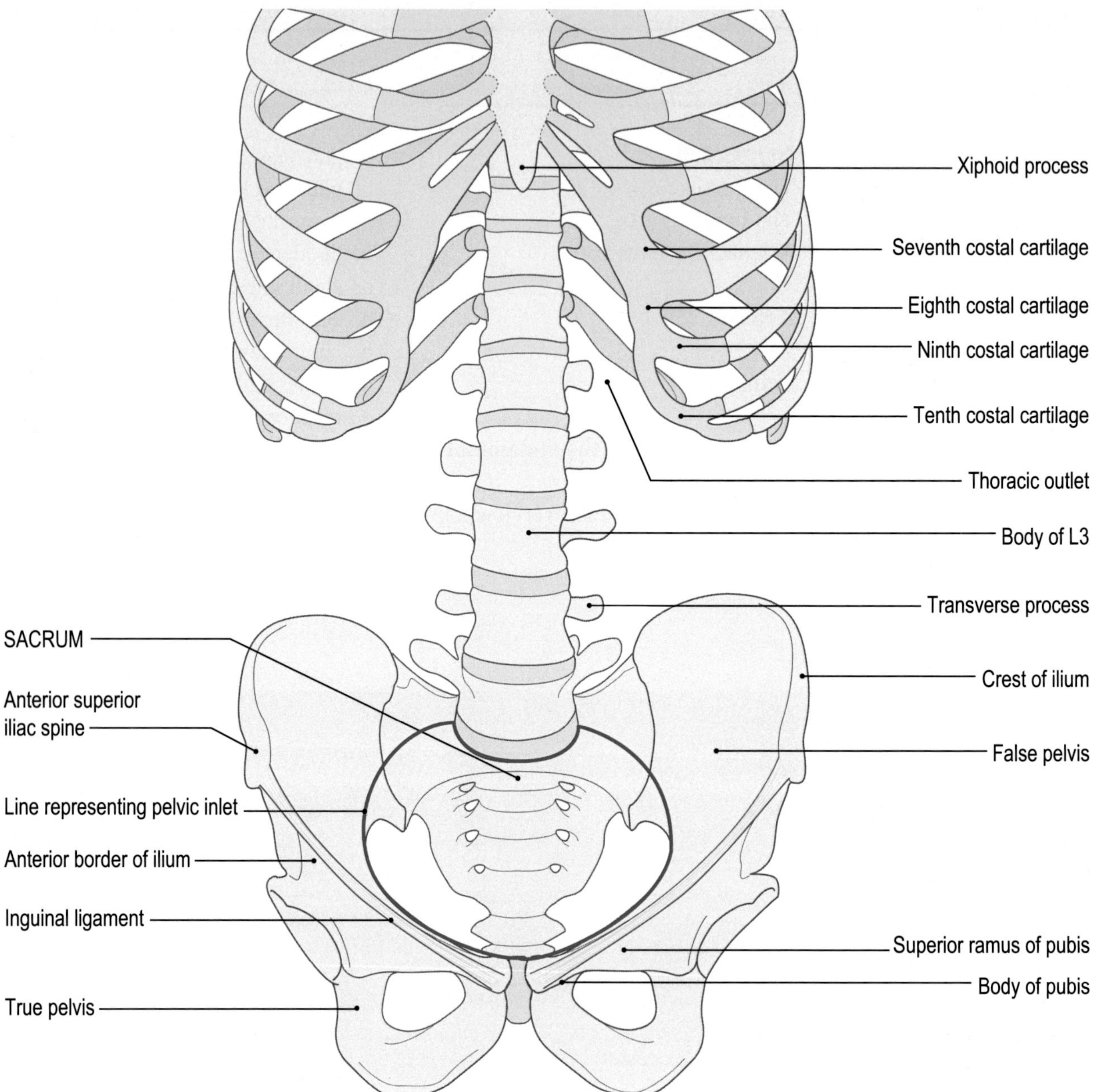

Fig. 6.1 (a) The bones surrounding the abdomen (anterior aspect)

BONES

The abdomen consists mainly of soft tissue contained with predominantly muscular walls. Its only bony features are:

- above: the **xiphoid process** at its centre in the front, the lower border of the **seventh**, **eighth**, **ninth** and **tenth costal cartilages**, the tip of the eleventh rib and the inferior border of the twelfth rib
- posteriorly: the body of the twelfth thoracic vertebra completes the ring
- below: the pelvic inlet comprises the pubis anteriorly, its **superior rami** on either side, the **anterior border** and the **crest of the ilium** and posteriorly the **base of the sacrum**
- the posterior boundary: the vertebral column.

It is, however, important to mark out these boundaries as they provide useful landmarks for some of the organs the abdomen contains.

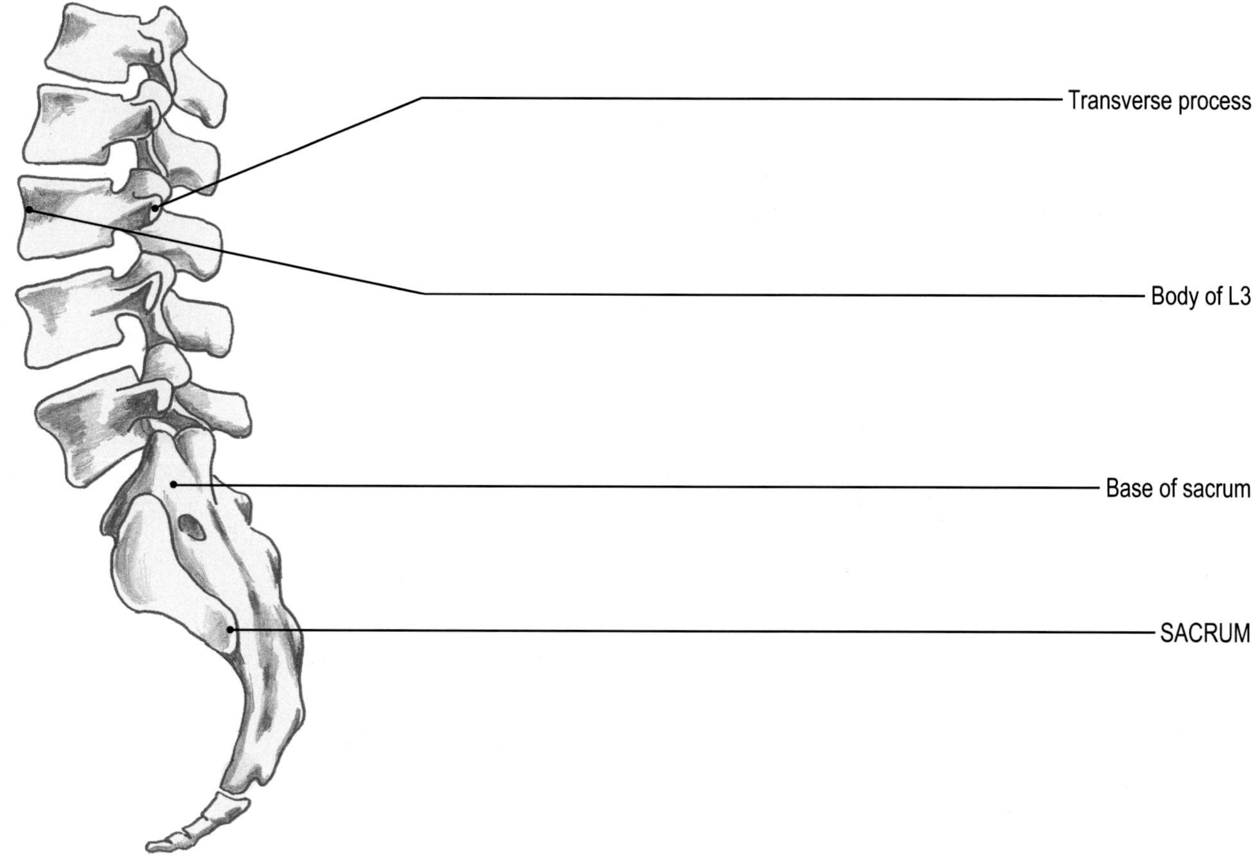

Fig. 6.1 (b) The bones surrounding the abdomen (lateral aspect, viewed from left)

The thoracic outlet (Fig. 6.1a, b)

Palpation

For palpation in this region, the model is in the supine lying position.

- The thoracic outlet. Find the xiphoid process, which is the most inferior portion of the sternum. Trace along the costal margin beyond the costal angle (the ninth costal cartilage) to its lowest extremity, which is normally the **tenth rib**. Continuing posteriorly, the eleventh rib becomes evident, with its tip just anterior to the mid-axillary line, with the tip of the twelfth rib slightly lower and just posterior. The tip of the twelfth rib normally lies on the same level as the spine of the first lumbar vertebra.

The pelvic girdle

Palpation

- The pelvic girdle. Identify the anterior superior iliac spine at the anterior extremity of the iliac crest. Trace the lateral lip of the iliac crest posteriorly, beyond the iliac tubercle to the posterior superior iliac spine and sacrum. Now, run the pads of your fingers down the central part of the abdominal wall to about 5 cm above the genitalia. The pubic tubercles become evident on either side, with each pubic crest running medially to a central space which marks the pubic symphysis. The bony ring is completed by the superior ramus of the pubis, which is difficult to palpate, and anterior border of the ilium, easily identifiable in its upper section. The inguinal ligament stretches above this region from the pubic tubercle to the anterior superior iliac spine.

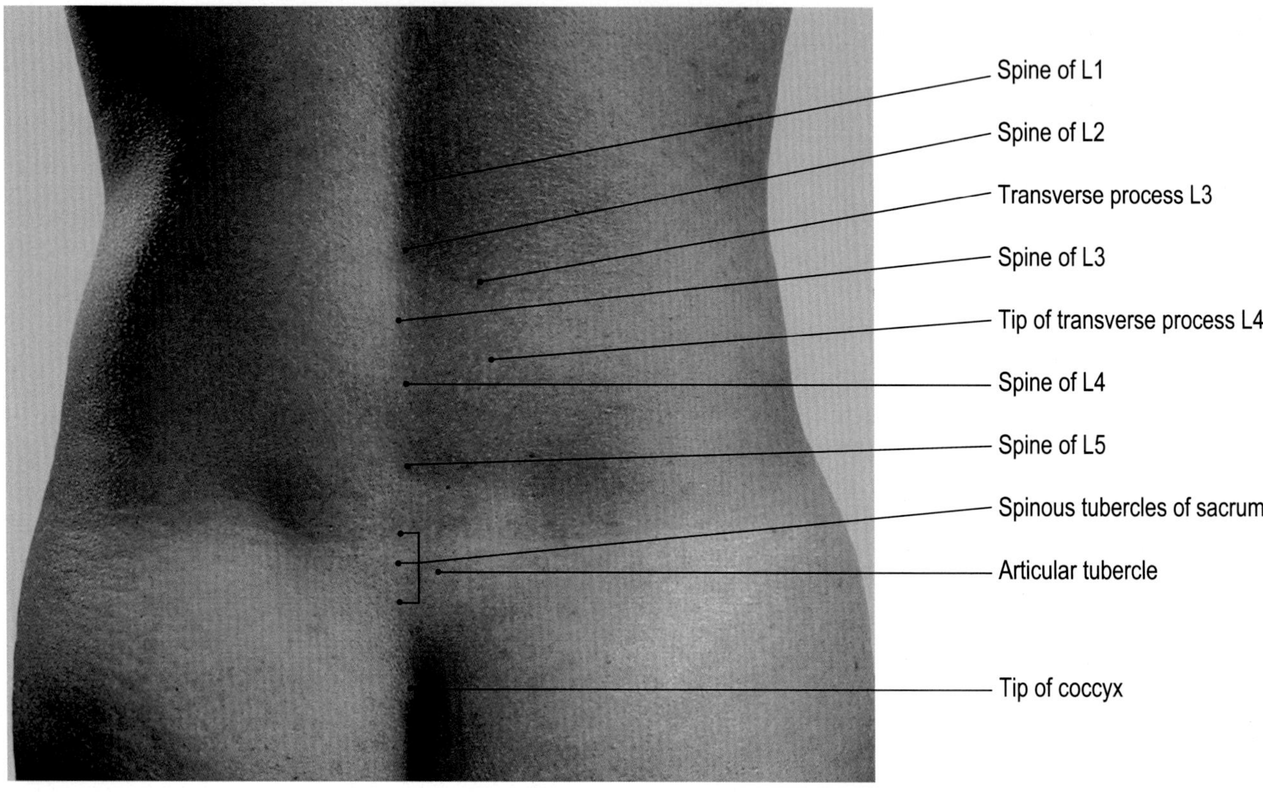

Fig. 6.1 (c) Lumbar vertebrae and sacrum (posterior aspect)

The lumbar vertebrae

There are five lumbar vertebrae, L1 being the smallest and L5 the largest. As in all other vertebrae, their bodies are anterior and their spines are posterior. Laterally, they present transverse processes, the fifth being much larger than the rest. Their upper articular processes face inwards and their lower facets face outwards, those of the fifth facing more anteriorly. There is a large neural canal in the lumbar region which is more triangular in shape.

Palpation

Posteriorly, the spines of the lumbar vertebrae project backwards and are individually identifiable.

For palpation in this region, the model is in the prone lying position.

- The lumbar vertebrae. Place a firm pillow under the abdomen which flattens the lumbar lordosis. This makes the spines of the lumbar vertebrae become more pronounced, appearing as a line of flattened edges forming a crest down the centre of the lumbar region (Fig. 6.1c, d). The spines are continuous with those of the sacrum below and the thoracic vertebrae above.
- The spines of the lumbar vertebrae. Immediately above the central part of the sacrum is a hollow, due to the spine of the fifth vertebra being shorter and the body being situated slightly more anterior than the rest. The small gaps between the spines tend to disappear when the vertebral column is flexed, owing to the tension of the supraspinous ligament.
- The transverse processes of the lumbar vertebrae. Apply deep pressure approximately 5 cm lateral to the vertebral spines beyond the bulk of the erector spinae muscles. Palpate the tips of the transverse processes.
- Note 1. The transverse process of the first lumbar vertebra is particularly easy to identify.
- Note 2. The transverse processes of the lumbar vertebrae are relatively thin compared with those of the thorax and may be tender to palpate.

The sacrum

The sacrum comprises five fused vertebrae, S1 being the largest and S5 being the smallest. The sacrum is triangular in shape with its base uppermost. Evidence of the separate vertebral bodies is still clear on the anterior surface. A line of spinous tubercles runs

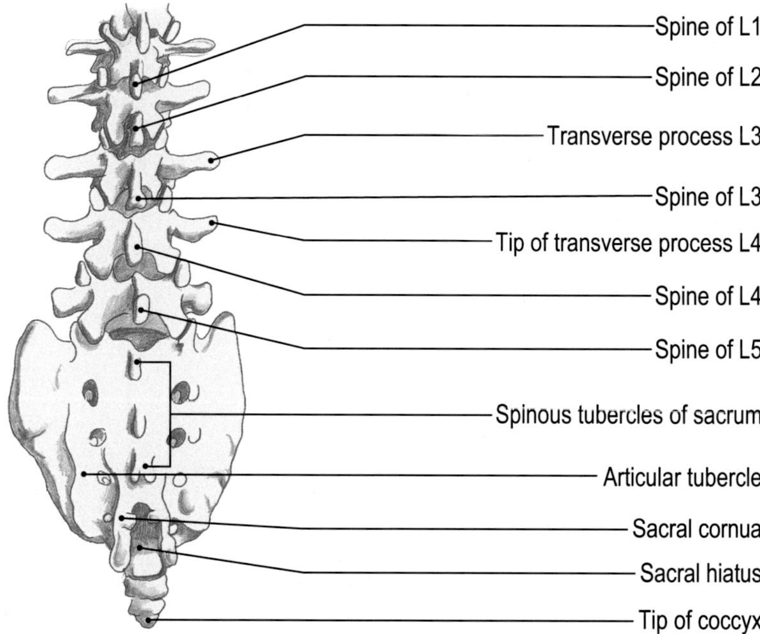

Fig. 6.1 (d) Lumbar vertebrae and sacrum (posterior aspect)

vertically down the centre of its posterior surface and it is marked on either side by **articular tubercles**. Laterally the sacrum presents large lateral masses beyond its neural foramina. The sacrum is tilted forwards above, with its lower section projecting backwards.

Palpation

- The sacrum. Identify the posterior surface of the sacrum between the posterior borders of the two ilia. Its lower section projects backwards and is easy to palpate. Its upper section (the base) lies more anterior and is more difficult to examine. Identify its central, vertical series of spinous tubercles which are in line with the lumbar spines and the coccyx. These are accompanied on either side by a row of articular tubercles which are all palpable (Fig. 6.1c, d).

The coccyx

The **coccyx** comprises three or four rudimentary vertebrae normally fused into one bone, the uppermost being the largest and the lowest being a very small tubercle of bone. Normally it is tilted, with its inferior tip pointing downwards and forwards.

Palpation

- **Note.** As the coccyx varies considerably in size and shape it may prove a little difficult to palpate. Several alternative methods can be employed:
  - Trace the spinous processes which run down the centre of the posterior surface of the sacrum to approximately 2.5 cm below the level of the posterior inferior iliac spines. At this point, palpate the pointed lower end of the coccyx.
  - Gently run your fingers up the cleft between the two gluteus maximus muscles until the hard bony tip of the coccyx is found.
  - Draw an equilateral triangle, with its base on the two posterior inferior iliac spines of the ilium and its apex downwards. This point should be on the tip of the coccyx.
- **Note.** In many subjects the coccyx is angled forwards and the finger must be pressed deep into the cleft to identify the shape. Care must be taken as pressure on the bone can cause pain, particularly if the joints between it and the sacrum have been damaged at any time.

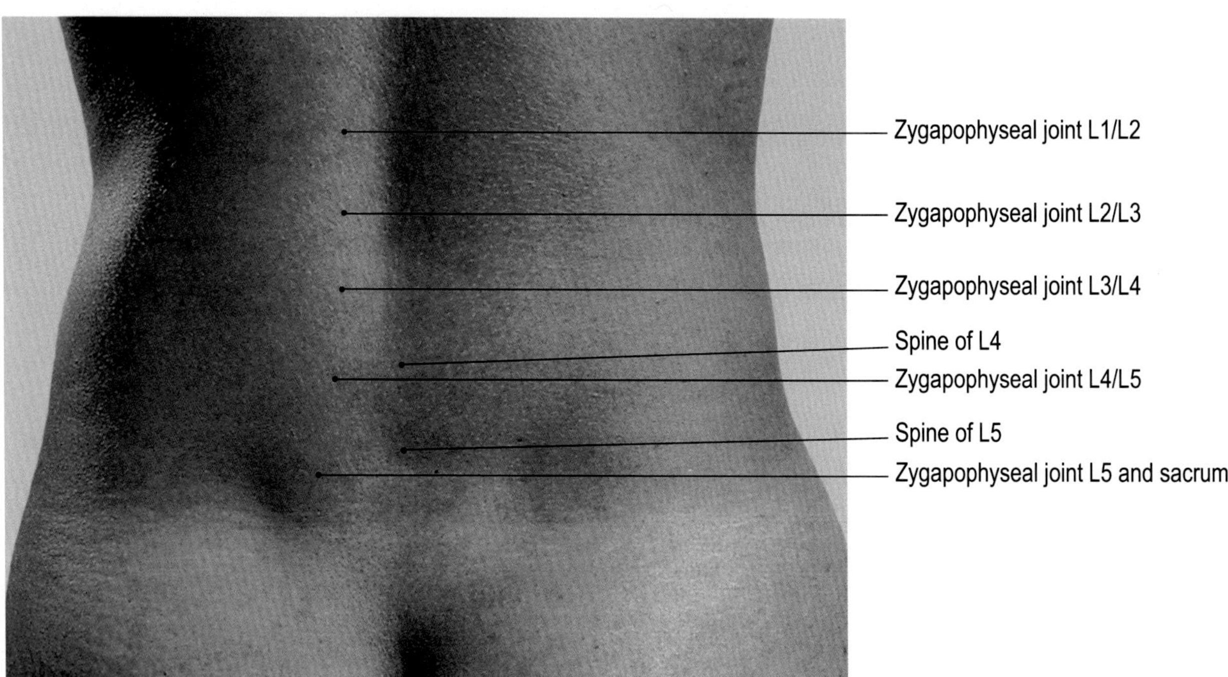

Fig. 6.2 (a) Zygapophyseal joints of lumbar spine (posterior view)

JOINTS

The lumbar spine (Fig. 6.2)

Palpation

The **zygapophyseal joints** are the most superficial in the lumbar region. They are nevertheless covered by thick, strong muscle, making the task of palpation extremely difficult.

For palpation in this region, the model is in the prone lying position.

- The zygapophyseal joints. Press your fingers between the sides of the **vertebral spines** and the parallel-running column of muscle (sacrospinalis). Identify the sides of each of the spines. In some subjects, it may also be possible to palpate the **laminae** of the vertebra. Each is a little higher than its corresponding spine, being almost totally hidden by the thick muscle layer.
- Posterior-anterior pressure. Using the tips of your thumbs, apply deep pressure through the muscle. This exerts pressure on the posterior aspect of the zygapophyseal joints, which lie 1 cm lateral and slightly lower than the vertebral spine. With great care and precision, this pressure can be targeted on to the upper articular pillar of the vertebra below by moving lateral to the joint, or on to the lower articular pillar of the vertebra above by moving just medial to the joint.
- **Note.** The lower facets of the vertebrae are convex anteriorly and fit snugly into the concave anterior edge of the upper facets of the vertebra below. Thus, anterior pressure on the lower vertebra causes its articular facet to glide forwards, slightly parting its anterior segments, whereas pressure on the upper vertebra pushes the lower facet into the socket, preventing any further movement (Fig. 6.2d, e).

Accessory movements

Palpation

- Distraction. Distraction (traction) of the joints of the lumbar spine is the only true accessory movement possible. All other movements of gliding, gapping and compression of the

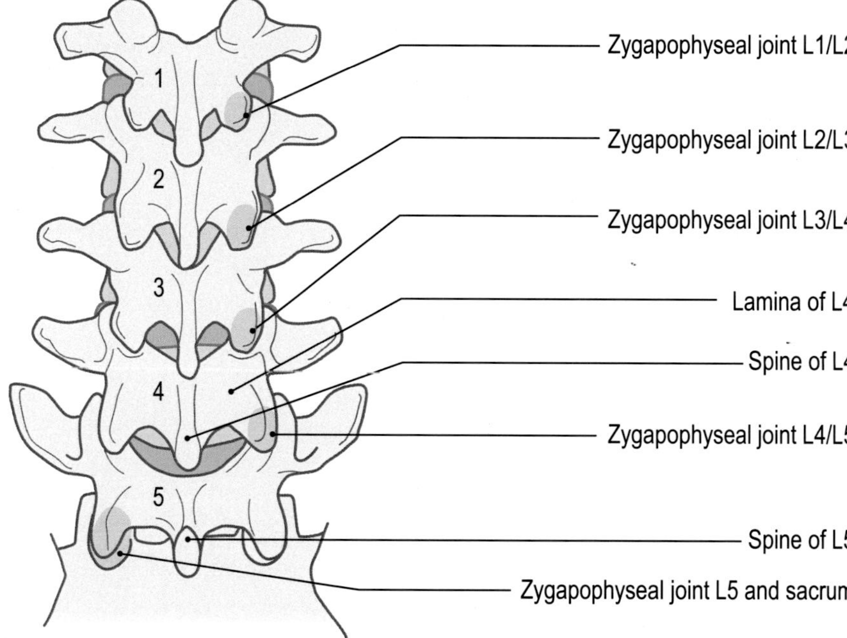

Fig. 6.2 (b) Zygapophyseal joints of lumbar spine (posterior view)

zygapophyseal joints, together with twisting and compression of the intervertebral discs, occur in the area during normal lumbar activities.

- Note 1. Traction can be applied to this area in many ways, either manually or mechanically. The lumbar column, however, can be placed in many different positions to achieve the therapeutic result required.
- Note 2. Extension of the lumbar spine tends to create a 'close-packed' position for the individual joints as the articular surfaces come into full contact and ligaments become taut. This, therefore, is not a desirable position in which to achieve traction. All other positions towards flexion allow space for the joint surfaces to part or glide. In full flexion, however, the ligaments again become taut, preventing the required movements. Traction in full flexion is almost impossible to apply.
- Note 3. The optimum position in which to apply traction is midway between extension and flexion.
- Note 4. Simple traction can be applied to the lumbar spine by applying a distraction force to either the pelvis or the lower limbs, with the subject lying either supine or prone. It is preferable to place a pillow under the abdomen in the latter position to prevent extension.
- Note 5. Manual traction can also be applied with the model sitting or standing. This is achieved by raising the upper trunk and allowing the pelvis and lower limbs to act as the traction force.
- Note 6. Mechanical traction can be applied in many positions of the lumbar spine, avoiding full extension and full flexion for the same reasons as outlined above. It may be applied continuously or intermittently over a set period of time. These therapeutic techniques are complex and need skill and knowledge of procedures and precautions. For further study, reference should be made to literature dedicated to this subject.

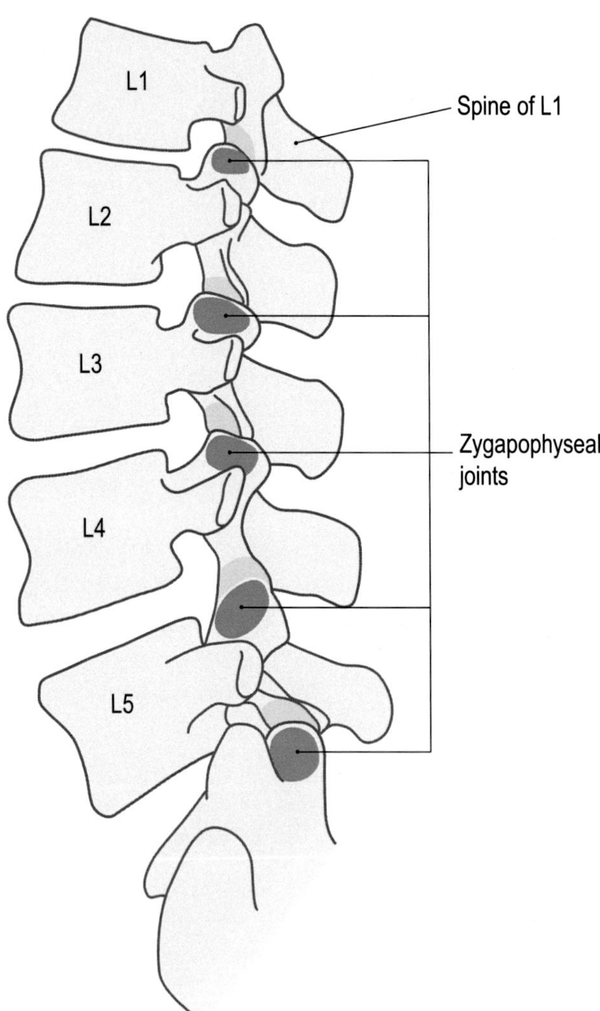

Fig. 6.2 (c) Zygapophyseal joints of the lumbar spine (lateral aspect from left)

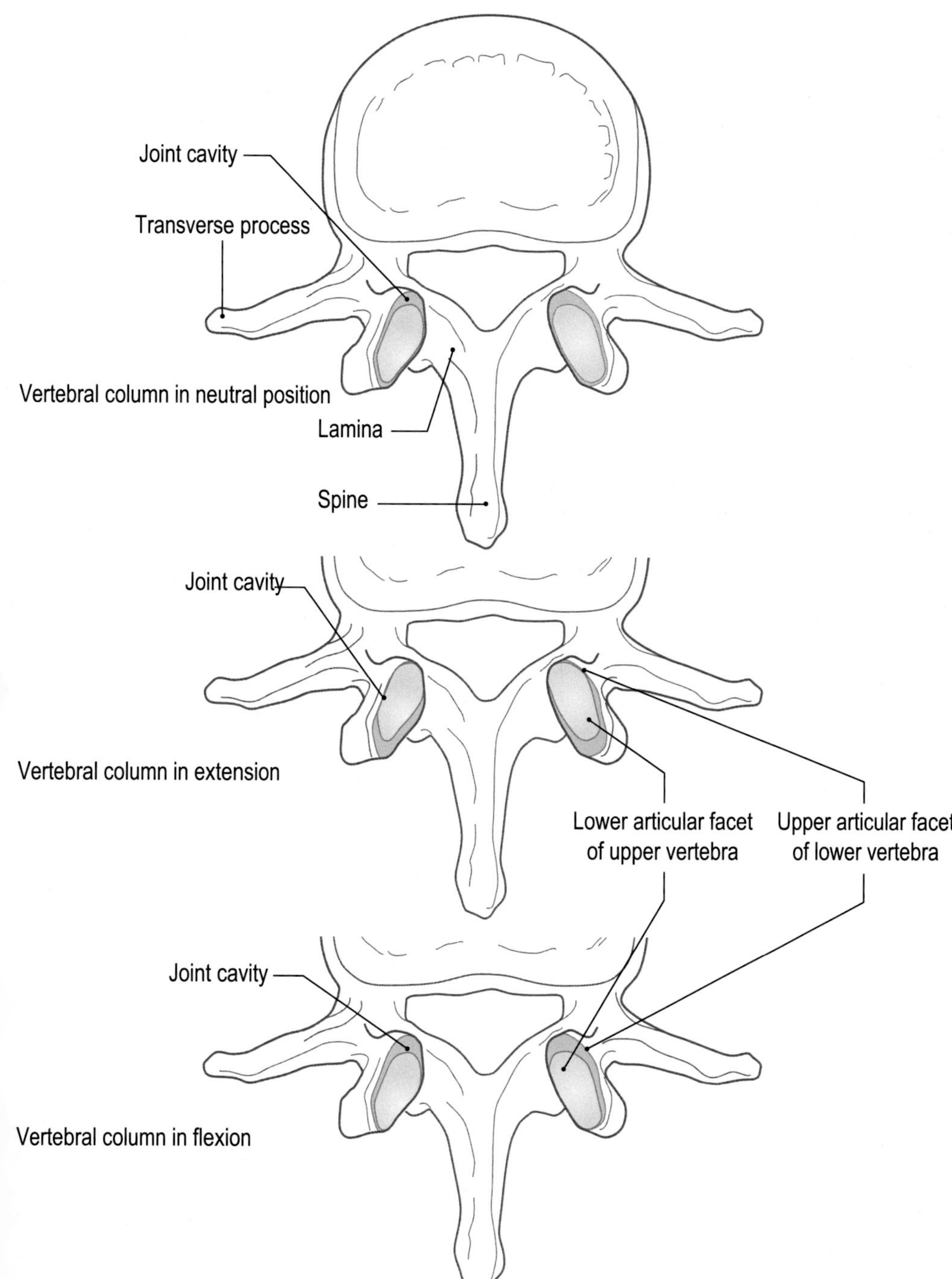

Fig. 6.2 (d)–(f) Zygapophyseal joints of lumbar section of vertebral column (viewed from above)

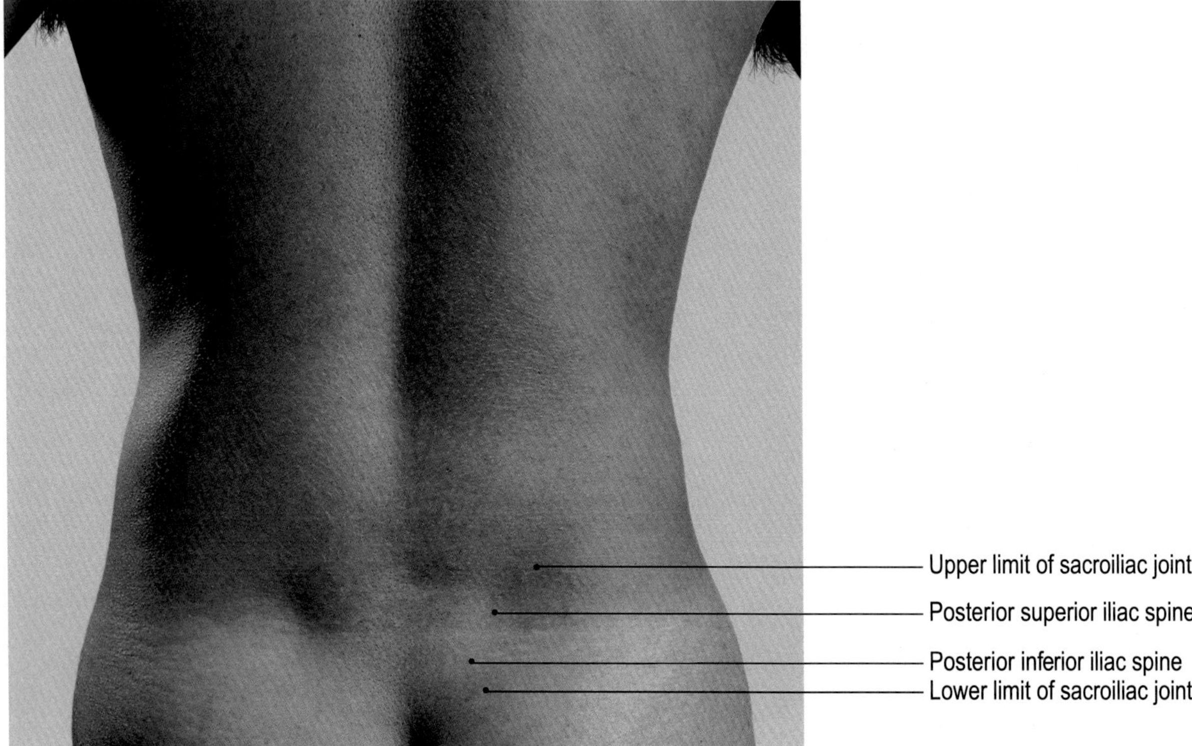

Fig. 6.3 (a) Sacroiliac joint (posterior aspect)

The pelvis (Figs 6.3 and 6.4)

Posteriorly, the sacrum articulates on either side with the ilium (innominate) bone at the sacroiliac joints (also discussed in Chapter 3). Anteriorly, the two pubic bodies articulate with each other at the pubic symphysis. The former is a very stable plane synovial joint supported by powerful interosseous and accessory ligaments. The latter is also stable, but is a secondary cartilaginous joint containing a modified disc of fibrocartilage. The sacroiliac joints allow a small degree of rotation of the sacrum, with respect to the innominate bones, about an axis through its interosseous ligament. Movement is more noticeable in young females, particularly during pregnancy and childbirth, reducing considerably after the third decade. In males, movement is negligible and virtually nil after the second decade.

The pubic symphysis allows a slight rocking and twisting movement which accompanies any movements occurring at the sacroiliac joints.

The sacroiliac joint

Palpation: surface marking

For palpation in this region, the model is in the prone lying position.

- The sacroiliac joint. Place a pillow under the abdomen. Now identify the posterior superior iliac spine. The sacroiliac joint can be identified, lying 1 cm lateral and 1 cm anterior to this spine. It lies on an oblique line which extends above and below for a further 2 cm. The joint can also be marked by an oblique line passing downwards and medially from a point 5 cm lateral to the spine of the fifth lumbar vertebra to a point just lateral to the posterior inferior iliac spine (Fig. 6.3b). It is impossible to palpate this joint.

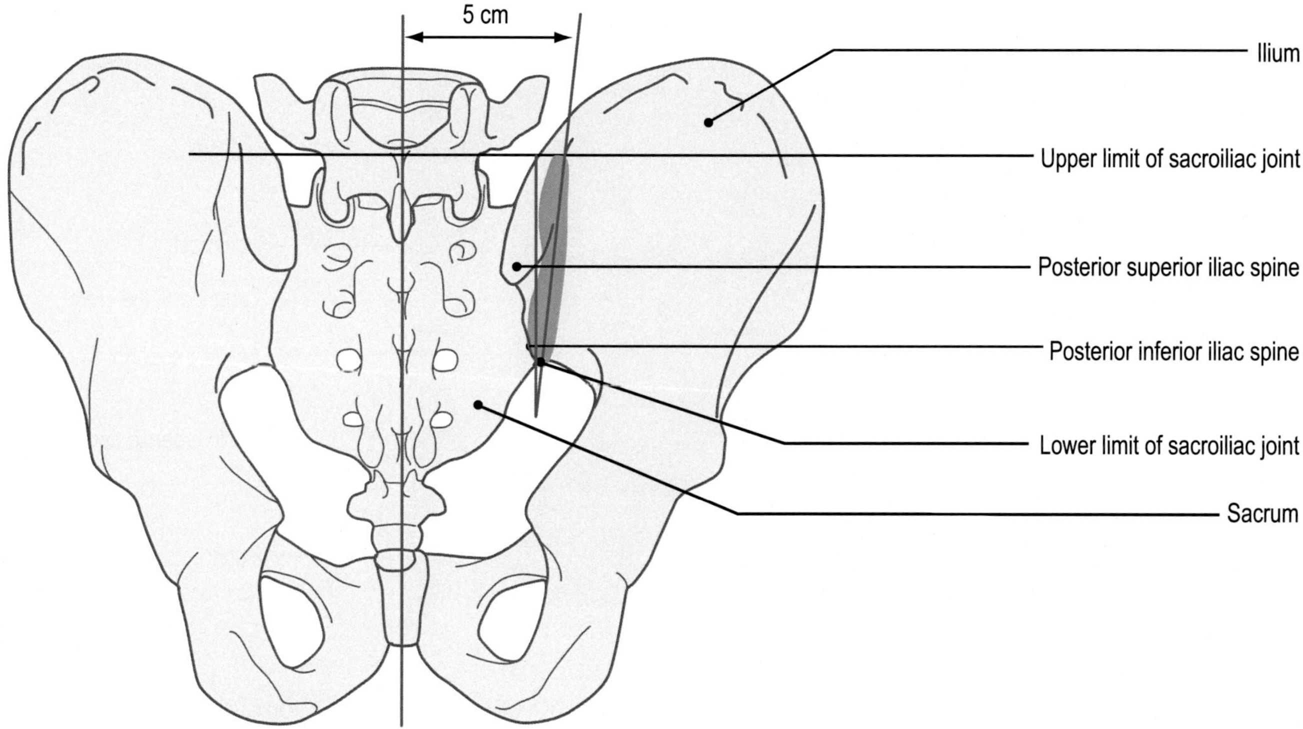

Fig. 6.3 (b) Sacroiliac joint (posterior aspect)

Accessory movements

Palpation

Little movement occurs at the sacroiliac joint. There is more movement in young females and less in middle-aged and elderly males (see above).

- Rocking. Rocking the sacrum around a frontal axis can be achieved. Place the heel of one hand over the apex and the heel of your other hand over the base of the sacrum. Now apply alternate pressure to the apex and base. This produces a slight rocking movement of the sacrum between the two innominate bones.
- Localization of movement. This movement can be increased locally on one side. Place one hand on the apex of the sacrum and the other on the posterior aspect of the crest of the ilium. The opposite movement can be produced if you place one hand on the base of the sacrum and the other on the ischial tuberosity.
- Note. The pressure applied to these two areas must be downwards and towards each other, in the same direction as the movement of each component. It is a difficult movement to obtain and some skill and practice are necessary before it can be achieved.
- Gapping. The model is in the supine lying position. In this position, the posterior aspect of the sacroiliac joint can normally be gapped or at least stressed by using the leverage of the femur. Flex the model's opposite knee and hip and roll the limb and pelvis towards you. When the pelvis is rotated approximately 45°, apply a downward and medial pressure towards the opposite hip joint to the femoral condyles.
- Note. This technique is used in the examination and treatment of sacroiliac problems and is covered in greater detail in the manipulation literature.

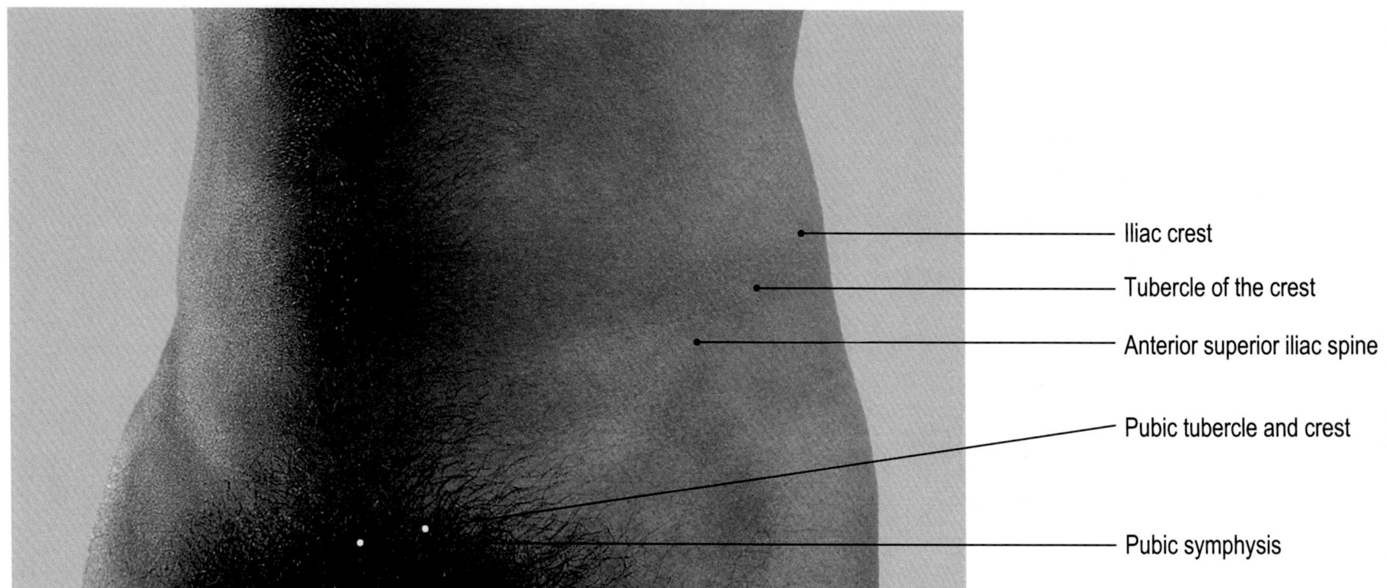

Fig. 6.4 (a) The pelvis (anterior view)

The pubic symphysis

This joint is situated centrally at the lower aspect of the abdomen between the two pubic bones and just above the external genitalia.

Palpation

For palpation in this region, the model is in the supine lying position.

- The pubic symphysis. Locate the pubic tubercles on the upper border of the body of the pubis on either side of the midline. Note that there is a depressed line between the two tubercles. Trace this line downwards for about 2.5 cm. This indicates the anterior marking of the pubic symphysis, being the medial surfaces of the pubic bones separated only by the intervening interarticular disc.

Accessory movements

Palpation

The slight twisting and gapping that occurs at this joint is due to stresses on the pelvis and sacrum which occur during movements at the sacroiliac and hip joint.

- Twisting and gapping. Apply pressure to the anterior surface of the pubic body on one side only. This will produce a slight gliding movement.
- Compression and stressing. The model is in the side lying position. Apply a downward compression force to the upper part of the ilium. This increases compression at the pubic symphysis while also stressing the posterior sacroiliac ligament.
- Lateral stressing. The model is in the supine lying position. The two ilia can be stressed laterally if you apply a downward and lateral pressure to the two iliac crests. This produces a distraction force to the pubic symphysis. In addition, it produces an anterior gapping and stress on the anterior ligament of the sacroiliac joint.

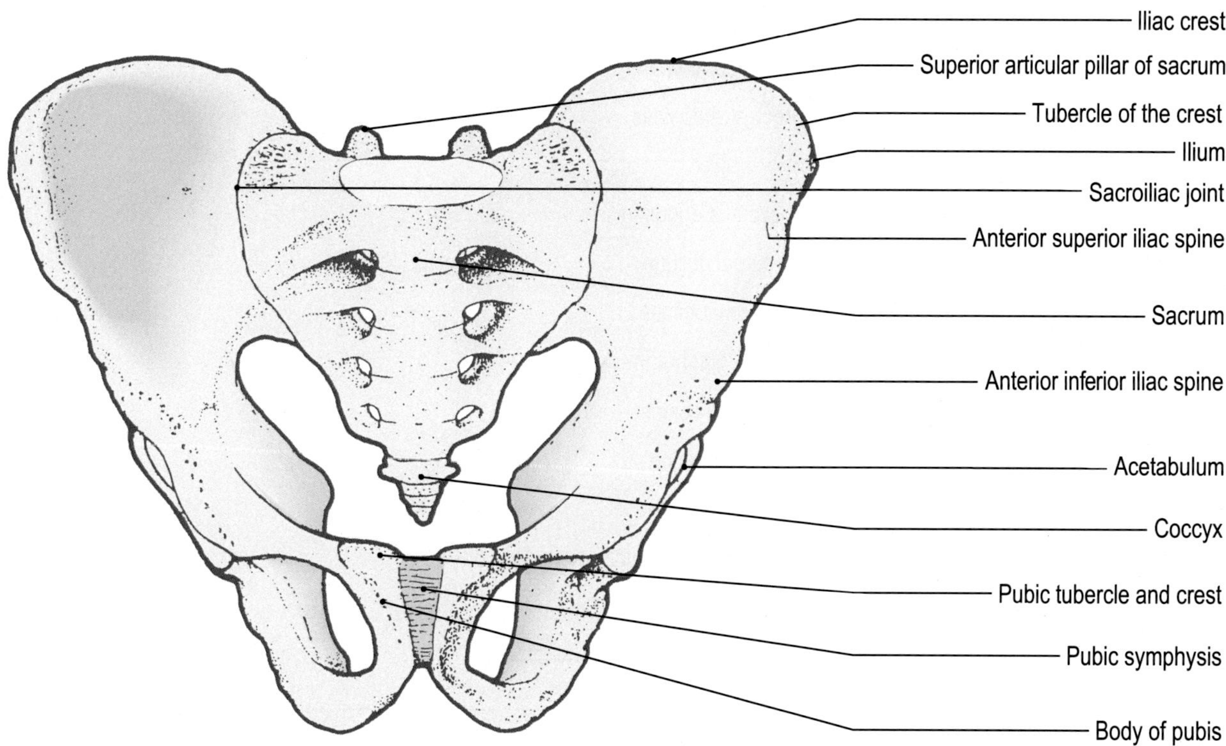

Fig. 6.4 (b) The pelvis (anterior view)

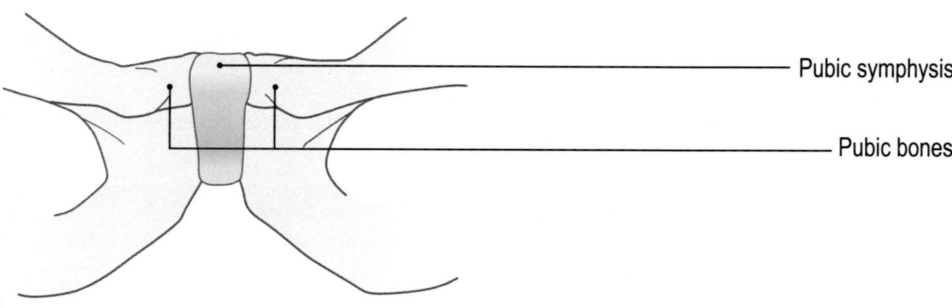

Fig. 6.4 (c) The pelvis (anterior view)

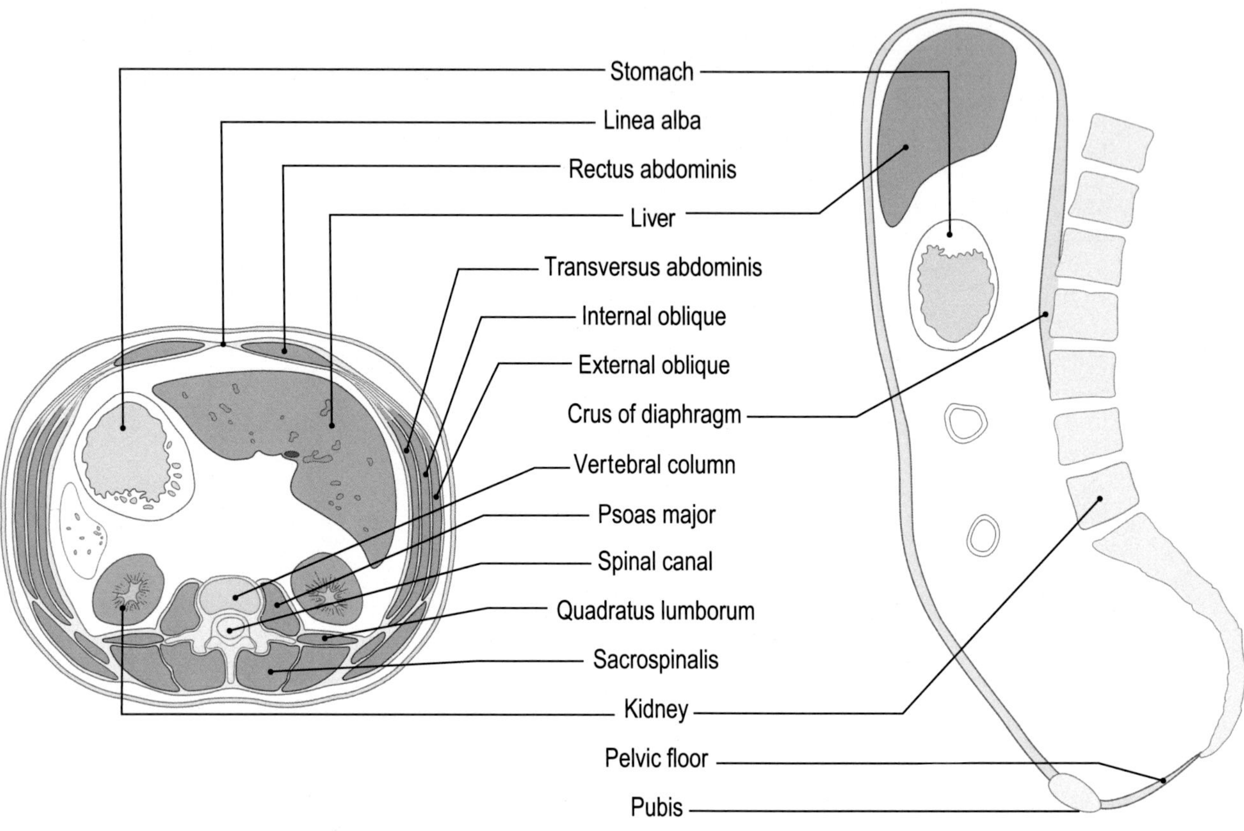

Fig. 6.5 (a), (b) The abdomen

MUSCLES

The abdominal muscles form a continuous wall around the abdominal viscera. The cavity so formed is enclosed:

- above: the **diaphragm**
- posteroinferiorly: the **vertebral column** and **psoas major**
- posterolaterally: **quadratus lumborum**
- anterolaterally: the **internal** and **external oblique** abdominal muscles
- anteriorly: the above muscles supported on their deep surface by **transversus abdominis**
- anteriorly: **rectus abdominis**
- inferiorly: the muscles which form the **pelvic floor** (i.e. levator ani and coccygeus).

Some of these muscles may be palpable when they are contracting, although they may not always appear distinct (Fig. 6.5).

Identification of structures and muscles in this area is dependent, to a certain extent, on the physique of the subject. Subcutaneous fat in the superficial fascia covering the abdomen can hinder accurate identification.

Palpation

For palpation in this region, the model is in the supine lying position.

- Rectus abdominus. Place both your hands on the central area of the abdomen, one above and one below the **umbilicus**. Now ask the model to raise the head. Palpate the column of muscle running down either side of the central depressed line (the **linea alba**) (Fig. 6.5a–d). These two columns of muscle are the left and right sections of the rectus abdominus muscle.
- **Note 1.** Each muscle is narrow inferiorly. It can be traced from the **pubic tubercle** and **crest** below to its broader superior attachment to the **fifth**, **sixth** and **seventh ribs**.
- **Note 2.** The upper attachment of rectus abdominus is V-shaped as the attachment to the fifth rib laterally is higher than that to

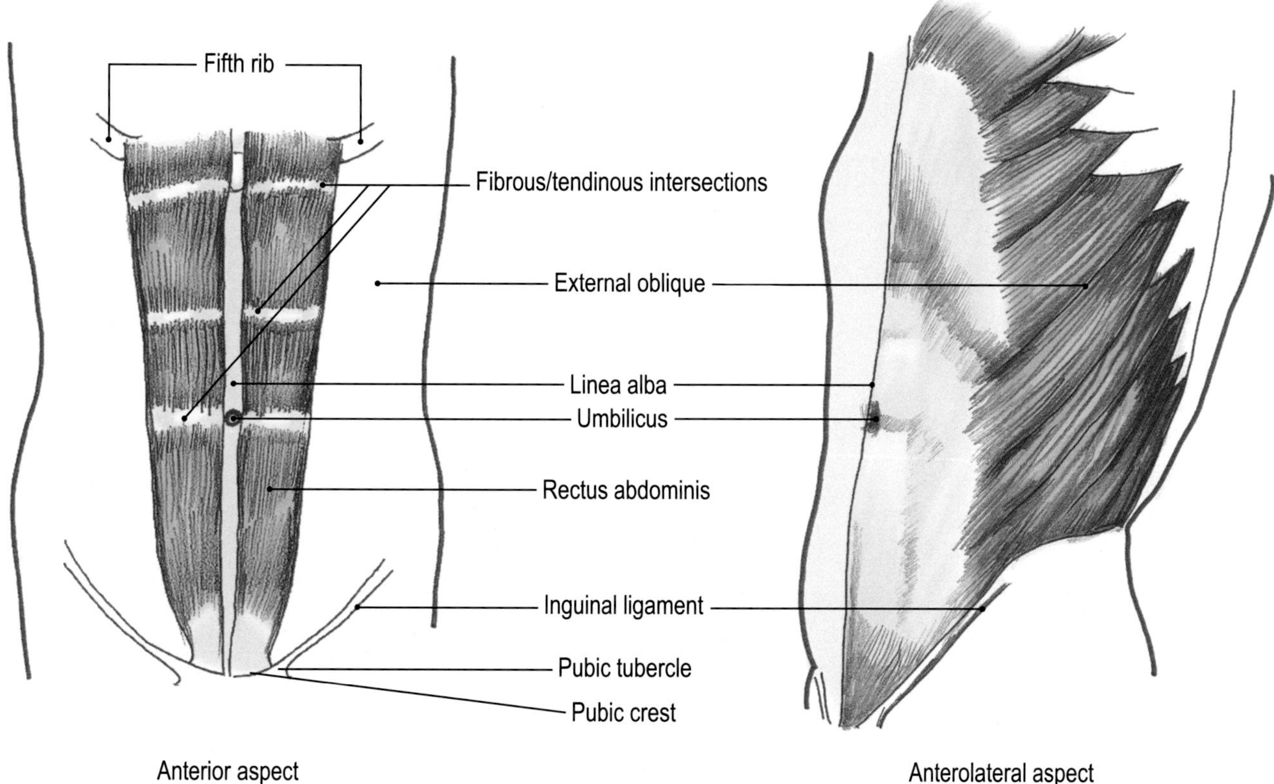

Fig. 6.5 (c), (d) Muscles of the abdomen

the seventh costal cartilage centrally. The lateral border of each muscle is convex. The muscle is interrupted by three transverse depressed **fibrous intersections**. These are at the level of the xiphoid, the umbilicus and midway between the two. These appear as transverse grooves across the muscles.

- The internal and external oblique muscles. Ask the model to flex the trunk. Palpate the contraction of both these muscles.
- **Note.** Each of these muscles can be identified more easily if its action is resisted.
- The right external oblique muscle. Stand on the model's left-hand side. Ask the model to rotate the trunk to the left against resistance. This will be easier if you apply resistance to the right shoulder, preventing the head and shoulder from being lifted and turned to the left. Palpate the contraction of the muscle. Contraction of the muscle tightens the aponeurosis just above its attachment to the right iliac crest.
- The left internal oblique. This muscle lies deep to the external oblique so that, if you repeat the technique described above (rotation of the trunk to the left) the left internal oblique also contracts. The contraction can be palpated between the left iliac crest and the umbilicus.
- Quadratus lumborum. The model is in the prone lying position. Ask the model to raise the head and shoulders. The muscle can be palpated on either side of the vertebral column, between the twelfth rib above and the posterior part of the iliac crest below. It mostly lies deep to latissimus dorsi, but its anterior border can be palpated just posterior to the mid-axillary line.

In this region sacrospinalis (erector spinae) lies close to the spinous processes of the lumbar vertebrae. These muscles form two firm columns passing from the posterior part of the iliac crest and sacrum below, to the angle of the ribs and transverse processes of the thoracic vertebrae.

- Sacrospinalis. Ask the model to raise the head and shoulders. Palpate the contraction of these muscles (also visible) lateral to the lumbar spines.

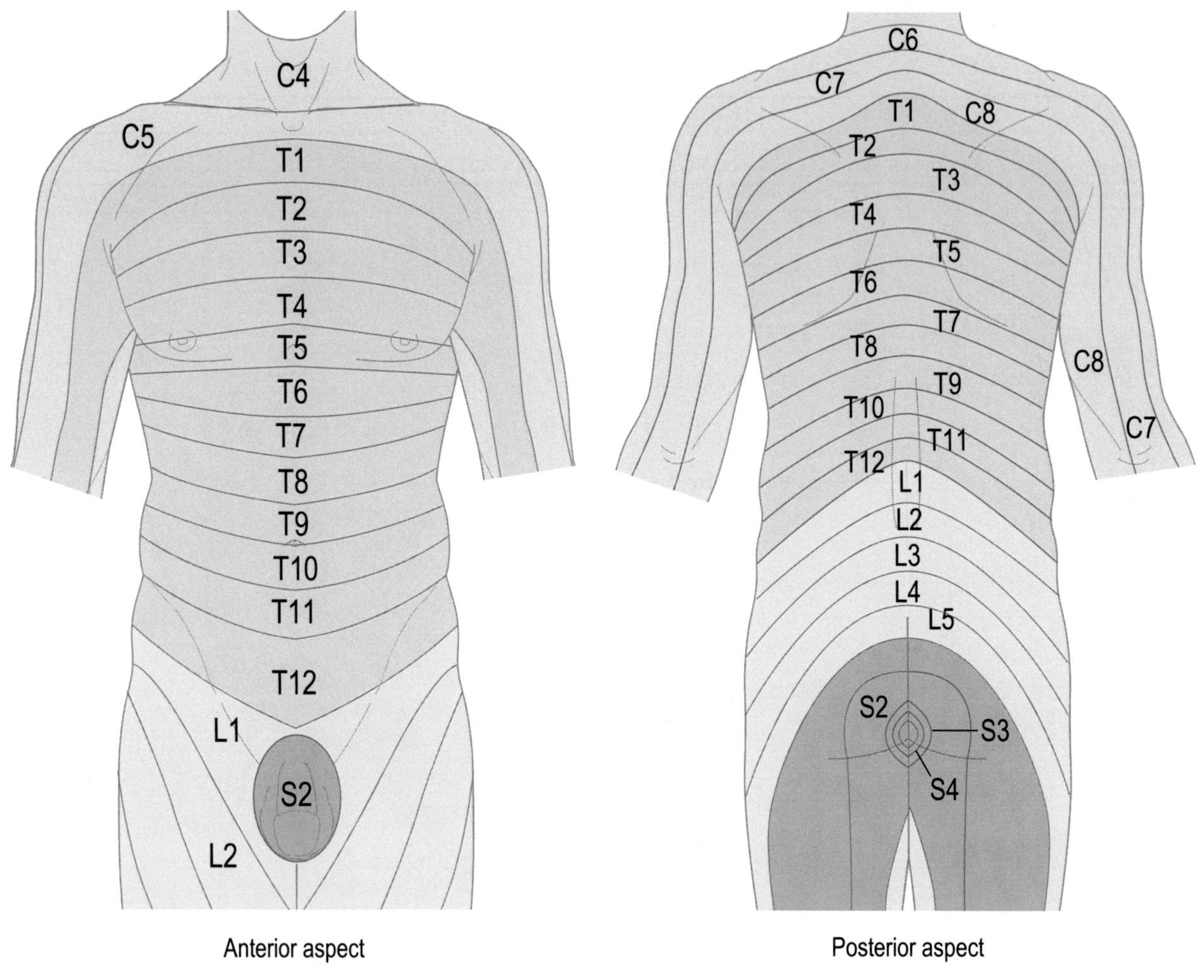

Fig. 6.6 (a), (b) The cutaneous nerve supply

NERVES (FIG. 6.6 A, B)

The nerve supply to the abdomen and lower limbs is derived from the T8–12, all five lumbar, all five sacral and the coccygeal nerve roots. The arrangement of these nerves is extremely complex (see Palastanga et al 2002) and is dealt with here in outline only.

The thoracic nerves

Nerve roots T8–11 behave in a similar manner to intercostal nerves, supplying muscles in intercostal spaces and anteriorly contributing to the supply to the abdominal muscles. Their cutaneous branches follow the same general direction, supplying a band of skin running downwards and forwards.

The lumbar plexus

This is formed by part of T12 and L1–4. It supplies muscles of the lower abdomen, pelvis and front and inner side of the thigh. Its cutaneous supply is to the lower back and running downwards and forwards to the lower abdomen and the front and inner side of thigh and the inner side of the leg and foot.

The sacral plexus

Deriving its fibres from the ventral rami of L4, L5 S1, S2, S3 and S4 the sacral plexus supplies the muscles of the gluteal region, hamstrings, leg and foot. Its cutaneous supply is the gluteal region, back of the thigh, anterior, lateral and posterior aspects of the leg and plantar and dorsal aspects of the foot.

The coccygeal plexus supplies an area of skin around the anus.

The larger nerves of this region are situated deeply within the abdomen. Those of the lumbar plexus are formed within psoas major, while those of the sacral plexus mainly lie in front of the sacrum. All nerves that reach the surface of the abdominal and lumbar areas are too small to palpate. Nevertheless, these cutaneous nerves often influence their areas of distribution, with palpable signs such as changes in temperature and sweating. It is therefore important to study the cutaneous distribution over the abdomen and lumbar areas. As in the costal area, there is an overlap of root supply, each nerve covering an area of skin above and below.

ARTERIES (FIG. 6.6C)

All the larger arteries of the abdomen are also situated deeply within the abdominal cavity and are difficult or impossible to find

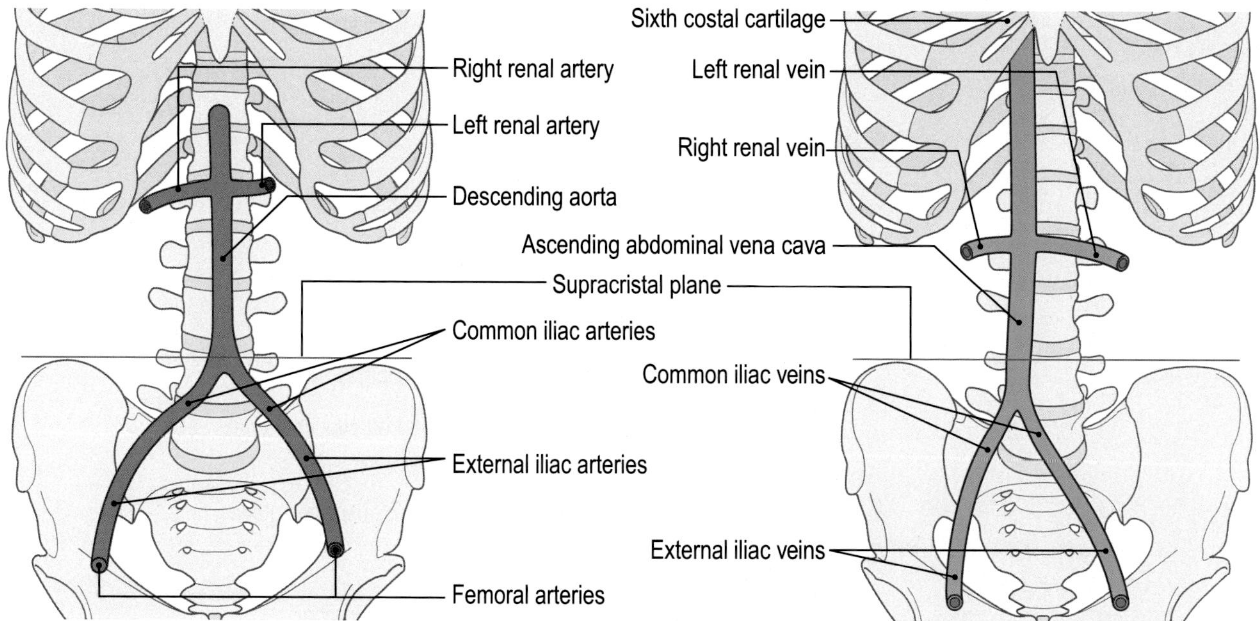

Fig. 6.6 **(c)** Abdominal aorta and common iliac arteries. **(d)** Ascending abdominal vena cava and common iliac veins

Palpation

For palpation in this region, the model is in the supine lying position.

- The pulsations of the **abdominal aorta**. Using your fingers, apply deep pressure to the left of the umbilicus. This compresses the abdominal aorta against the lumbar vertebral bodies.
- **Note.** This technique is unpleasant. It can be improved by encouraging the model to relax the abdominal muscles.
- The surface marking of the abdominal aorta. Draw a line vertically from a point on the midline 2.5 cm above the transpyloric plane (see Fig. 6.7b) to a point just to the left of the midline 2.5 cm below the **supracristal plane** (Fig. 6.6c).
- The **common iliac arteries**. At this point, the aorta divides into the common iliac arteries. These diverge from each other at an angle of approximately 37° to bifurcate again one vertebra below (lower border of the fifth lumbar vertebra) into the internal and external iliac arteries.
- The **external iliac artery**. This artery can be marked as it passes to the mid point of the inguinal ligament to be continued below the ligament as the **femoral artery**.

VEINS (FIG. 6.6D)

Again, all the large veins of the abdomen are deep within the cavity and impossible to palpate. It is, however, quite important to know where the **abdominal** portion of the **inferior vena cava** commences and leaves the abdominal cavity.

Palpation: surface marking

For palpation in this region, the model is in the supine lying position.

- The abdominal portion of the inferior vena cava. This vein commences at the junction of the two **common iliac veins** at the level of the fourth lumbar vertebra. It progresses upwards and slightly to the right. It is initially accompanied on its left by the abdominal aorta. It leaves the abdominal cavity by passing behind the liver and through the diaphragm at the level of the spine of T8 (Fig. 6.6d).
- The inferior vena cava. Draw a line 2.5 cm wide, commencing at a point just to the right of the midline 2.5 cm below the **supracristal plane** (lower body of the fourth lumbar vertebra), to a point just above the **sixth costal cartilage** on the right, where it passes through the vena caval opening in the tendinous portion of the diaphragm (Fig. 6.6d).

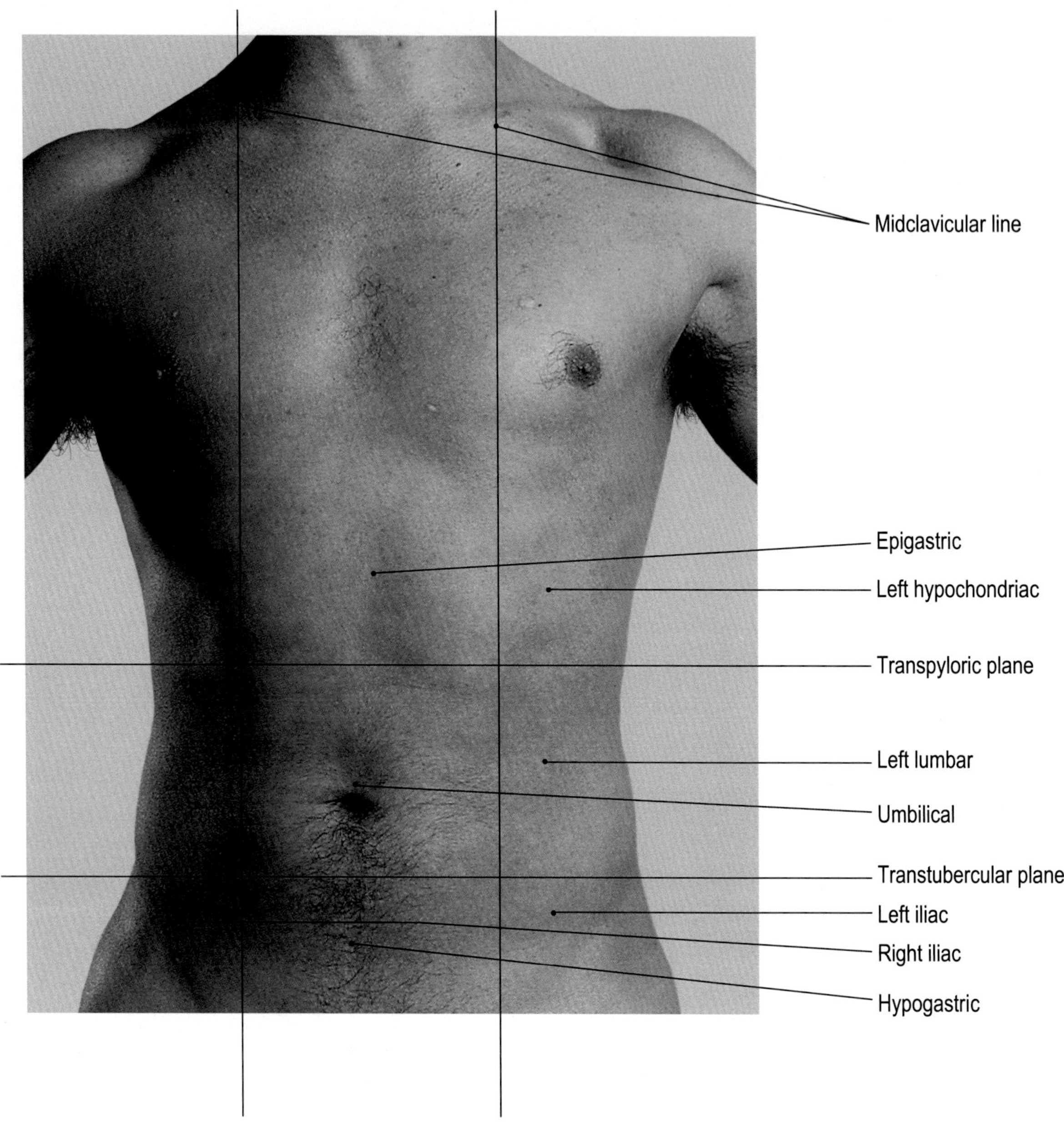

Fig. 6.7 (a) Regions of the abdomen

STRUCTURES WITHIN THE ABDOMINAL CAVITY

For convenient location of viscera, the abdomen may be divided into nine regions by two vertical and two horizontal lines (Fig. 6.7a, b). Other methods of dividing the abdomen into regions also exist but will not be covered here (Keogh and Ebbs 1984).

Palpation: surface marking

For surface markings in this region, the model is in the supine lying position.

- The **mid-clavicular lines**. Trace the two vertical lines as follows. They pass superiorly from the mid-inguinal point, which is halfway between the anterior superior iliac spine and the pubic tubercle, to the mid point of the clavicle. They are usually referred to as the mid-clavicular lines.
- The upper horizontal line and the transpyloric plane. This is drawn level with the tip of the ninth costal cartilage. It crosses the tip of the twelfth rib and the spine of the first lumbar vertebra. This is known as the transpyloric plane as it also passes through the pylorus of the stomach.
- The lower horizontal line and the transtubercular plane. This is drawn across the abdomen between the tubercle of the crest of each ilium and is known as the **transtubercular plane** (Fig. 6.7a, b). It crosses the vertebral column level with the upper portion of the body of L5. It may serve as a useful landmark when identification of lumbar vertebrae is necessary.

The three regions above the transpyloric plane are the **right** and **left hypochondriac**, with the **epigastric** centrally. The three regions between the transpyloric and transtubercular planes are

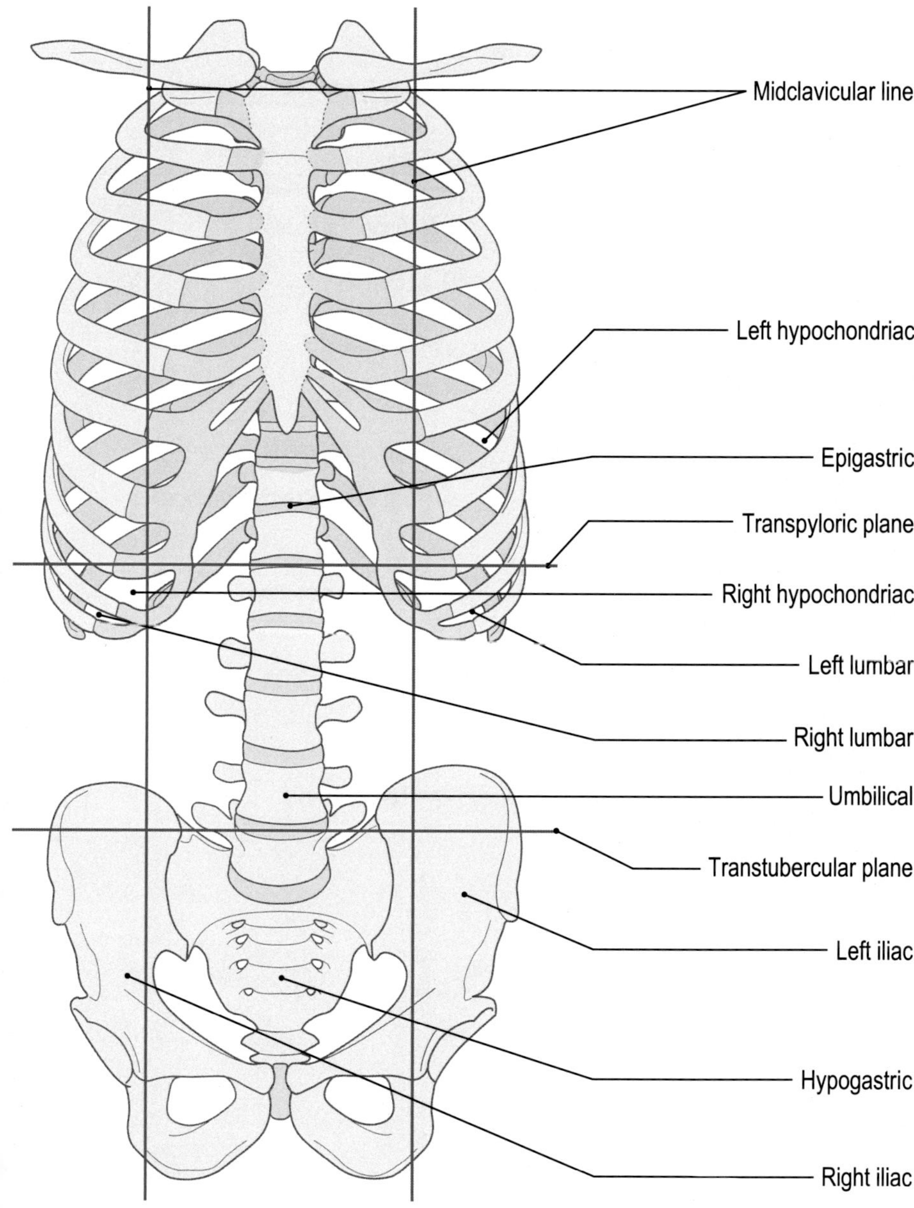

Fig. 6.7 (b) Regions of the abdomen

the right and left lumbar, with the umbilical centrally. The three lower regions are the right and left iliac, with the hypogastric centrally.

Organs in the abdominal cavity are normally quite movable, some changing their shape and size according to their contents. This makes surface marking difficult and often unreliable. It is, however, important to be able to mark the areas in which the particular organ lies and note any fixed sites where markings are constant.

General locations and overview

- The liver. This organ lies mainly in the right hypochondriac and epigastric areas.
- The spleen. This organ is located mainly in the left hypochondriac and extends posteriorly into the epigastric area.
- The pancreas. This organ lies on the transpyloric plane between the epigastric and umbilical areas.
- The gall bladder. This organ lies on the transpyloric plane where it crosses the right mid-clavicular line.
- The stomach. The stomach varies considerably in size but is normally in the left hypochondriac and umbilical areas.
- The duodenum. This organ lies partly in the umbilical and partly in the epigastric areas, the transpyloric plane passing through its second part.
- The small intestine. This organ lies mainly in the hypogastric area.
- The caecum and appendix. These organs lie in the right iliac region.
- The large intestine. This organ passes through the right iliac and lumbar, umbilical, left lumbar and iliac areas and passes down through the hypogastric area.
- The kidneys. These organs lie partly in the epigastric and partly in the umbilical areas.
- The bladder. This organ lies behind the two pubic bones and pubic symphysis.

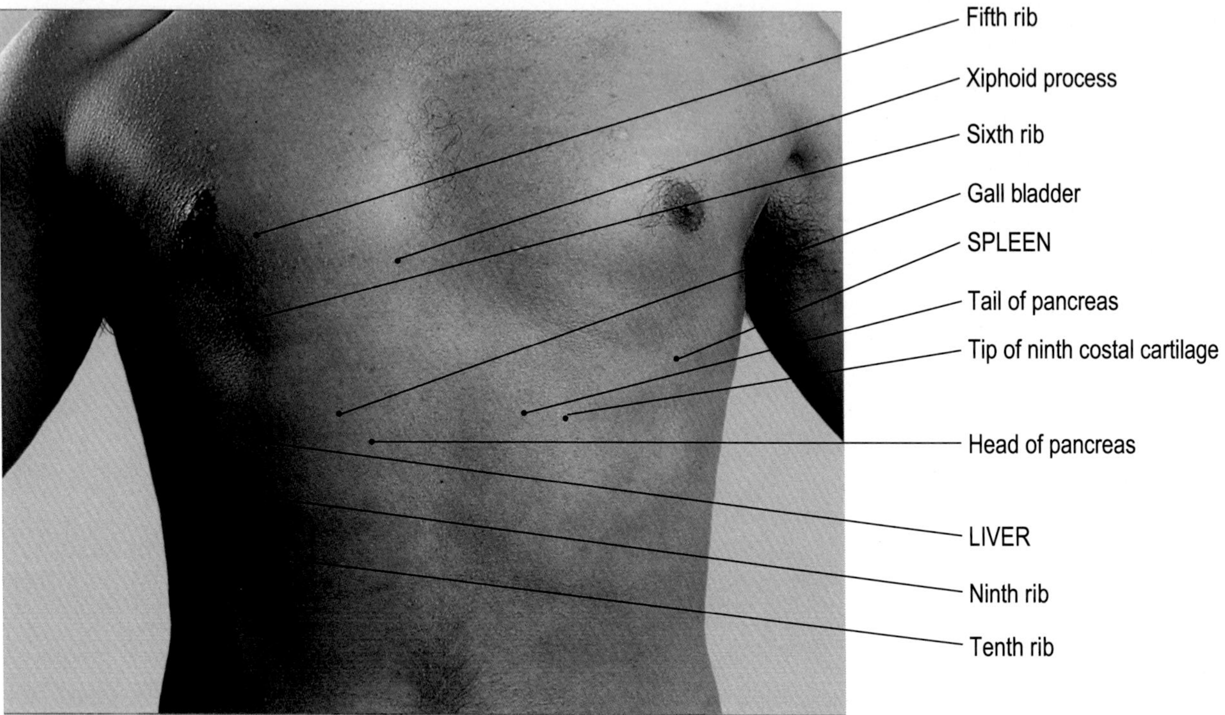

Fig. 6.7 (c) The liver and spleen (anterior aspect)

The liver (Fig. 6.7c, d)

The liver is a large wedge-shaped organ situated mainly in the right hypochondriac and epigastric regions of the abdomen just below the diaphragm. Its upper surface is moulded by the undersurface of the diaphragm. The right side is thicker, narrowing as it passes towards the left. Posteriorly, it is grooved by the inferior vena cava.

Palpation: surface marking

- Note. For identification of the following organs, the model is either in the supine or prone lying position.
- The liver. The model is in the supine lying position. The position of the liver is fairly constant in healthy subjects. Mark its upper boundary by drawing a line horizontally at the level of the xiphisternal joint, extending some 7 cm to the left of the midline and all the way round the right side of the thoracic cage. Mark its lower border by drawing an oblique line beginning 7 cm to the left of the midline, crossing the left costal margin at the eighth costal cartilage, reaching the right costal margin at the ninth costal cartilage and continuing around the costal margin.

The spleen (Fig. 6.7c, d)

The spleen [*splen* (L) = spleen] is a reservoir for blood. It is soft and highly vascular and is just deep to the lower left ribs below the diaphragm and behind the stomach. In addition to the storage of blood, it is part of the reticuloendothelial system. It contains phagocytes which engulf microorganisms, foreign particles and damaged cells. It is involved with the manufacture of white blood cells and in the infant it will also produce red blood cells.

The spleen lies under cover of the ribs, although it is an abdominal organ. This is due to the domes of the diaphragm rising into the thorax from its costal attachments.

Palpation: surface marking

- The spleen. The model is in the supine lying position. The spleen lies posteriorly on the left side of the body. It is situated deep to the ninth, tenth and eleventh ribs and extends as far forwards as the mid-axillary line. It is approximately 10 cm long, 7 cm deep and 3–4 cm thick. Although it occasionally projects just below the costal margin, the spleen cannot usually be palpated unless it is enlarged to approximately three times its normal size.

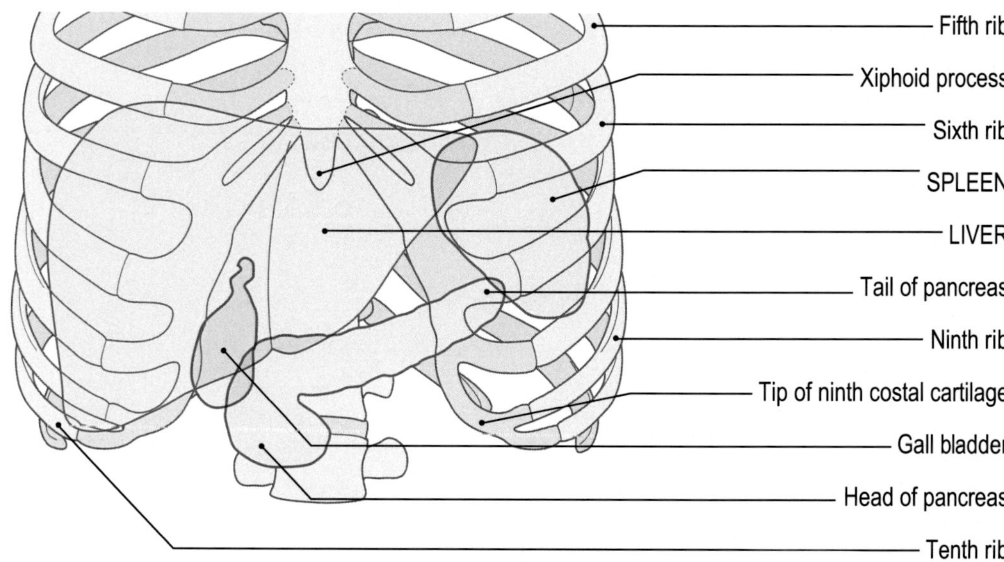

Fig. 6.7 (d) The liver and spleen (anterior aspect)

- Note 1. The spleen is often ruptured in severe accidents where the chest is crushed and may well be overlooked. This will lead to large amounts of blood escaping into the abdominal cavity.
- Note 2. The spleen can be removed without affecting the human body too seriously.

The pancreas (Fig. 6.7c, d)

The pancreas [*pan* (Gk) = all, *keras* (Gk) = flesh] is a strangely shaped gland resembling a large tadpole, having a head to the right with a body and tail which narrows as it passes to the left.

Palpation: surface marking

- The pancreas. The model is in the prone lying position. The organ is approximately 10 cm long and 4 cm broad at its head. It is situated anterior to the vertebral column, level with the body of the first lumbar vertebra. The head is surrounded by the four sections of the duodenum, the pylorus of the stomach lying anterior to the body. The pancreatic duct passes from the head to the right, emptying into the second part of the duodenum at a point on the transpyloric plane 2 cm to the right of the median line (Fig. 6.7c, d). Behind the body lie the superior mesenteric and splenic veins; just below, they form the portal vein. The head is related posteriorly with the inferior vena cava and the right crus of the diaphragm. The body lies just in front of the abdominal aorta. The tail is related to the spleen at its far left and with the stomach anteriorly. The pancreas is not palpable in the normal subject.

The gall bladder (Fig. 6.7c, d)

The gall bladder is a small reservoir, approximately 3 cm in diameter, with a short tail passing posteriorly.

Palpation: surface marking

- The gall bladder. The model is in the supine lying position. The organ is situated below the centre of the anterior border of the liver, projecting a little below the right costal margin deep to the costal angle level with the ninth costal cartilage (Fig. 6.7c, d). In the normal subject, the gall bladder is difficult to palpate. It discharges bile through the bile duct into the second part of the duodenum, which aids in the breakdown of fatty foods during digestion.
- Note. Sometimes stones are formed in the gall bladder and are passed down the tortuous and sometimes narrowing tubes of the cystic and bile ducts. The blockage of these tubes causes acute pain and often irritates other structures in this area. If this is a recurring problem, the gall bladder can be removed (cholecystectomy).

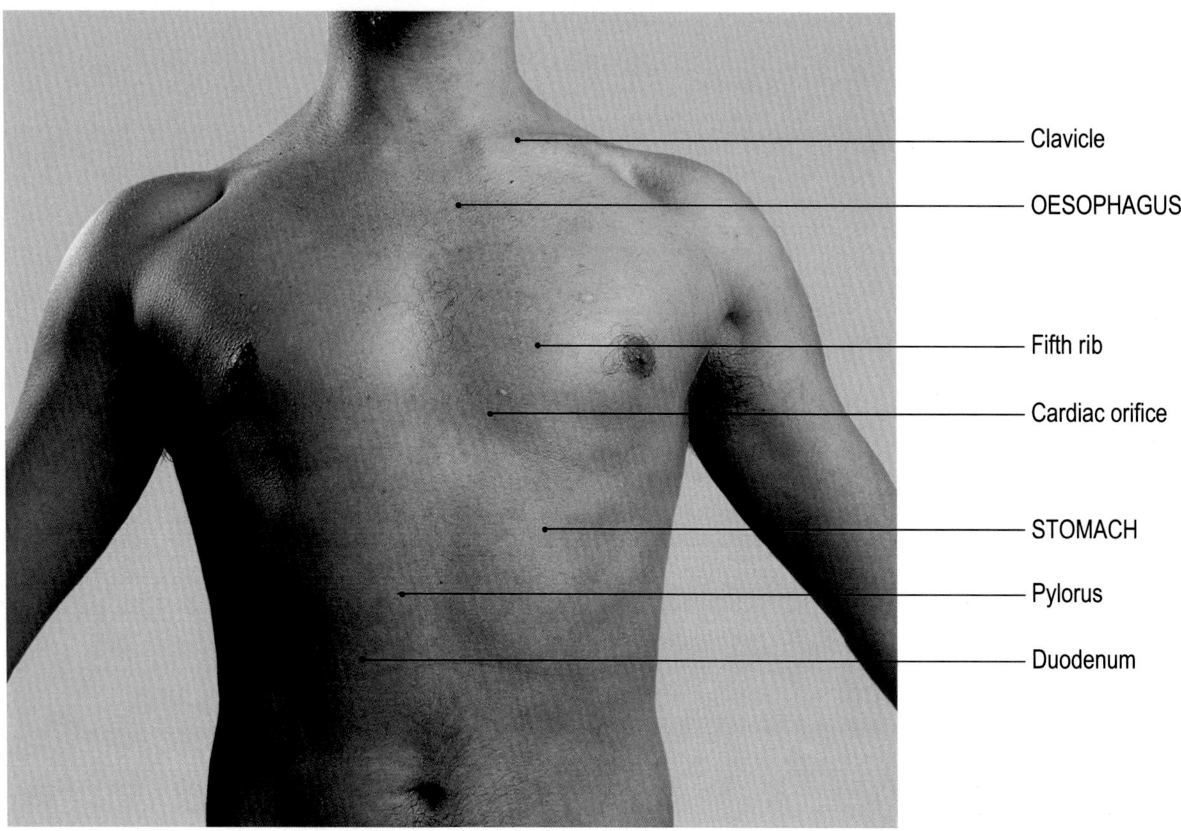

Fig. 6.8 (a) The oesophagus, stomach and duodenum

The stomach (Fig. 6.8)

The **stomach** [*stomachos* (Gk) = the Greeks used this word for the gullet and the oesophagus; later, they used 'gaster' to denote its lower end]. This is a mobile, muscular, highly vascular organ. Its function is as a container in the digestive system. It is situated deep to the lower left rib cage, below the diaphragm, to the left of the liver and in front of the spleen. It receives food from the **oesophagus** [*oiso* (Gk) = I carry, *phagein* (Gk) = food] through its **cardiac orifice** into its upper part (the **fundus**). After passing through the **body of the stomach**, the partially digested food is passed on through the **pylorus** and **pyloric orifice** into the first part of the **duodenum**. The stomach varies enormously in shape and size according to its contents. It is basically J-shaped, its upper section being thicker and more expanded. Its lower end becomes narrower as it passes medially and slightly upwards, continuing as the first part of the duodenum.

Palpation: surface marking

- The stomach. The model is in the supine lying position. Although the central section of the stomach varies in shape and size, its two openings – the cardiac and pyloric orifices – remain comparatively fixed.
- The cardiac orifice. Mark this orifice by drawing a short oblique line, approximately 2 cm long, along the seventh costal cartilage, 2.5 cm to the left of the midline, where it is level with the tip of the xiphoid process.
- The pyloric orifice. This orifice can be identified lying on the transpyloric plane, 1.5 cm to the right of the midline.

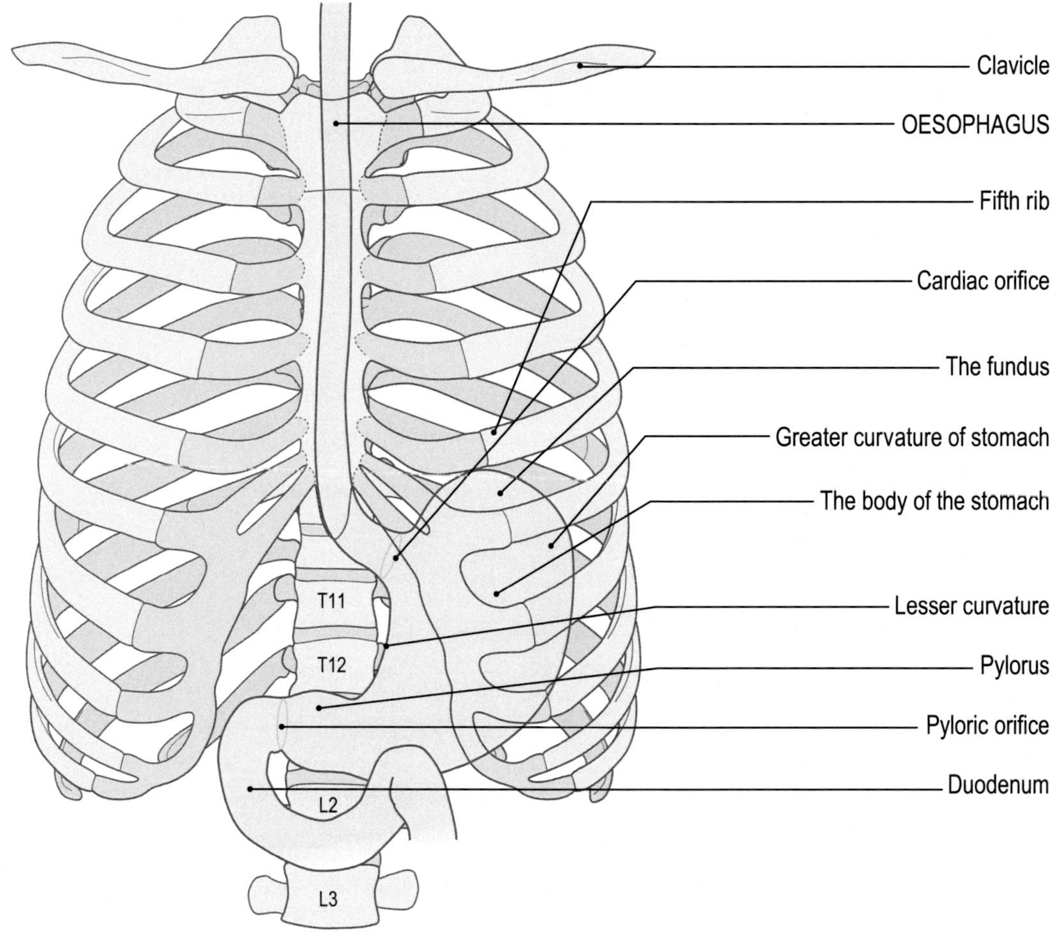

Fig. 6.8 (b) The oesophagus, stomach and duodenum

- The fundus. The fundus, or upper part of the stomach, may rise up as far as the fifth intercostal space, 7 cm left of the midline, or as far down as the tenth costal cartilage.
- The **lesser curvature** of the stomach. Mark this area by drawing a curved line, concave to the right, joining the cardiac and pyloric openings.
- The **greater curvature** of the stomach. Mark this area by drawing a line, convex to the left, joining the upper limit of the stomach at the fifth intercostal space to approximately the tenth costal cartilage (Fig. 6.8a, b).

The duodenum (Fig. 6.8)

The **duodenum** [*duoden arius* (L) = continuing twelve. Herophilus in 344 BC measured the duodenum as twelve finger breadths] is the continuation of the digestive tract beyond the pylorus of the stomach.

Palpation: surface marking

- The duodenum. The model is in the supine lying position. The duodenum is approximately 25 cm long.
- First part. Initially, the duodenum passes upwards, backwards and to the right for 5 cm as far as the costal margin.
- Second part. This passes downwards to the left for 7.5 cm, to reach the level of the tenth costal cartilage across the front of the body of L3.
- Third part. This passes upwards and to the left for approximately 10 cm.
- Fourth part. This finally ascends for 2.5 cm to become continuous with the jejunum at the duodenojejunal flexure at the level of L2, 2 cm left of the mid line.
- **Note.** The common bile duct and pancreatic duct drain into the duodenum midway along its second part.

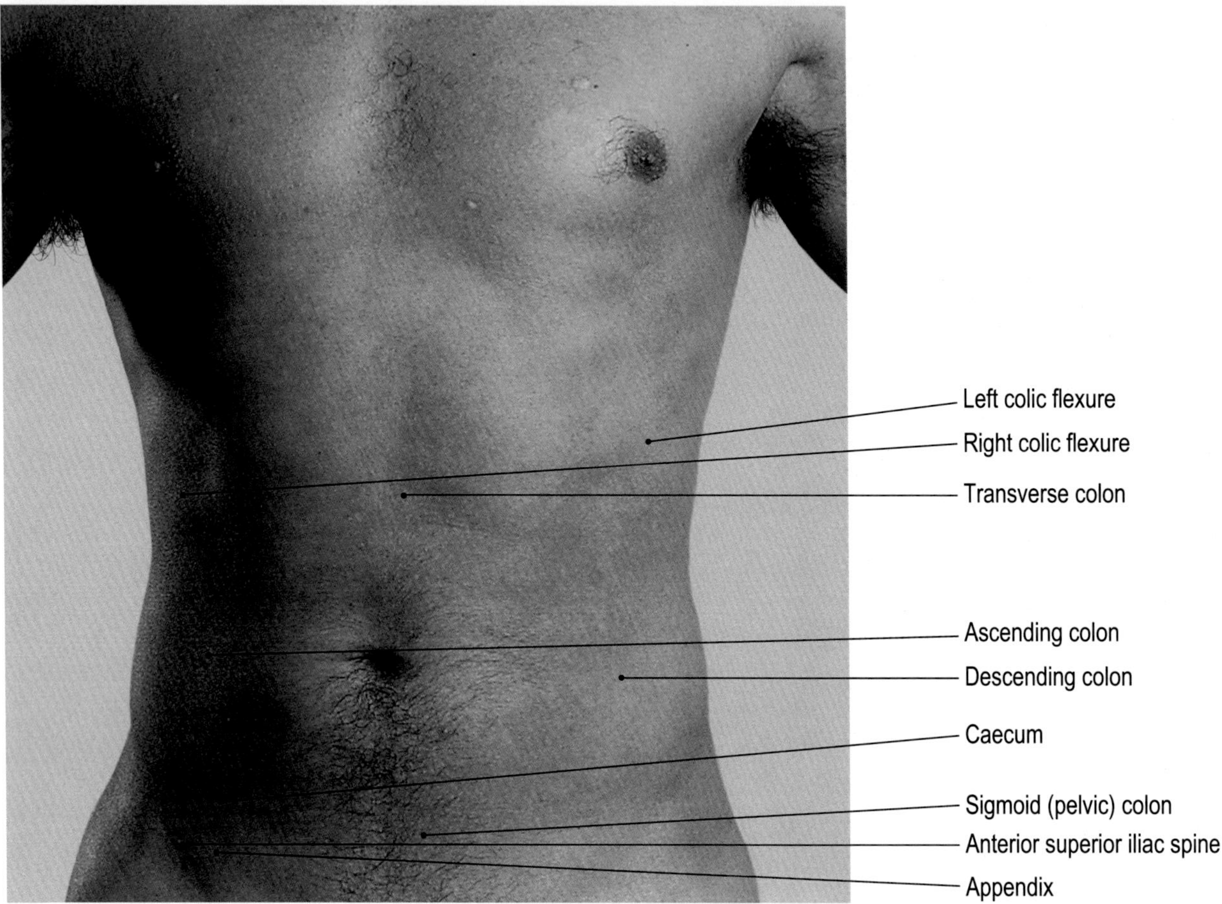

Fig. 6.9 (a) The large bowel

The small intestine

The small intestine is described in two parts, the first being termed the jejunum and the second, the ileum.

Palpation: surface marking

- The jejunum. The model is in the supine lying position. The jejunum begins as a continuation of the duodenum (Fig. 6.8a, b). It starts at the level of L2, 2 cm to the left of the midline and continues as the ileum.
- The ileum. This ends at its junction with the **caecum** (Fig. 6.9a, b) at the junction of the right mid-clavicular line with the transtubercular plane (drawn through the tubercles of the crest of the ilium). Each end is fixed in its position.
- **Note.** The central portion, which may be up to 8 m long, is continually mobile. It is, however, contained within the confines of the large bowel.

The caecum (Fig. 6.9a, b)

The caecum [*caecus* (L) = blind. Galen confused the caecum with the appendix]. This is the first section of the large intestine and receives the contents of the small intestine.

Palpation: surface marking

- The caecum. The model is in the supine lying position. The caecum fills the right iliac region of the abdomen. It lies above the lateral half of the right inguinal ligament.
- The **appendix**. This organ lies in the mid-clavicular line 1.5 cm medial to the **anterior superior iliac spine**.
- **Note.** The caecum and appendix are not palpable, but pressure applied to this region can be extremely painful, particularly if the appendix is inflamed.

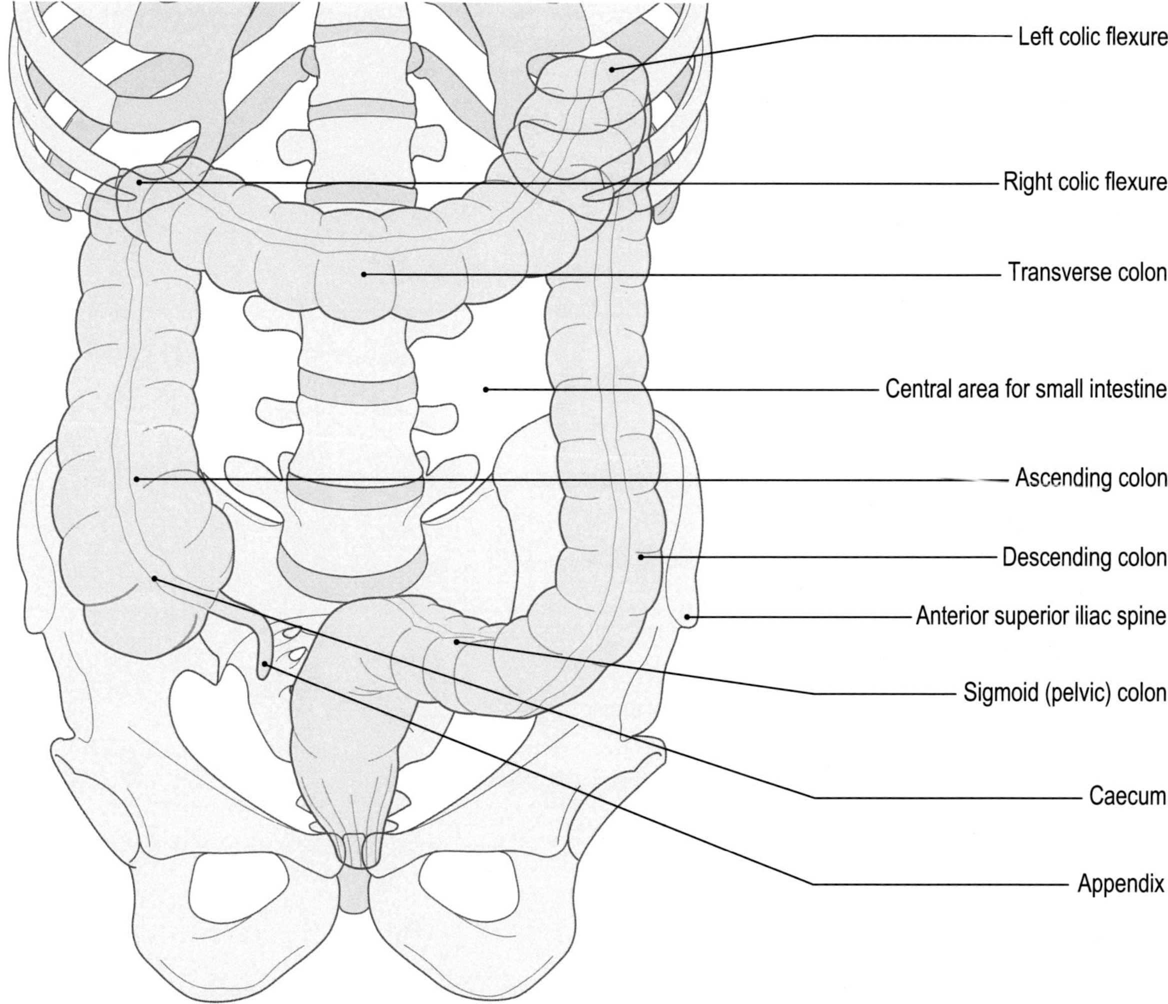

Fig. 6.9 (b) The large bowel

The large intestine (large bowel) (Fig. 6.9a, b)

For descriptive purposes, the large intestine is normally divided into four sections: **ascending**, **transverse**, **descending** and **sigmoid** (pelvic). It can be represented by a band, approximately 5 cm wide, but varies considerably according to its contents.

Palpation: surface marking

- The ascending colon. The model is in the supine lying position. The ascending colon commences in the right iliac region at the caecum. It ascends through the right lumbar region, deep to the costal margin, to the level of the transpyloric plane. At the transpyloric plane it arches backwards and to the left, forming the **right colic** (hepatic) [*hepar* (Gk) = liver] **flexure**.
- The transverse colon. This section passes from the colic flexure, across the umbilical region below the liver towards the spleen. There it turns downwards, forming the **left colic** (splenic) flexure just above the transpyloric plane.
- The descending colon. This section passes through the left lumbar and iliac regions. It turns backwards at the inguinal ligament to become the **sigmoid** [*sigma* (Gk) = letter S, *-oeides* (Gk) = shape, form] **colon**.
- The sigmoid colon. This section passes backwards and downwards in an S-shaped curve to pass vertically downwards in front of the sacrum, becoming the rectum. This is continuous with the anal canal and reaches the surface at the anus.

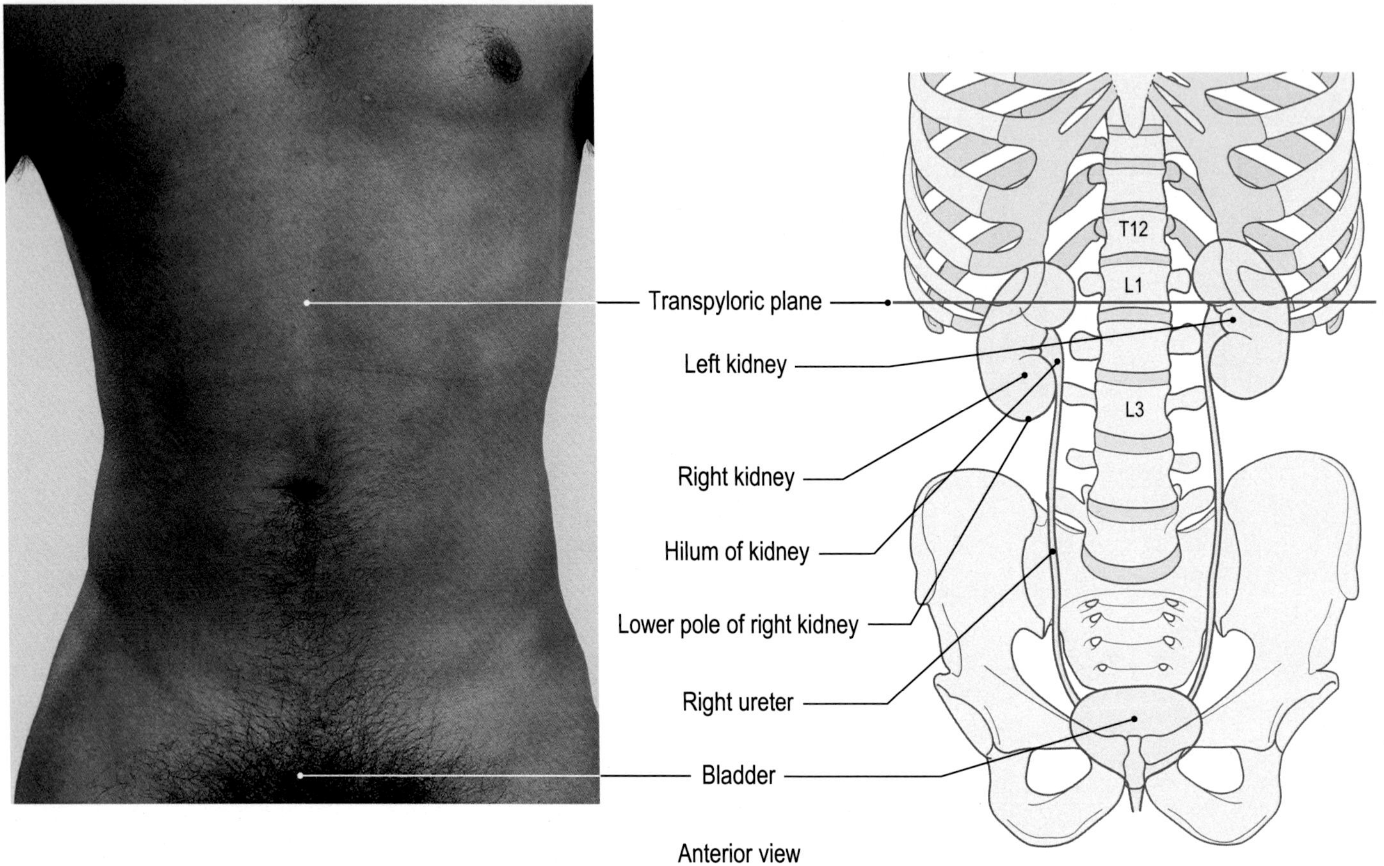

Fig. 6.10 (a), (b) The kidneys, ureters and bladder

The kidneys (Fig. 6.10)

The kidneys are situated on the posterior abdominal wall anterior to quadratus lumborum behind the peritoneum. Each kidney lies obliquely with its anterior surface facing slightly laterally. The anterior relations of the right kidney are the right suprarenal gland and liver superiorly, the duodenum and right colic flexure infero-medially. The left kidney has the left suprarenal gland above, the tail of the pancreas and splenic vessels, the stomach and left colic flexure anteriorly, with the spleen postero-superiorly. Each kidney is related posteriorly to quadratus lumborum, the diaphragm and the medial and lateral arcuate ligaments. The right kidney lies mainly in front of the twelfth rib, while the left lies anterior to the eleventh rib. Each kidney is approximately 11 cm in length, 6 cm wide and 3 cm thick. The hilum lies level with the spine of the first lumbar vertebra (the transpyloric plane), the right normally slightly lower than the left.

Palpation: surface marking

- The kidneys: general points. The model is in the prone lying position. Each kidney can be located between two horizontal and two vertical lines, forming a rectangle on either side of the vertebral column. The upper and lower limits of both kidneys lie between horizontal lines through the upper margin of T12 above and L3 below.
- The kidneys. To facilitate the location of these lines, first draw a horizontal line through the lower edge of the spine of L1 Now draw a second line 5.5 cm above this (i.e. level with the upper border of T12). Then draw a third line 5.5 cm below (i.e level with L3).
- Note. Because the two kidneys lie obliquely, the two vertical lines enclosing them are closer together than the width of the organ. Draw two vertical lines, one 3 cm and one 6.5 cm

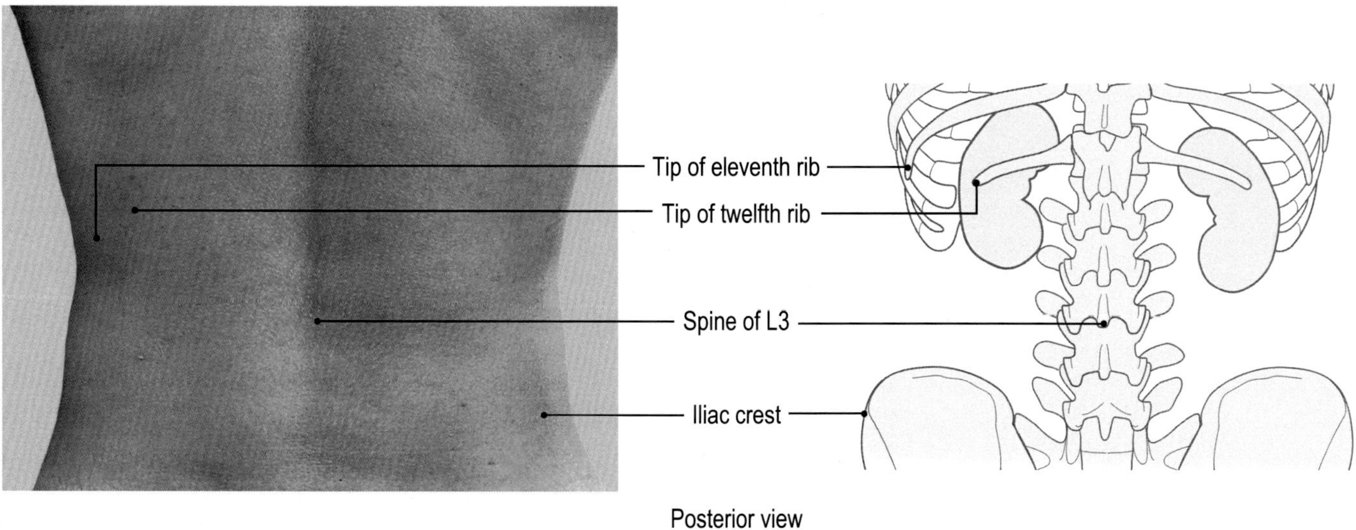

Fig. 6.10 (c), (d) The kidneys

lateral to the lumbar spines. These represent the medial and lateral margins of the kidneys.

Palpation

The kidneys are well protected, lying anterior to the lower ribs and strong back muscles, below the diaphragm. The vertebral column, with the attachments of the crura of the diaphragm, lies between the two kidneys and psoas major and minor lie behind them. The kidneys are protected in front by the large and small bowel and the powerful abdominal muscles. They are thus virtually impossible to palpate.

- The lower pole of the right kidney. The **lower pole of the right kidney** can be palpated with difficulty. You will need to apply deep pressure through a relaxed abdominal wall at a point just lateral to the vertical mid-clavicular line and just below the level of the tenth rib.

The bladder (Fig. 6.10a, b)

The **bladder** is a thin-walled muscular reservoir which varies in size according to the volume of fluid it contains. It is estimated that it is able to hold about 250 mL of urine before having to be emptied, but this estimate appears to be a little on the low side practically. Its volume obviously grows according to the frequency it is filled with large quantities of fluid.

- The bladder. The model is in the prone lying position. The bladder is situated directly behind the two pubic bones and pubic symphysis, with its upper border reaching to the crest on either side. When full, however, it rises above the pubic rami by up to 5 cm.
- **Note.** The empty bladder is not palpable in the normal subject but when full it can be felt as a soft swelling just above the pubic symphysis.

7 Conclusion

Although the major part of this book is devoted to encouraging readers to acquire anatomical knowledge through familiarization with the surface markings of underlying tissues, its principal aim is to promote the development of manual skills to improve clinical practice. If the suggested manoeuvres have been carried out, a thorough knowledge of the surface markings will have been gained together with an increased awareness of the sense of touch and the consequent improvement of palpation techniques. This knowledge will be invaluable to all practitioners during their subsequent clinical practice.

These palpation skills will, of course, be developed further with regular practice in which exploration of the basic techniques can take place. Regular evaluation and modification of all techniques will be crucial if improvement in performance is to be achieved. Indeed, the benefits of continually upgrading palpation skills extend far beyond the clinical setting. The activities of many skilled craftspeople provide excellent examples of highly developed manual skills. It may be useful to consider the following examples in which observation of the activities of craftspeople confirms their awareness of the importance of tactile input and the high level of skill in manual dexterity:

- the care with which a carpenter approaches the task of preparing and working on a piece of wood
- the attention to detail demonstrated by a dressmaker when selecting appropriate material prior to creating a particular garment
- the respect of a potter for a piece of clay
- the fine dexterity of the gardener's fingers when pricking out seedlings
- the careful smoothing and moulding carried out by a tailor when fitting a suit
- the care with which a hairdresser handles the hair of a client.

It is evident from the above examples that these craftspeople have great reverence for the materials with which they work. In the case of the hairdresser, the recipient gains something from the interaction which is far more subtle and psychologically significant than the experience of physical contact would initially suggest.

This is also true within the clinical context. Observation of the care and sensitivity with which a physiotherapist handles a painful limb confirms the intrinsic value of acquiring expertise in manual techniques. Most recipients acknowledge the importance of, and pleasure associated with, this physical contact and many recognize and express appreciation of its psychological benefits. The value of such non-verbal communication can never be underestimated. The gripping of a hand, an arm around the shoulder or a touch on the elbow can all be comforting to a person who is under some stress. All convey empathy and understanding and sometimes represent the only means by which such feelings can be effectively conveyed to the recipient.

As stated in Chapter 1, the art of palpation involves a combination of the appropriate use of touch, the application of methodical investigatory techniques, accurate interpretation of sensory feedback (based upon sound general knowledge), the ability to draw on previous experience, to reflect, critically, upon findings and arrive at a reasoned conclusion. The acquisition of this skill provides the therapist with valuable supplementary information to that which can be obtained through observation and verbal questioning and is crucial to arriving at a meaningful clinical diagnosis. Not until the practitioner becomes skilled at being able to 'read' the patient, however, can this art be regarded as having been fully developed. In order to help those with whom professionals have the privilege to come into contact, clinicians need to strive towards making conscious those processes which, in so many practitioners, often remain unconscious. By developing the sense of touch through the practise of palpation skills, we come closer to attaining this ideal.

The objective of this book is to inspire readers to improve their clinical practice by developing an expertise in palpation skills. All too often, evidence suggests that these skills remain underused and undervalued by professionals involved in the care and treatment of patients, not forgetting animals. Our experience confirms that the benefits of pursuing this form of study far outweigh the perceived drawbacks in terms of time and effort. Communication through touch has the potential to reveal information that may otherwise remain undiscovered: its power should never be underestimated and its status in relation to therapeutic practice should never be undermined.

References and further reading

Bayne, R., Nicolson, P., Horton, I. (Eds.), 1998. Counselling and Communication Skills for Medical and Health Practitioners. BPS Books, Leicestershire.

Chaitow, L., 2003. Palpation and Assessment Skills: Assessment and Diagnosis through Touch, second ed. Churchill Livingstone, Edinburgh.

Charman, R. (Ed.), 2000. Complementary Therapies for Physical Therapists. Butterworth-Heinemann, Oxford.

Christensen, N., Jones, M., Edwards, I., 2004. Clinical reasoning in the diagnosis and management of spinal pain. In: Boyling, J., Jull, G. (Eds.), Grieve's Modern Manual Therapy: the Vertebral Column, third ed. Churchill Livingstone, Edinburgh, pp. 391–403.

Dennis, M., Jones, C., Holey, E., 1995. Complementary medicine. In: Everett, T., Dennis, M., Ricketts, E. (Eds.), Physiotherapy in Mental Health: a Practical Approach. Butterworth-Heinemann, Oxford, pp. 252–280.

Evans, D., 2000. The reliability of assessment parameters: accuracy and palpation techniques. In: Boyling, J., Palastanga, N. (Eds.), Grieve's Modern Manual Therapy: the Vertebral Column, second ed. Churchill Livingstone, Edinburgh, pp. 539–546.

Everett, T., 1997. Psychological treatment in physiotherapy practice. In French, S. (Ed.), Physiotherapy: a Psychosocial Approach, second ed. Butterworth-Heinemann, Oxford, pp. 421–432.

Field, E.J., Harrison, R.J., 1974. Anatomical Terms: Their Origin and Derivation. W. Heffer & Sons, Cambridge.

Grieve, G., 1986. Modern Manual Therapy of the Vertebral Column. Churchill Livingstone, Edinburgh.

Guyton, A.C., 1991. Medical Physiology, sixth ed. W.B. Saunders, Philadephia, pp. 605–606.

Hengeveld, E., Banks, K. (Eds.), 2005. Maitland's Peripheral Manipulation, fourth ed. Elsevier, Edinburgh.

Hinkle, C., 1997. Fundamentals of Anatomy and Movement: a Workbook and Guide. Mosby, St. Louis.

Keogh, B., Ebbs, S., 1984. Normal Surface Anatomy. Heinemann, London.

Krieger, D., 1986. The Therapeutic Touch: How to Use Your Hands to Help or Heal. Prentice Hall, New York.

Krieger, D., 1993. Accepting Your Power to Heal: the Personal Practice of Therapeutic Touch. Bear, Vermont.

Krieger, D., 1997. Therapeutic Touch: Inner Workbook. Bear, New Mexico.

Krieger, D., 2002. Therapeutic Touch as Transpersonal Healing. Lantern Books, New York.

Macrae, J., 1987. Therapeutic Touch: a Practical Guide. Alfred A. Knopf, New York.

MacWhanell, 1992. Communication in physiotherapy. In: French, S., (Ed.), Physiotherapy: a Psychosocial Approach. Butterworth-Heinemann, Oxford.

Magee, D., 1997. Orthopedic Physical Assessment, third ed. W.B. Saunders, Philadelphia.

Maitland, A.D., 1991. Peripheral Manipulation, third ed. Butterworth-Heinemann, Oxford.

Mason, A., 1985. Something to do with touch. Physiotherapy 71, 167–169.

Montague, A., 1978. Touching: the Human Significance of Skin, second ed. Harper & Row, New York.

Nathan, B., 1999. Touch and Emotion in Manual Therapy. Churchill Livingstone, Edinburgh.

Owen Hutchinson, J., 2004. Health, health education and physiotherapy practice. In: French, S., Sim, J. (Eds.), Physiotherapy: a Psychosocial Approach, third ed. Elsevier, Edinburgh, pp. 25–43.

Owen Hutchinson, J., Atkinson, K., Orpwood, J., 1998. Breaking Down Barriers: Access to Further and Higher Education for Visually Impaired Students. Stanley Thornes, Gloucestershire.

Palastanga, N., Field, D., Soames, R., 2002. Anatomy and Human Movement: Structure and Function, fourth ed. Elsevier, Edinburgh.

Phillips, N., 2004. Motor learning. In: Trew, M., Everett, T. (Eds.), Human Movement: an Introductory Text, fourth ed. Churchill Livingstone, Edinburgh, pp. 129–141.

Poon, K., 1995. Touch and handling. In: Everett, T., Dennis, M., Ricketts, E. (Eds.), Physiotherapy in Mental Health: a Practical Approach. Butterworth-Heinemann, Oxford, pp. 91–101.

Porter, S., 2002. The Anatomy Workbook. Butterworth-Heinemann, Oxford.

Ramsden, E. (Ed.), 1999. The Person as Patient: Psychological Perspectives for the Health Care Professional. W.B. Saunders, London.

Sayre-Adams, J., Wright, S., 2001. Therapeutic Touch. Churchill Livingstone, Edinburgh.

Standring, S. (Ed.), 2004. Gray's Anatomy: the Anatomical Basis of Clinical Practice, thirty-ninth ed. Churchill Livingstone, Edinburgh.

Stevenson, C., Grieves, M., Stein-Parbury, J., 2004. Patient and Person: Empowering Interpersonal Relationships in Nursing. Elsevier, Oxford.

Sunderland, S., 1978. Nerves and Nerve Injuries, second ed. Churchill Livingstone, Edinburgh, p. 355.

Subject Index

Page numbers followed by 'f' indicate figures, 'b' indicate boxes.

Printed in the United States
By Bookmasters